EXAM ✓ CRAM

NCLEX-RN®

Third Edition

Wilda Rinehart, Diann Sloan, Clara Hurd

800 East 96th Street, Indianapolis, Indiana 46240 USA

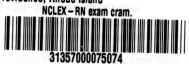
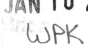
WPK

...ored in a retrieval system, or trans-
...cording, or otherwise, without writ-
...d with respect to the use of the
information contained herein. Although every precaution has been taken in the preparation of this
book, the publisher and author assume no responsibility for errors or omissions. Nor is any liability
assumed for damages resulting from the use of the information contained herein.

ISBN-13: 978-0-7897-4482-1
ISBN-10: 0-7897-4482-1

Library of Congress Cataloging-in-Publication Data

Rinehart, Wilda.
  NCLEX-RN exam cram / Wilda Rinehart, Diann Sloan, Clara Hurd. -- 3rd
ed.
      p. ; cm.
  Includes index.
  ISBN-13: 978-0-7897-4482-1 (pbk.)
  ISBN-10: 0-7897-4482-1 (pbk.)
  1. Nursing--Examinations, questions, etc. 2. National Council
Licensure Examination for Registered Nurses--Study guides. I. Sloan,
Diann. II. Hurd, Clara. III. Title.
  [DNLM: 1. Nursing--Examination Questions. WY 18.2]
  RT55.R563 2011
  610.73076--dc22
                                    2010038176
Printed in the United States of America

First Printing: November 2010

Trademarks

All terms mentioned in this book that are known to be trademarks or service marks have been
appropriately capitalized. Pearson IT Certification cannot attest to the accuracy of this information.
Use of a term in this book should not be regarded as affecting the validity of any trademark or service mark.

NCLEX® is a registered trademark of the National Council of State Boards of Nursing, Inc.
(NCSBN), which does not sponsor or endorse this product.

Warning and Disclaimer

Every effort has been made to make this book as complete and as accurate as possible, but no war-
ranty or fitness is implied. The information provided is on an "as is" basis. The author and the publisher shall have neither liability nor responsibility to any person or entity with respect to any loss or
damages arising from the information contained in this book or from the use of the CD or programs
accompanying it.

Bulk Sales

Pearson IT Certification offers excellent discounts on this book when ordered in quantity for bulk
purchases or special sales. For more information, please contact

U.S. Corporate and Government Sales
1-800-382-3419
corpsales@pearsontechgroup.com

For sales outside of the U.S., please contact

International Sales
international@pearsoned.com

Publisher
Paul Boger

Associate Publisher
David Dusthimer

Acquisitions Editor
Betsy Brown

**Senior Development
Editor**
Christopher Cleveland

Managing Editor
Sandra Schroeder

Project Editor
Mandie Frank

Indexer
Angie Martin

Proofreader
Leslie Joseph

Technical Editor
Maura Cappiello

Publishing Coordinator
Vanessa Evans

Multimedia Developer
Dan Scherf

Designer
Gary Adair

Page Layout
Bronkella Publishing

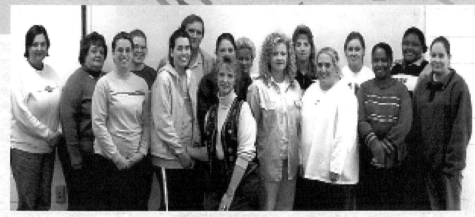

Contents at a Glance

Table of Contents

About the Authors

Wilda Rinehart received an Associate Degree in Nursing from Northeast Mississippi Community College in Booneville, Mississippi. After working as a staff nurse and charge nurse, she became a public health nurse and served in that capacity for a number of years. In 1975, she received her nurse practitioner certification in the area of obstetrics-gynecology from the University of Mississippi Medical Center in Jackson, Mississippi. In 1979, she completed her Bachelor of Science degree in Nursing from Mississippi University for Women. In 1980, she completed her Master of Science degree in Nursing from the same university and accepted a faculty position at Northeast Mississippi Community College, where she taught medical-surgical nursing and maternal-newborn nursing. In 1982, she founded Rinehart and Associates Nursing Consultants. For the past 26 years, she and her associates have worked with nursing graduates and schools of nursing to assist graduates to pass the National Council Licensure Exam for Nursing. She has also worked as a curriculum consultant with faculty to improve test construction. Ms. Rinehart has served as a convention speaker throughout the southeastern United States and as a reviewer of medical-surgical and obstetric texts. She has co-authored materials used in seminars presented by Rinehart and Associates Nursing Review. As the president of Rinehart and Associates, she serves as the coordinator of a company dedicated to improving the quality of health through nursing education.

Dr. Diann Sloan received an Associate Degree in Nursing from Northeast Mississippi Community College, a Bachelor of Science degree in Nursing from the University of Mississippi, and a Master of Science degree in Nursing from Mississippi University for Women. In addition to her nursing degrees, she holds a Master of Science in Counseling Psychology from Georgia State University and a Doctor of Philosophy in Counselor Education, with minors in both Psychology and Educational Psychology from Mississippi State University. She has completed additional graduate studies in healthcare administration at Western New England College and the University of Mississippi. Dr. Sloan has taught pediatric nursing, psychiatric mental health nursing, and medical surgical nursing in both associate degree and baccalaureate nursing programs. As a member of Rinehart and Associates Nursing Review, Dr. Sloan has conducted test construction workshops for faculty and nursing review seminars for both registered and practical nurse graduates. She has co-authored materials used in the item-writing workshops for nursing faculty and Rinehart and Associates Nursing Review. She is a member of Sigma Theta Tau nursing honor society.

Clara Hurd received an Associate Degree in Nursing from Northeast Mississippi Community College in Booneville, Mississippi (1975). Her experiences in nursing are clinically based, having served as a staff nurse in medical-surgical nursing. She has worked as an oncology, intensive care, orthopedic, neurological, and pediatric nurse. She received her Bachelor of Science degree in Nursing from the University of North Alabama in Florence, Alabama, and her Master of Science degree in Nursing from the Mississippi University for Women in Columbus, Mississippi. Ms. Hurd is a certified nurse educator. She currently serves as a nurse educator consultant and an independent contractor. Ms. Hurd has taught in both associate degree and baccalaureate degree nursing programs. She was a faculty member of Mississippi University for Women; Austin Peay State University in Clarksville, Tennessee; Tennessee State University in Nashville, Tennessee; and Northeast Mississippi Community College. Ms. Hurd joined Rinehart and Associates in 1993. She has worked with students in preparing for the National Council Licensure Exam and with faculty as a consultant in writing test items. Ms. Hurd has also been a presenter at nursing conventions on various topics, including item-writing for nursing faculty. Her primary professional goal is to prepare the student and graduate for excellence in the delivery of healthcare.

About the Technical Editor

Maura Cappiello received her bachelor's degree from Boston College and her master's degree in healthcare administration from Seton Hall University. She is also a certified case manager. Maura has worked as a staff RN in the NICU and the pediatric home care environment. Currently, she works as the Director for Staff Development for Alere, a case management company.

Dedication

We would like to thank our families for tolerating our late nights and long hours. Also, thanks to Gene Sloan for his help without pay. Special thanks to all the graduates who have attended Rinehart and Associates Review Seminars. Thanks for allowing us to be a part of your success.

Acknowledgments

Our special thanks to our editors, support staff, and nurse reviewers for helping us to organize our thoughts and experiences into a text for students and practicing professionals. You made the task before us challenging and enjoyable.

We Want to Hear from You!

As the reader of this book, *you* are our most important critic and commentator. We value your opinion and want to know what we're doing right, what we could do better, what areas you'd like to see us publish in, and any other words of wisdom you're willing to pass our way.

As an associate publisher for Pearson, I welcome your comments. You can email or write me directly to let me know what you did or didn't like about this book—as well as what we can do to make our books better.

Please note that I cannot help you with technical problems related to the topic of this book. We do have a User Services group, however, where I will forward specific technical questions related to the book.

When you write, please be sure to include this book's title and author as well as your name, email address, and phone number. I will carefully review your comments and share them with the author and editors who worked on the book.

Email: feedback@pearsonitcertification.com.

Mail: David Dusthimer
          Associate Publisher
          Pearson
          800 East 96th Street
          Indianapolis, IN 46240 USA

Reader Services

Visit our website and register this book at www.pearsonitcertification.com/register for convenient access to any updates, downloads, or errata that might be available for this book.

Introduction

Welcome to the NCLEX-RN® Exam Cram

Often when we are studying for a very important exam such as the NCLEX®, we feel overwhelmed by the amount of content there is to master. This book will help you organize your knowledge and get ready to take and pass the Licensure Exam for Registered Nurses. This introduction discusses the NCLEX® exam in general and how the *Exam Cram* can help you prepare for the test. It doesn't matter whether this is the first time you're going to take the exam or if you have taken it previously; this book gives you the necessary information and techniques to obtain licensure.

Exam Cram books help you understand and appreciate the subjects and materials you need to pass. The books are aimed at test preparation and review. They do not teach you everything you need to know about the subject of nursing. Instead they present you with materials you are likely to encounter on the exam. Using a simple approach, we will help you understand the need-to-know information. First, you will learn medical-surgical content, psychiatric content, obstetric content, and pediatric content, with an emphasis on pharmacology, skills, and treatment of these disorders. In a well-organized format, you will learn the pathophysiology of the most common problems affecting clients, the treatment of these disorders, and the nursing care.

The NCLEX-RN® consists of questions from the cognitive levels of knowledge, comprehension, application, and analysis. The majority of questions are written at the application and analysis levels. Questions incorporate the five stages of the nursing process (assessment, diagnosis, planning, implementation, and evaluation) and the four categories of client needs. Client needs are divided into subcategories that define the content within each of the four major categories. These categories and subcategories are

- Safe, effective care environment:
    - Management of care: 16–22%
    - Safety and infection control: 8–14%
- Health promotion and maintenance: 6%–12%
- Psychosocial integrity: 6%–12%

▶ Physiological integrity:

    ▶ Basic care and comfort: 6%–12%

    ▶ Pharmacological and parenteral therapy: 13%–19%

    ▶ Reduction of risk: 10%–16%

    ▶ Physiological adaptation: 11%–17%

Taking the Computerized Adaptive Test

Computerized Adaptive Testing offers the candidate several advantages. The graduate can schedule the exam at a time that is convenient for him. The Pearson VUE Testing group is responsible for administering the exam. Because you might not be familiar with the Pearson testing centers, we recommend that you arrive at least 30 minutes early. If you are late, you will not be allowed to test. Bring two forms of identification with you, one of which must be a picture ID. Be sure that your form of identification matches your application. You will be photographed and fingerprinted on entering the testing site, so don't let this increase your stress. The allotted time is six hours. The candidate can receive results within approximately seven days (in some states even sooner). Remember that the exam is written at approximately the 10th-grade reading level, so keep a good dictionary handy during your studies.

The Cost of the Exam

The candidate wishing to write the licensure exam must fill out two applications: one to the National Council and one to the state in which she wants to be licensed. A separate fee must accompany each application. The fee required by the National Council is $200. State licensing fees vary from state to state. Licensure applications can be obtained on the National Council's website at www.ncsbn.org. Several states are members of the multistate licensure compact. This means that, if you are issued a multistate license, you pay only one fee. This information can be obtained by visiting the National Council's website as well.

How to Prepare for the Exam

Judicious use of this book, either alone or with other books such as the *NCLEX® Exam Prep* book by the same authors, and a review seminar such as the one provided by Rinehart and Associates, will help you achieve your goal of becoming a registered nurse. As you review for the NCLEX® Exam, we suggest that you find a location where you can concentrate on the material each day. A minimum of two hours per day for at least two weeks is suggested. We have provided you with exam alerts, tips, notes, and sample questions—both multiple-choice and alternative items. These questions will acquaint you with the types of questions you will see during the exam. We have also formulated a mock exam with those difficult management and delegation questions that you can score to determine your readiness to test. Pay particular attention to the exam alerts and the Cram Sheet. Using them will help you gain and retain knowledge and reduce your stress as you prepare to test.

How to Use This Book

Each topical *Exam Cram* chapter follows a regular structure, along with cues about important or useful information. Here's the structure of a typical chapter:

- ▶ **Opening hotlists**—Each chapter begins with a list of terms and concepts you must learn and understand before you can know the subject matter. The hotlists are followed by an introductory section that sets the stage for the rest of the chapter.

- ▶ **Topical coverage**—After the opening hotlists, each chapter covers a series of topics related to the chapter's subject title. Throughout this section, we highlight topics or concepts that are likely to appear in the exam.

Even though the book is structured to the exam, these flagged items are often particularly important:

- ▶ **Exam alerts**—An exam alert stresses concepts, terms, or activities that are likely to relate to one or more test questions. For that reason, we think any information in an alert is worthy of unusual attentiveness on your part. A special exam alert layout is used like this:

EXAM ALERT

This is what an exam alert looks like. Remember to pay particular attention to these items!

- ▶ **Notes**—Throughout each chapter, additional information is provided that, although not directly related to the exam itself, is still useful and will aid your preparation. A sample note is shown here:

NOTE

This is how notes are formatted. Notes direct your attention to important pieces of information that relate to nursing and nursing certification.

▶ **Tips**—A tip might tell you another way of accomplishing something in a more efficient or time-saving manner. An example of a tip is shown here:

> **TIP**
>
> This is how tips are formatted. Keep your eyes open for these, and you'll learn some interesting nursing tips!

▶ **Exam prep questions**—Although we talk about test questions and topics throughout the book, the section at the end of each chapter presents a series of mock test questions and explanations of both correct and incorrect answers.

▶ **Practice exams**—Practice Exam I and Practice Exam II provide additional practice questions. Use these to gauge your learning and to build the confidence needed to move forward to the real exam.

▶ **Glossary**—At the end of the book you will find a glossary that defines critical nursing terms we cover in this book.

▶ **CD**—The CD includes a testing engine with many practice questions that you should use repeatedly to practice your test-taking skills and to measure your level of learning. You should be able to correctly answer more than 90% of the questions on the practice tests before taking the real exam.

▶ **Cram Sheet**—At the very beginning of the book is a tear card we call the Cram Sheet. This is a helpful tool that gives you distilled, compressed facts. It is a great tool for last-minute study and review.

About the Book

The topics in this book have been structured using the systems approach to nursing. We believe that the simple way to learn the disease process, treatments, and diagnostic studies is the best way. You will review material from each system and the related skills, diagnostics, diets, and so on with each system as we move through the content. You will also consider cultural and religious concerns when caring for the client experiencing threats or deprivations.

Aside from being a test preparation book, this book is also useful if you are brushing up on your nursing knowledge. It is an excellent quick reference for the licensed nurse.

Contact the Authors

The authors of this text are interested in you and want you to pass on the first attempt. If, after reviewing with this text, you would like to contact the authors, you can do so at Rinehart and Associates, PO Box 124, Booneville, MS 38829 or by visiting our website at www.nclexreview.net.

Self-Assessment

Before you take the exam, you might have some concerns, such as

- ▶ Am I required to answer all 265 questions to pass?

  No. If you run out of time, the computer looks at the last portion of the exam and determines whether you are consistently above or below the pass point.

- ▶ What score do I have to make to pass the NCLEX-RN® Exam?

  There is not a set score. When you were in nursing school, you might have been required to score 75% or 80% to pass and progress onto the next level. The licensure exam is not scored in percentages. The computer is looking for consistency above or below the pass point. When the candidate shows this consistency, the computer stops asking questions.

- ▶ How do they develop the test plan?

  Every three years a survey is sent out to 4,000 newly licensed nurses. These nurses are asked questions based on the "Activity Statement" for nursing practice. Based on the results of the survey, the test plan is set by the National Council and members of the Licensure Committee. These members are appointed from representative states.

- ▶ What types of questions will I be asked?

  The majority of questions are multiple-choice. A small number of the questions may be *alternative items*. These items are identify picture, put on ear phones and identify sound such as breath sounds, identify grafts, fill-in-the-blanks, identify-a-diagram, place-in-sequence, or check-all-that-apply questions. Some examples of alternative items are:

  - ▶ Figure the 8-hour intake and output.

  - ▶ Identify the area where the mitral valve is heard the loudest.

  - ▶ Place in sequence the tasks you would use in the skill of washing your hands.

  - ▶ Work the math problem.

  - ▶ Check all that apply to the care of the client after a cardiac catheterization.

▶ Will I have a calculator for math problems?

Yes, a drop-down calculator is provided.

▶ Will I have something to write on in the testing area?

Yes, a dry erase board or paper will be provided. Don't worry about the test givers thinking that you are cheating. They clean and secure the area after each candidate.

▶ What if I get sick and cannot take my exam?

You have a period of time allowed during which you can cancel your appointment and reschedule. If, however, you do not contact the Pearson VUE group in that allotted time and do not attend to take the exam, you forfeit your money and have to reapply.

▶ Can I carry a purse or bag into the testing center?

No, there will be lockers for your use in the testing center. (Also, dress warmly because the area is usually cool.) Any suspicious behavior can cause you to forfeit the opportunity to complete your test so be sure to leave any paper or notes in your car.

▶ Can I take breaks?

Yes, there are optional breaks throughout the test.

▶ If I should fail, when could I retest?

The required time to wait before you can rewrite is 45 days in most states; however, some states require that you wait 90 days. Should you be unsuccessful, you should contact the state where you want to obtain licensure for its required retest time.

Testing Your Exam Readiness

First and foremost, you obviously must have completed or be very close to completing your RN classes at the college level. The better you did in your college work, the better your chances are of doing well on this exam. However, there are no guarantees on the NCLEX-RN® exam, so you should prepare specifically for this exam using your college class work as a foundation.

Whether you attend a formal review seminar or use written material such as this book, or a combination of both, preparation is essential. Costing as much as $400 a try—pass or fail—you want to do everything you can to pass on your first attempt. Spend time each day studying and taking exam questions. The more questions you take, the more prepared you will be. I recommend that you score at least 90% on our practice questions consistently before you attempt to take the exam. With these facts in mind, let's get ready to take the NCLEX-RN® exam. Good luck!

CHAPTER ONE

Preparing for the National Council Exam for Registered Nurses

Terms you'll need to understand

✓ Alternative items

✓ Client needs

✓ Computerized Adaptive Testing (CAT)

✓ Distracters

✓ National Council of State Boards of Nursing

✓ Nursing process

✓ Options

✓ Stem

✓ Test item

Preparing for the Exam

As you prepare to take the National Council Licensure Examination, you might feel overwhelmed and frustrated. There is so much material to review and so many decisions to make. Where do I begin? Most graduates feel that way. This chapter will help you to become aware of the NCLEX test plan and to know the types of questions you will encounter on the exam.

The CAT Exam

Computerized Adaptive Testing (CAT) provides a means of individualized testing of each candidate seeking licensure as a registered professional nurse. Selecting from a large test bank, the computer chooses questions based on the candidate's ability and competence as demonstrated on the prior question.

The minimum number of questions is 75, and the maximum number is 265. The average candidate's exam is comprised of 160 items. You must answer the question that appears on the screen before another question is given and you can neither skip questions nor return to a previous question. It is imperative that you read each question carefully before selecting a response. We suggest that you cover the answers with your nondominant hand and read the stem completely before looking at the answers.

As you might have read in the introduction to this book, the NCLEX-RN® consists of questions from the cognitive levels of knowledge, comprehension, application, and analysis. The majority of questions are written at the application and analysis levels. Questions incorporate the five stages of the nursing process.

- ▸ Assessment
- ▸ Analysis
- ▸ Planning
- ▸ Implementation
- ▸ Evaluation

There are also questions from the four categories of client needs. Client needs are divided into subcategories that define the content within each of the four major categories. According to www.NCSBN.org, these categories and subcategories, as well as the percentages of questions allocated to each area, are as shown in the following table.

A. Safe, Effective Care Environment
- ▶ Management of Care   16%–22%
- ▶ Safety and Infection Control   8%–14%

B. Health Promotion and Maintenance   6–12%

C. Psychosocial Integrity   6–12%

D. Physiological Integrity
- ▶ Basic Care and Comfort   6%–12%
- ▶ Pharmacological and Parenteral Therapies   13%–19%
- ▶ Reduction of Risk Potential   10%–16%
- ▶ Physiological Adaptation   11%–17%

Computerized Adaptive Testing (CAT) offers the candidate several advantages over the former paper and pencil exam. The test questions, which are stored in a large test bank and classified by test plan areas and level of difficulty, are administered to the candidate. Depending on the answer given by the graduate, the computer presents another question that is either more difficult or less difficult. This allows the computer to determine the candidate's knowledge of the subject matter more concisely.

The pass/fail decision is not based on how many questions the candidate answers correctly, but on the difficulty of the questions answered correctly. Even though candidates might answer different questions and different numbers of questions, the test plan remains the same. All NCLEX-RN examinations conform to this test plan. Each time you answer a question correctly the next question gets harder until you miss a question; then an easier question is given until you answer correctly. This way the computer concludes if a candidate has met the passing standard. If you are clearly above the passing standard at 75 questions, the computer stops asking questions. If you are clearly below the passing standard, the computer stops asking questions. If your ability estimate is close to the passing standard, the computer continues to ask questions until either the maximum number of questions is asked or time expires. The CAT exam offers another advantage. The candidate can schedule the exam at a time that is convenient. The candidate usually receives test results in seven days or sooner. The candidate can retake the exam after 45 days in most states. We suggest that you review this text and others, and, if needed, take a review seminar prior to taking the NCLEX. Allow at least two weeks to study and prepare for the exam. Remember: You want to take the exam only one time.

Testing Strategies

After learning the materials, you may want to utilize a number of testing strategies. These strategies are intended to provide you with additional skills and are not to be considered as a substitute for good study habits or an adequate knowledge of the content. Although some candidates attempt to commit information to memory, it has been shown that merely memorizing facts is of little help because few test items rely on simple recall. Most questions that appear as test items above the pass point require the graduate to pull together information from a variety of sources. If you have a thorough knowledge of the content measured, use good testing skills, and can apply this knowledge, you will pass the exam. Remember that testing skills, like any other skill, improve with practice.

Before discussing strategies for successful test taking, you should be familiar with the following terms:

▸ **Test item**—This is the entire question.

▸ **Stem**—These are portions of the test item that ask a question or propose the problem.

▸ **Options**—These are potential answers.

▸ **Alternative item**—These are items utilizing a diagram, listing in order of priority, checking all that apply, calculating math or intake and output, or filling in blanks.

Read the Question Carefully

Exam scores are often affected by reading ability and careful reading of exam questions. Before selecting an answer, ask the following questions:

▸ What is the question asking?

▸ Are there keywords?

▸ Is there relevant information in the stem?

▸ How would I ask this question (in my own words)?

▸ How would I answer this question (in my own words)?

After answering these questions, see if there is an option similar to your answer. Is this option the best or most complete answer to the question?

Look for Keywords

Keywords in the stem should alert you to use care in choosing an answer. Avoid selecting answers that include keywords such as *always, never, all, every, only, must, no, except,* and *none.* Answers that contain these keywords are seldom correct because they limit and qualify potentially correct answers.

Watch for Specific Details

Careful reading of details in the stem can provide important clues to the correct option. For example, if the item seeks information on a short-term goal, look for something to be accomplished within the hospital; if the item seeks information on a long-term goal, look for something to be accomplished in the home or community.

Eliminate Options That Are Clearly Wrong or Incorrect

By eliminating those answers that are clearly incorrect, you increase the probability of selecting the correct option. With the elimination of each distracter, you increase the probability of selecting the correct option by 25%.

Look for Similar Options

If a test item contains two or more options that are similar in meaning, look for an umbrella term or phrase that encompasses the other correct options. The following list gives you hints about how to read the question and its options to accurately identify the correct answer:

- **Look at the parts of the options**—If an answer contains two or more parts, you can reduce the number of possible correct answers by identifying one part as incorrect.

- **Identify specific determiners**—Look for the same or similar words in the stem and in the options. The word in the stem that clues you to a similar word in the option or that limits potential options is referred to as a *specific determiner*. The option with the specific determiner is often the correct answer.

- **Identify words in the option that are closely associated with, but not identical to, words in the stem**—An option that contains words closely associated with words appearing in the stem is often the correct answer.

- **Be alert for grammatical inconsistencies**—The correct option must be consistent with the form of the question. If the item demands a response in the singular, look for an option in the singular, meaning an option in the plural would be incorrect.

- **Use relevant information from an earlier question**—Test writers often provide information that can be used in subsequent questions. For example, you might be asked several questions on the topic of diabetes mellitus. Write on the paper or slate provided in the testing area information that you remember on this topic. The information can help you later during the test if you are asked a similar question.

- **Look for the answer that is different from the other options**—This testing strategy is called *odd answer out*. An example of this type of question follows:

  The nurse is attempting to evaluate the client's knowledge of diabetes mellitus. Which statement made by the client indicates a need for further teaching?

  A. The client states that he will check his blood glucose levels prior to meals.

  B. The client selects a 10 oz. steak from his menu.

  C. The client can demonstrate how he will give himself insulin.

  D. The client verbalizes understanding of ways to improve circulation.

Answer B is correct. Answers A, C, and D all indicate a knowledge of diabetes mellitus. Answer B indicates that the client lacks understanding because the correct portion size for a steak is 3 oz.

Look for Opposite Answers

When you see opposites, one of these options is usually correct. An example of this testing strategy is shown here:

▶ The pediatric client with hemophilia is admitted with bleeding in the right knee. Which action by the nurse indicates an understanding of hemophilia?

    A. The nurse applies heat to the knee.

    B. The nurse applies ice to the knee.

    C. The nurse offers to perform passive range of motion.

    D. The nurse positions the extremity lower than the heart.

Answer B is correct. Applying ice to the knee will help to vasoconstrict. This action will decrease the bleeding into the knee. (Notice that answer A is opposite to answer B.) Answers A, C, and D are incorrect because they will increase bleeding.

Remember Legalities

Remember that, when dealing with legalities of nursing practice, assign the most critical to the registered nurse and the most stable to the nursing assistant. If skilled nursing care is required, assign the stable client to the licensed practical nurse and self-assign the most critical. When organizing client care, visit the most critical first. Remember the ABCs: airway, breathing, and circulation.

Remember Infection Control

Infection control is an important part of nursing practice. The nurse should be aware of potential transmission based on precautions. This information can be found in detail in Appendix A, "Things You Forgot." Do not co-assign or assign to a room clients who have active infections with surgical or immune-compromised clients.

Exam Prep Questions

The following exam prep questions allow you to practice the testing strategies we have discussed in this chapter. These questions include content you have learned in school. We will discuss the content in later chapters.

1. The client with leukemia who has had a bone marrow transplant should be instructed to avoid which of the following flavor enhancers?

   ○ **A.** Salt

   ○ **B.** Pepper

   ○ **C.** Lemon juice

   ○ **D.** Lime juice

2. The most important information for the nurse to have when planning care for the client with diabetes is the client's:

   ○ **A.** Family medical history

   ○ **B.** Blood glucose history

   ○ **C.** 24-hour dietary history

   ○ **D.** Medical history

3. The nurse has just received the shift report. Which one of the following clients should be seen first?

   ○ **A.** A 14-year-old one day post-appendectomy with a WBC of 6500

   ○ **B.** A 5-year-old three days post-fracture of the right tibia with a temperature of 100.1° Fahrenheit

   ○ **C.** A 10-year-old admitted during the previous shift with dehydration and a hematocrit of 44%

   ○ **D.** An 8-week-old admitted four hours earlier with substernal retractions and an oxygen saturation of 90%

4. Which client should receive a private room if only one is available?

   ○ **A.** A client with diabetes mellitus

   ○ **B.** A client with Cushing's disease

   ○ **C.** A client with Graves' disease

   ○ **D.** A client with gastric ulcers

5. The nurse is making assignments for the day. The staff consists of an RN, an LPN, and a nursing assistant. Which client should be assigned to the nursing assistant?

   ○ **A.** A client with a laparoscopic cholecystectomy

   ○ **B.** A client with viral pneumonia

   ○ **C.** A client with suspected ectopic pregnancy

   ○ **D.** A client with intermittent chest pain

6. The nurse knows that the client with peripheral vascular disease understands instructions in ways to improve circulation if the client states:

   ○ **A.** "I will massage my legs three times a day."

   ○ **B.** "I will elevate the foot of my bed on blocks."

   ○ **C.** "I will take a brisk walk for 20 minutes each day."

   ○ **D.** "I will prop my feet up when I sit to watch TV."

7. Which action by the client best indicates acceptance of his recent amputation?

   ○ **A.** He verbalizes acceptance.

   ○ **B.** He looks at the operative site.

   ○ **C.** He asks for information regarding prosthesis.

   ○ **D.** He remains silent during dressing changes.

8. The client with cancer of the larynx is admitted to the unit with pneumonia. Which nursing diagnosis should receive priority?

   ○ **A.** Alteration in oxygen perfusion

   ○ **B.** Alteration in comfort/pain

   ○ **C.** Alteration in mobility

   ○ **D.** Alteration in sensory perception

9. Treatment of sickle cell crisis involving the joints includes the application of:

   ○ **A.** A heating pad to the joints

   ○ **B.** An ice pack to the joints

   ○ **C.** A CPM device to the lower leg

   ○ **D.** A TENS unit to the back

10. The client is admitted to the intensive care unit with severe chest pain. Which information provides the nurse with the most data that can be utilized in planning care?

     ○ **A.** The blood pressure

     ○ **B.** The vital signs

     ○ **C.** The pulse oximetry

     ○ **D.** The electroencephalography

Answer Rationales

1. Answer B is correct. The client with a bone marrow transplant is maintained on immunosuppressants. Pepper is unprocessed and contains bacteria, so it should be avoided. Notice the opposites in the choices. Salt is another type of seasoning, but is allowed. Lemon and lime juices are also allowed. The testing strategy is to look for opposite answers.

2. Answer B is correct. The most objective finding is the blood glucose history. Answers A, C, and D are more subjective, therefore they are incorrect. This information is reported data.

3. Answer D is correct. There is nothing in answer A that indicates the client is unstable. Answer B is a good choice, but the client three days post-fracture may have a slight temperature, so he should be evaluated after the client with substernal retraction. Answer C is also a good choice, but if the child is dehydrated, the hematocrit will be increased due to a decreased blood volume and hemoconcentration.

4. Answer C is correct. Graves' disease is hyperthyroidism. These clients have insomnia and any noise will wake them. Lack of sleep makes their condition worse. Answer B is a good choice, but if you answered B you are reading into the question because the question does not say that the client should be placed in a room with a client who is infected. Answers A and D are vague answers; stay away from vague answers. The answer does not tell us if they are in the hospital for diagnostic studies or for complications of their diseases.

5. Answer A is correct. The client with a laparoscopic cholecystectomy has three or four very small incisions and is the most stable client. Answers B, C, and D are all more critical clients and should be assigned to a licensed practical or registered nurse.

6. Answer C is correct. Walking increases peripheral circulation. Answer A is wrong. If this is done, a clot may be present that can become a pulmonary embolus. Answers B and D are similar, but they both can be eliminated because they assist in returning blood to the heart, but not increasing circulation to the extremities.

7. Answer B is correct. Any time that there is a change in body image looking at the operative site is the *best* indicator of acceptance. Simply stating that he accepts the change in body image is not the best indicator of acceptance, so answer A is incorrect. Answer C is incorrect because asking for information is not an accurate indicator of acceptance. Answer D is incorrect because remaining silent is not an indicator of acceptance.

8. Answer A is correct. Remember the ABCs: Airway or oxygenation is always first. B, C, and D are incorrect because they do not take priority in this situation.

9. Answer A is correct. The treatment for sickle cell crisis is heat, hydration, oxygenation, and pain relief.

10. Answer B is correct. Notice that answer B, taking the vital signs, includes answer A, taking the blood pressure. This is an example of an umbrella answer. C is incorrect because a pulse oximetry does not provide the most information. D is incorrect because a electroencephalogram does not give information related to chest pain.

CHAPTER TWO

Pharmacology

Terms you'll need to understand

- ✓ Adverse reactions
- ✓ Agonist
- ✓ Allergic response
- ✓ Antagonists
- ✓ Buccal
- ✓ Contraindications
- ✓ Enteral administration
- ✓ Enteric coating
- ✓ FDA
- ✓ Intradermal
- ✓ Intramuscular
- ✓ Nursing implication

- ✓ Oral
- ✓ Peak drug level
- ✓ Pharmacodynamics
- ✓ Pharmacokinetics
- ✓ Pharmacotherapeutics
- ✓ Side effects
- ✓ Spansules
- ✓ Subcutaneous
- ✓ Synergistic
- ✓ Toxicity
- ✓ Trough drug level

Nursing skills you'll need to master

- ✓ Drug calculations
- ✓ Administering oral medication
- ✓ Administering parenteral medication

- ✓ Administering suppositories
- ✓ Interpreting normal lab values

For a number of years, I have searched for a way to help students understand and apply knowledge of pharmacology to nursing practice. The graduate nurse is frequently responsible for instructing the client and the client's family regarding the safe administration of medications. The study of pharmacology is constantly changing as new drugs are constantly being approved for public use by the Food and Drug Administration (FDA). The recent test plan approved by the National Council Licensure Exam devotes 13%–19% of the Physiological Integrity section to pharmacology. This chapter contains useful information to help you look at the classification and generic name of drugs. If you can remember the drug classification, frequently you can understand why the drug was ordered.

Three Areas of Pharmacology

It is important to note that the study of pharmacology includes three areas:

- **Pharmacokinetics:** This is the study of how drugs are absorbed, distributed, metabolized, and excreted by the body. Elderly clients and clients with renal or liver disease frequently have difficulty metabolizing and excreting medications. These clients can develop drug toxicity more easily than those with no renal or liver impairment.

- **Pharmacodynamics:** This is the study of how drugs are used by the body. For example, pharmacodynamics of oral hypoglycemics explain how the blood glucose is reduced by stimulating the pancreatic beta cells to produce more insulin, by also making insulin receptor sites more sensitive to insulin, and by increasing the number of insulin receptor cells. These drugs are effective only if the client's pancreas is producing some insulin.

- **Pharmacotherapeutics:** This is the study of how the client responds to the drug. A client might experience side effects such as gastrointestinal symptoms to a number of medications, including antibiotics. Side effects might cause discomfort but are usually not severe enough to warrant discontinuation of the medication. Demerol (meperidine HCl) is a narcotic analgesic that can cause nausea and vomiting. To prevent these side effects, the physician frequently orders an antiemetic called Phenergan (promethazine) to be given with Demerol. These drugs have a synergistic effect that provides pain relief while preventing the discomfort of side effects.

Adverse effects of medications result in symptoms so severe that it is necessary to reduce the dosage or discontinue the medication completely. Antituberculars and anticonvulsants are two categories of medications that can have adverse effects on the liver. The nurse should carefully assess the client's liver function studies as well as assess for signs of jaundice that indicate drug-related hepatitis, in which case the medication will be discontinued.

How Nurses Work with Pharmacology

Nurses are expected to utilize their knowledge of pharmacology to:

- ▶ Recognize common uses, side effects, and adverse effects of the client's medication
- ▶ Challenge medication errors
- ▶ Meet the client's learning needs

Generally, the medication the nurse is expected to administer depends on the area of practice and the assigned client. The following medication classifications are commonly prescribed for adult clients within a medical/surgical setting:

- ▶ **Anti-infectives:** Used for the treatment of infections. Common side effects include GI upset.

- ▶ **Antihypertensives:** Lower blood pressure and increase blood flow to the myocardium. Common side effects include orthostatic hypotension. Other side effects are specific to types of antihypertensive prescribed.

- ▶ **Antidiarrheals:** Decrease gastric motility and reduce water content in the intestinal tract. Side effects include bloating and gas.

- ▶ **Diuretics:** Decrease water and sodium absorption from the loop of Henle (loop diuretics) or inhibit antidiuretic hormone (potassium-sparing diuretics). Side effects of non–potassium-sparing diuretics include hypokalemia.

- ▶ **Antacids:** Reduce hydrochloric acid in the stomach. A common side effect of calcium- and aluminum-based antacids is constipation. Magnesium-based antacids frequently cause diarrhea.

- ▶ **Antipyretics:** Reduce fever.

- ▶ **Antihistamines:** Block the release of histamine in allergic reactions. Common side effects of antihistamines are dry mouth, drowsiness, and sedation.

- ▶ **Bronchodilators:** Dilate large air passages and are commonly prescribed for clients with asthma and chronic obstructive lung disease. A common side effect of these is tachycardia.

- ▶ **Laxatives:** Promote the passage of stool. Types of laxatives include stool softeners, cathartics, fiber, lubricants, and stimulants.

- ▶ **Anticoagulants:** Prevent clot formation by decreasing vitamin K levels and blocking the clotting chain or by preventing platelet aggregation.

▶ **Antianemics:** Increase factors necessary for red blood cell production. Examples of antianemics include B12, iron, and Epogen (erythropoetin).

▶ **Narcotics/analgesics:** Relieve moderate to severe pain. Medications in this category include opioids (morphine and codeine), synthetic opioids (meperidine), and NSAIDs (ketorolac).

▶ **Anticonvulsants:** Used for the management of seizure disorder and the treatment of bipolar disorder. Medications used as anticonvulsants include phenobarbital, phenytoin (Dilantin), and lorazepam (Ativan).

▶ **Anticholinergics:** Cause the mucous membranes to become dry; therefore, oral secretions are decreased. Anticholinergics such as atropine are often administered preoperatively.

▶ **Mydriatics:** Dilate the pupils. Mydriatics are used in the treatment of clients with cataracts.

▶ **Miotics:** Constrict the pupil. Miotics such as pilocarpine HCl are used in the treatment of clients with glaucoma.

Time-released Drugs

The following abbreviations indicate to the nurse that the drug is time-released. These preparations should not be crushed or opened:

▶ **Dur** = Duration

▶ **SR** = Sustained release

▶ **CR** = Continuous release

▶ **SA** = Sustained action

▶ **Contin** = Continuous action

▶ **LA** = Long acting

Enteric-coated tablets and caplets are those coated with a thick shell that prevents the medication from being absorbed in the upper GI tract, allowing the medication to be absorbed more slowly. *Spansules* are capsules containing time-released beads that are released slowly. The nurse should not alter the preparation of these types of medications. The physician should be notified to obtain an alternative preparation if the client is unable to swallow a time-released preparation.

Administering Medications

When preparing to administer medications, the nurse must identify the client by reviewing the physician's order. She must also administer the medication by the right route. Many medications are supplied in various preparations. The physician orders the method of administration. The choice of medication administration is dependent on several factors, including the desired blood level, the client's ability to swallow, and the disease or disorder being treated.

The Seven Rights of Administering Medication

The nurse is expected to use the seven rights when administering medications to the client. These include five rights of drug administration, plus two from the Patient's Bill of Rights.

The Patient's Bill of Rights was enacted to protect the client's well-being, both mentally and physically. The client has the right to refuse treatment, which can include medications. The nurse must document any treatment provided to the client. Documentation of care given must be made promptly to prevent forgetting any details and to ensure that another nurse does not duplicate medication administration.

The seven rights of medication administration are

- ▶ **Right client:** Identification of the client must be done by asking the client to state his name and checking the identification band.

- ▶ **Right route:** The physician orders the prescribed route of administration.

- ▶ **Right drug:** Checking both the generic and trade names with the physician's order ensures that the right drug is administered. If the client's diagnosis does not match the drug category, the nurse should further investigate the ordered medication.

- ▶ **Right amount:** The nurse is expected to know common dosages for both adults and children.

- ▶ **Right time:** The nurse can administer the medication either 30 minutes before the assigned time or 30 minutes after.

- ▶ **Right documentation (from the Patient's Bill of Rights and legality issues in nursing):** This right is different from the others in that it must be done to prevent duplicating drug administration.

- ▶ **Right to refuse treatment (from the Patient's Bill of Rights):** The client has the right to refuse medication or treatment.

Understanding and Identifying the Various Drugs

It is important to know that drugs generally have several names. The following list explains these different names for you:

- ▶ **Chemical name:** This is often a number or letter designation that tells you the chemical makeup of the drug. This name is of little value to the nurse in practice.

- ▶ **Generic name:** This is the name given by the company that developed the drug, and it remains the same even after the patent is released and other companies are allowed to market the medication.

- ▶ **Trade name:** This is the name given to the drug by the originating company. After the drug has been released to the market for approximately four years, a trade-named medication can be released by an alternative company. The trade name will be different, while the generic name will remain the same.

It is much safer for the nurse to remember the *generic name* rather than the trade name because the trade name will probably change.

> **EXAM ALERT**
>
> On the NCLEX exam, both the generic and trade names of medications might be included for clarification. The generic name will be given.

Approximately 80% of the time generic drugs in the same category have common syllables. If you can identify the commonality within the generic names, you can more easily learn the needed information for the NCLEX. The sections that follow look at some commonly given categories of drugs and help you to recognize the commonalities in the names. As you will see, each drug has a common part in its name, which will help you to quickly identify a particular drug by the common part of the name for that drug category.

Angiotensin-Converting Enzyme Inhibitors

This category of drugs is utilized to treat both primary and secondary hypertension. These drugs work by inhibiting conversion of angiotensin I to angiotensin II. Notice that all the generic names include the syllable *pril*. When you see these letters, you will know that they are angiotensin-converting enzyme (ACE) inhibitors. Table 2.1 highlights these in more depth.

TABLE 2.1   Angiotensin-Converting Enzyme Inhibitors

Action/Use	Drug Name*
Antihypertensives	Benazepril (Lotensin)
	Lisinopril (Zestril)
	Captopril (Capoten)
	Enalapril (Vasotec)
	Fosinopril (Monopril)
	Moexipril (Univas)
	Quinapril (Accupril)
	Ramipril (Altace)

*The generic name is listed first with the trade name in parentheses.

When working with angiotensin-converting enzyme inhibitors, it is important to know the potential side effects. The following list details the possible side effects/adverse reactions with this drug category:

- ▶ Hypotension
- ▶ Hacking cough
- ▶ Nausea/vomiting
- ▶ Rashes
- ▶ Angioedema

The following items are nursing considerations to know when working with ACE inhibitors:

- ▶ Monitor the vital signs frequently.
- ▶ Monitor the white blood cell count.
- ▶ Monitor the potassium and creatinine levels.
- ▶ Monitor the electrolyte levels.

Beta Adrenergic Blockers

Beta adrenergic blockers are drugs that help lower blood pressure, pulse rate, and cardiac output. They are also used to treat migraine headaches and other vascular headaches. Certain preparations of the beta blockers are used to treat glaucoma and prevent myocardial infarctions. These drugs act by blocking the sympathetic vasomotor response.

Notice the syllable *olol*. When you see these letters, you will know that these drugs are beta blockers. Table 2.2 highlights these beta blockers in more detail.

TABLE 2.2 Beta Adrenergic Blockers

Action/Use	Drug Name*
Act by blocking sympathetic vasomotor response	Acebutolol (Monitan, Rhotral, Sectral)
	Atenolol (Tenormin, Apo-Atenol, Nova-Atenol)
	Carvedilol (Coreg)
	Esmolol (Brevibloc)
	Propanolol (Inderal)
	Toprol-XL (Metoprolol)

*The generic name is listed first with the trade name in parentheses.

The potential side effects/adverse reactions of beta adrenergic blockers are listed here:

► Orthostatic hypotension

► Bradycardia

► Nausea/vomiting

► Diarrhea

► May mask hypoglycemic symptoms

The following list gives you some nursing interventions for working with clients using beta adrenergic blockers:

► Monitor the client's blood pressure, heart rate, and rhythm.

► Monitor the client for signs of edema. The nurse should assess lung sounds for rales and rhonchi.

► Monitor the client for changes in lab values (protein, BUN, creatinine) that indicate nephrotic syndrome.

► Teach the client to:

  ► Rise slowly

  ► Report bradycardia, dizziness, confusion, depression, or fever

  ► Taper off the medication

Anti-Infectives (Aminoglycosides)

Anti-infective drugs include bactericidals and bacteriostatics. They interfere with the protein synthesis of the bacteria, causing the bacteria to die. They are active against most aerobic gram-negative bacteria and against some gram-positive organisms.

Notice that these end in *cin*, and many of them end in *mycin*. So, when you see either of these syllables, you know these are anti-infectives. Table 2.3 explains the various anti-infectives.

TABLE 2.3   Anti-Infective Drugs

Action/Use	Drug Name*
Interfere with the protein synthesis of the bacteria, causing the bacteria to die	Gentamicin (Garamycin, Alcomicin, Genoptic)
	Kanamycin (Kantrex)
	Neomycin (Mycifradin)
	Streptomycin (Streptomycin)
	Tobramycin (Tobrex, Nebcin)
	Amikacin (Amikin)

*The generic name is listed first with the trade name in parentheses.

The following list highlights some possible side effects/adverse reactions from the use of anti-infectives (aminoglycosides):

▶ Ototoxicity

▶ Nephrotoxicity

▶ Seizures

▶ Blood dyscrasias

▶ Hypotension

▶ Rash

The following are nursing interventions you need to be aware of when working with clients using anti-infectives (aminoglycosides):

▶ Obtain a history of allergies.

▶ Monitor intake and output.

▶ Monitor vital signs during intravenous infusion.

▶ Maintain a patent IV site.

- ▶ Monitor for therapeutic levels.

- ▶ Monitor for signs of nephrotoxicity.

- ▶ Monitor for signs of ototoxicity.

- ▶ Teach the client to report any changes in urinary elimination.

- ▶ Monitor peak and trough levels.

TIP

Tests on peak and trough levels are done to obtain a blood level and determine the dosage needed for the client. They should be done 30–60 minutes after the third or fourth IV dose or 60 minutes after the third or fourth IM dose. Trough levels should be drawn 5 minutes before the next dose if possible. The client should be taught to report any change in renal function or in hearing because this category can be toxic to the kidneys and the auditory nerve.

CAUTION

These drugs are frequently used to treat super-infections such as methicillin-resistant staphylococcus aureus (MRSA). Clients with MRSA can exhibit the following symptoms: fever, malaise, redness, pain, swelling, perineal itching, diarrhea, stomatitis, and cough.

Benzodiazepines (Anticonvulsants/Antianxiety)

These drugs are used for their antianxiety or anticonvulsant effects.

Notice that all these contain the syllable *pam*, *pate*, or *lam*. Table 2.4 gives you a breakdown of these drug types.

TIP

Not all the benzodiazepines contain *pam*; some of them contain *pate* and *lam*, as in *aprazolam* (Xanax). However, they all contain *azo* or *aze*.

TABLE 2.4   Benzodiazepines (Anticonvulsants/Sedative/Antianxiety) Drugs

Action/Use	Drug Name*
Sedative-hypnotic; also used as anticonvulsants; have antianxiety effects	Clonazepam (Klonopin)
	Diazepam (Valium)
	Chlordiazepoxide (Librium)
	Lorazepam (Ativan)
	Flurazepam (Dalmane)

*The generic name is listed first with the trade name in parentheses.

The following list gives you some possible side effects and adverse reactions from the use of this classification of drugs:

- ▶ Drowsiness
- ▶ Lethargy
- ▶ Ataxia
- ▶ Depression
- ▶ Restlessness
- ▶ Slurred speech
- ▶ Bradycardia
- ▶ Hypotension
- ▶ Diplopia
- ▶ Nystagmus
- ▶ Nausea/vomiting
- ▶ Constipation
- ▶ Incontinence
- ▶ Urinary retention
- ▶ Respiratory depression
- ▶ Rash
- ▶ Urticaria

The following are some nursing interventions to know when working with the client taking benzodiazepines:

- ▶ Monitor respirations.
- ▶ Monitor liver function.
- ▶ Monitor kidney function.
- ▶ Monitor bone marrow function.
- ▶ Monitor for signs of chemical abuse.

Phenothiazines (Antipsychotic/Antiemetic)

These drugs are used as antiemetics or neuroleptics. These drugs are also used to treat psychosis in those clients with schizophrenia. Some phenothiazines, such as Phenergan (promethazine) and Compazine (prochlorperzine), are used to treat nausea and vomiting.

CAUTION

Because they are irritating to the tissue, Z-track method should be used when administering phenothiazines by intramuscular injection. If the client is allergic to one of the phenothiazines, she probably is allergic to all of them. If the client experiences an allergic reaction or extrapyramidal effects, a more severe reaction, she should be given Benadryl (diphenhydramine hydrochloride) or Cogentin (benztropine mesylate).

Notice that all these contain the syllable *zine* (see Table 2.5).

TABLE 2.5 Phenothiazines (Antipsychotic/Antiemetic) Drugs

Action/Use	Drug Name*
Used as antiemetics or major tranquilizers	Chlopromazine (Thorazine)
	Prochlorperazine (Compazine)
	Trifluoperazine (Stelazine)
	Promethazine (Phenergan)
	Hydroxyzine (Vistaril)
	Fluphenazine (Prolixin)

*The generic name is listed first with the trade name in parentheses.

The following list gives you some possible side effects and adverse reactions from the use of phenothiazines:

▶ Extrapyramidal effects

▶ Drowsiness

▶ Sedation

▶ Orthostatic hypotension

▶ Dry mouth

▶ Agranulocytosis

▶ Photosensitivity

▶ Neuroleptic malignant syndrome

The following are some nursing interventions to know when working with a client taking phenothiazines:

▶ Protect the medication from light.

▶ Do not mix the liquid forms of Prolixin (Fluphenazine HCL) with any beverage containing caffeine, tannates, or pectin due to physical incompatibility.

▶ Monitor liver enzymes.

▶ Monitor renal function.

▶ Protect the client from overexposure to the sun.

Glucocorticoids

These drugs are used in the treatment of conditions requiring suppression of the immune system or to decrease inflammatory response. They are also used in Addison's disease, chronic obstructive pulmonary disease (COPD), and immune disorders. These drugs have anti-inflammatory, anti-allergenic, and anti-stress effects. They are used for replacement therapy for adrenal insufficiency (Addison's disease); as immunosuppressive drugs in post-transplant clients; and to reduce cerebral edema associated with head trauma, neurosurgery, and brain tumors.

Notice that all these contain *sone* or *cort* (see Table 2.6).

TABLE 2.6 Glucocorticoid Drugs

Action/Use	Drug Name*
Used to decrease the inflammatory response to allergies and inflammatory diseases or to decrease the possibility of organ transplant rejection	Prednisolone (Delta-Cortef, Prednisol, Prednisolone)
	Prednisone (Apo-Prednisone, Deltasone, Meticorten, Orasone, Panasol-S)
	Betamethasone (Celestone, Selestoject, Betnesol)
	Dexamethasone (Decadron, Deronil, Dexon, Mymethasone, Dalalone)
	Cortisone (Cortone)
	Hydrocortisone (Cortef, Hydrocortone Phosphate, Cortifoam)
	Methylprednisolone (Solu-cortef, Depo-Medrol, Depopred, Medrol, Rep-Pred)
	Triamcinolone (Amcort, Aristocort, Atolone, Kenalog, Triamolone)

*The generic name is listed first with the trade name in parentheses.

The following list gives you some possible side effects and adverse reactions from the use of this drug type:

- ▶ Acne
- ▶ Poor wound healing
- ▶ Leukocytosis
- ▶ Ecchymosis
- ▶ Bruising
- ▶ Petechiae
- ▶ Depression
- ▶ Flushing
- ▶ Sweating
- ▶ Mood changes (depression), insomnia, hypomania
- ▶ Hypertension
- ▶ Osteoporosis
- ▶ Diarrhea
- ▶ Hemorrhage

CAUTION

These drugs can cause Cushing's syndrome. Signs of Cushing's syndrome include moon faces, edema, elevated blood glucose levels, purple straie, weight gain, buffalo hump, and hirsutism.

The following are nursing interventions used when working with a client taking glucocorticoids:

- ▶ Monitor glucose levels.
- ▶ Weigh the client daily.
- ▶ Monitor blood pressure.
- ▶ Monitor for signs of infection.

Antivirals

These drugs are used for their antiviral properties. They inhibit viral growth by inhibiting an enzyme within the virus. Herpetic lesions respond to these drugs. Clients with acquired immune deficiency syndrome (AIDS) are often treated with this category of drugs either alone or in combination with other antiviral drugs. These drugs are also used to treat herpetic lesions (HSV-1, HSV-2), varicella infections (chickenpox), herpes zoster (shingles), herpes simplex (fever blisters), encephalitis, cytomegalovirus (CMV), and respiratory syncytial virus (RSV).

Notice that all these drug names contain *vir*. Table 2.7 lists some of these drug types.

TABLE 2.7   Antiviral Drugs

Action/Use	Drug Name*
Used for their antiviral effects	Acyclovir (Zovirax)
	Ritonavir (Norvir)
	Saquinovir (Invirase, Fortovase)
	Indinavir (Crixivan)
	Abacavir (Ziagen)
	Cidofovir (Vistide)
	Ganciclovir (Cytovene, Vitrasert)

*The generic name is listed first with the trade name in parentheses.

The following list gives some side effects and adverse effects that are usually associated with this drug category:

▶ Nausea

▶ Vomiting

▶ Diarrhea

▶ Oliguria

▶ Proteinuria

▶ Vaginitis

▶ Central nervous side effects (these are less common):

    ▶ Tremors

    ▶ Confusion

    ▶ Seizures

    ▶ Severe, sudden anemia

The following nursing interventions are used when working with a client taking antivirals:

▶ Tell the client to report a rash because this can indicate an allergic reaction.

▶ Watch for signs of infection.

▶ Monitor the creatinine level frequently.

▶ Monitor liver profile.

▶ Monitor bowel pattern before and during treatment.

Cholesterol-Lowering Agents

This drug type is used to help the client lower cholesterol and triglyceride levels and to decrease the potential for cardiovascular disease. Notice that all these contain the syllable *vas-tatin*. It should be noted that many advertisements call these "statin" drugs. These drugs should not be confused with the statin drugs used for their antifungal effects. These can include nystatin (trade name Mycostatin or Nilstat). Table 2.8 lists some of the cholesterol-lowering agents.

TABLE 2.8   Cholesterol-Lowering Drugs

Action/Use	Drug Name*
Used to lower cholesterol	Atorvastatin (Lipitor)
	Fluvastatin (Lescol)
	Lovastatin (Mevacor)
	Pravastatin (Pravachol)
	Simvastatin (Zocor)
	Rosuvastatin (Crestor)

*The generic name is listed first with the trade name in parentheses.

CAUTION

This category should not be taken with grapefruit juice and should be taken at night. The client should have regular liver studies to determine the presence of liver disease.

Here is a list of side effects and adverse reactions that could occur with the use of cholesterol-lowering agents:

▶ Rash

▶ Alopecia

▶ Dyspepsia

▶ Liver dysfunction

▶ Muscle weakness (myalgia)

▶ Headache

CAUTION

Rhabdomyolysis, a muscle-wasting syndrome, has been linked with the use of cholesterol-lowering agents. The client should be instructed to report cola-colored urine and unexplained muscle soreness and weakness to the physician because these can be signs of rhabdomyolysis.

The following nursing interventions are used when working with a client taking cholesterol-lowering agents:

▶ Include a diet low in cholesterol and fat in therapy.

▶ Monitor cholesterol levels.

▶ Monitor liver profile.

▶ Monitor renal function.

▶ Monitor for muscle pain and weakness.

Angiotensin Receptor Blockers

These drugs block vasoconstrictor- and aldosterone-secreting angiotensin II. They are used to treat primary or secondary hypertension and are an excellent choice for clients who complain of the coughing associated with ACE inhibitors. Notice that all these contain *sartan*. Table 2.9 lists some of these drugs.

TABLE 2.9 Angiotensin Receptor Blocker Drugs

Action/Use	Drug Name*
Used to lower blood pressure and increase cardiac output	Valsartan (Diovan)
	Candesartan (Atacand)
	Losartan (Cozaar)
	Telmisartan (Micardis)

*The generic name is listed first with the trade name in parentheses.

The following list gives some side effects and adverse effects that accompany the use of angiotensin receptor blockers:

▶ Dizziness

▶ Insomnia

▶ Depression

▶ Diarrhea

▶ Nausea/vomiting

▶ Impotence

▶ Muscle cramps

▶ Neutropenia

▶ Cough

The following nursing interventions are used when working with a client taking angiotensin receptor blocker agents:

▶ Monitor blood pressure.

▶ Monitor BUN.

▶ Monitor creatinine.

▶ Monitor electrolytes.

▶ Tell the client to check edema in feet and legs daily.

▶ Monitor hydration status.

Histamine 2 Antagonists

These drugs are used in the treatment of gastroesophageal reflux disease (GERD), acid reflux, and gastric ulcers. They inhibit histamine 2 (H2) release in the gastric parietal cells, therefore inhibiting gastric acids.

Notice that all these contain the syllable *tidine* (see Table 2.10).

TABLE 2.10   Histamine 2 Antagonist Drugs

Action/Use	Drug Name*
Block histamine 2 receptor sites, decreasing acid production; used to treat gastric ulcers and GERD	Cimetidine (Tagamet)
	Famotidine (Pepcid)
	Nizatidine (Axid)
	Rantidine (Zantac)

*The generic name is listed first with the trade name in parentheses.

The following list gives some side effects and adverse effects associated with histamine 2 antagonists:

▶ Confusion

▶ Bradycardia/tachycardia

▶ Diarrhea

▶ Psychosis

▶ Seizures

▶ Agranulocytosis

▶ Rash

▶ Alopecia

▶ Gynecomastia

▶ Galactorrhea

Following are some nursing interventions when working with a client taking H2 antagonists:

▶ Monitor the blood urea nitrogen levels.

▶ Administer the medication with meals.

▶ If the client is taking the medication with antacids, make sure he takes antacids one hour before or after taking these drugs.

▶ Cimetidine can be prescribed in one large dose at bedtime.

▶ Sucralfate decreases the effects of histamine 2 receptor blockers.

Proton Pump Inhibitors

These drugs suppress gastric secretion by inhibiting the hydrogen/potassium ATPase enzyme system. They are used in the treatment of gastric ulcers, indigestion, and GERD.

Notice that all these drugs contain the syllable *prazole* and should be given prior to meals. Table 2.11 highlights proton pump inhibitor drugs.

TABLE 2.11   Proton Pump Inhibitors

Action/Use	Drug Name*
Used in the treatment of GERD, gastric ulcers, and esophagitis	Esomeprazole (Nexium)
	Lansoprazole (Prevacid)
	Pantoprazole (Protonix)
	Rabeprazole (AciPhex)

*The generic name is listed first with the trade name in parentheses.

The following list gives some side effects and adverse effects associated with proton pump inhibitors:

- Headache

- Insomnia

- Diarrhea

- Flatulence

- Rash

- Hyperglycemia

Some nursing interventions to use when working with a client taking proton pump inhibitors are as follows:

- Do not crush pantoprazole (Protonix). Use a filter when administering IV pantoprazole.

- Advise the client to take proton pump inhibitors before meals for best absorption.

- Monitor liver function.

Anticoagulants

These drugs are used in the treatment of thrombolytic disease. These drugs are used to treat pulmonary emboli, myocardial infarction, and deep-vein thrombosis; after coronary artery bypass surgery; and for other conditions requiring anticoagulation.

Notice that all these drugs contain the syllable *parin* and are heparin derivatives. The client should have a PTT check to evaluate the bleeding time when giving heparin. The antidote for heparin is protamine sulfate. Table 2.12 lists some common anticoagulants.

TABLE 2.12 Anticoagulant Drugs

Action/Use	Drug Name*
Used to treat clotting disorders and to thin the blood	Heparin sodium (Hepalean)
	Enoxaparin sodium (Lovenox)
	Dalteparin sodium (Fragmin)

*The generic name is listed first with the trade name in parentheses.

The following list gives side effects and adverse effects of heparin derivatives:

▶ Fever

▶ Diarrhea

▶ Stomatitis

▶ Bleeding

▶ Hematuria

▶ Dermatitis

▶ Alopecia

▶ Pruritus

Nursing interventions to use in caring for a client taking an anticoagulant (heparin derivative) include the following:

▶ Blood studies (hematocrit and occult blood in stool) should be checked every three months.

▶ Monitor PTT often for heparin (therapeutic levels are 1.5–2.0 times the control). There is no specific bleeding time done for enoxaparin (Lovenox); however, the platelet levels should be checked for thrombocytopenia.

▸ Monitor platelet count.

▸ Monitor for signs of bleeding.

▸ Monitor for signs of infection.

More Drug Identification Helpers

These are some of the commonly given medications that allow you to utilize the testing technique of commonalities. Looking at these similarities will help you manage the knowledge needed to pass the NCLEX and better care for your clients.

Here are some other clues that can help you in identifying drug types:

▸ **Caine** = anesthetics (LidoCAINE)

▸ **Mab** = monoclonal antibodies (PalivazuMAB)

▸ **Ceph or cef** = cephalosporins (CEFatazime)

▸ **Cillin** = penicillins (AmpiCILLIN)

▸ **Cycline** = tetracycline (TetraCYCLINE)

▸ **Stigmine** = cholinergics (PhyoSTIGMINE)

▸ **Phylline** = bronchodilators (AminoPHYLLINE)

▸ **Cal** = calciums (CALcimar)

▸ **Done** = opioids (MethoDONE)

CAUTION

Do not give tetracycline to pregnant women or small children. It stains the child's teeth dark and stunts the growth of small children.

Herbals

Herbals are not considered by some to be medications. They are not regulated by the FDA and can be obtained without a prescription. They do, however, have medicinal properties. Herbals are included on the NCLEX in the category of pharmacology. The list that follows includes some common herbals used by clients as well as some associated nursing precautions:

▸ **Feverfew:** This is used to prevent and treat migraines, arthritis, and fever. This herbal should not be taken with Coumadin, aspirin, NSAIDs, thrombolytics, or antiplatelet medications because it will prolong the bleeding time.

▶ **Ginseng:** This is used as an anti-inflammatory. It has estrogen effects, enhances the immune system, and improves mental and physical abilities. This herbal decreases the effects of anticoagulants and NSAIDs. It also should not be taken by clients taking corticosteroids because the combination of these two can result in extremely high levels of corticosteroids. High doses cause liver problems. A client with hypertension and bipolar disorder should be cautioned regarding the use of ginseng because this herbal can interfere with medications used to treat these disorders.

▶ **Ginkgo:** This improves memory and can be used to treat depression. It also improves peripheral circulation. Ginkgo should not be taken with MAO inhibitors, anticoagulants, or antiplatelets. It increases the bleeding time in clients taking NSAIDs, cephalosporins, and valproic acid. Clients with seizure disorders should not take ginkgo because it can exacerbate seizure activity.

▶ **Echinacea:** This is used to treat colds, fevers, and urinary tract infections. This herbal can interfere with immunosuppressive agents, methotrexate, and ketoconizole.

▶ **Kava-kava:** This herb is used to treat insomnia and mild muscle aches and pains. It increases the effects of central nervous system (CNS) suppressants and decreases the effects of levodopa. It can also increase the effect of MAOIs and cause liver damage.

▶ **St. John's Wort:** This is used to treat mild to moderate depression. This herbal increases adverse CNS effects when used with alcohol or antidepressant medications.

▶ **Ma Huang:** This is used to treat asthma and hay fever, for weight loss, and to increase energy levels. It increases the effect of MAOIs, sympathomimetics, theophylline, and cardiac glycosides.

Drug Schedules

It is important for the nurse to be aware of the drug schedules because several questions might be asked on the NCLEX exam regarding safety. The list that follows characterizes the various drug schedules:

▶ **Schedule I:** Research use only (for example, LSD). These drugs are not medically safe to take and have a high potential for abuse.

▶ **Schedule II:** Requires a written prescription for each refill. No telephone renewals are allowed (for example, narcotics, stimulants, and barbiturates).

▶ **Schedule III:** Requires a new prescription after six months or five refills; it can be a telephone order (for example, codeine, steroids, and antidepressants).

▶ **Schedule IV:** Requires a new prescription after six months (for example, benzodi-azepines).

▶ **Schedule V:** Dispensed as any other prescription or without prescription if state law allows (for example, antidiarrheals and antitussives).

Pregnancy Categories for Drugs

These drug categories might also be included on the NCLEX exam. It is important for the nurse to know which categories the pregnant client should avoid:

▶ **Category A:** No risk to fetus.

▶ **Category B:** Insufficient data to use in pregnancy.

▶ **Category C:** Benefits of medication could outweigh the risks.

▶ **Category D:** Risk to fetus exist, but the benefits of the medication could outweigh the probable risks.

▶ **Category X:** Avoid use in pregnancy or in those who may become pregnant. Potential risks to the fetus outweigh the potential benefits.

Exam Prep Questions

1. Which instruction should be given to the client taking alendronate sodium (Fosamax)?

   ○ **A.** Take the medication before arising.

   ○ **B.** Force fluids while taking this medication.

   ○ **C.** Remain upright for 30 minutes after taking this medication.

   ○ **D.** Take the medication in conjunction with estrogen.

2. The client is discharged from the unit with a prescription for Evista (raloxifene HCl). Which of the following is a side effect of this medication?

   ○ **A.** Leg cramps

   ○ **B.** Hot flashes

   ○ **C.** Urinary frequency

   ○ **D.** Cold extremities

3. An elderly diabetic who has been maintained on metformin (Glucophage) is scheduled for a cardiac catheterization. Which instruction should be given to the client?

   ○ **A.** Take the medication as ordered prior to the exam.

   ○ **B.** Limit the amount of protein in the diet prior to the exam.

   ○ **C.** Discontinue the medication prior to the exam.

   ○ **D.** Take the medication with only water prior to the exam.

4. The client's mother contacts the clinic regarding medication administration stating, "My daughter can't swallow this capsule. It's too large." Investigation reveals that the medication is a capsule marked *SR*. The nurse should instruct the mother to:

   ○ **A.** Open the capsule and mix the medication with ice cream.

   ○ **B.** Crush the medication and administer it with 8 oz. of liquid.

   ○ **C.** Call the pharmacist and request an alternative preparation of the medication.

   ○ **D.** Stop the medication and inform the physician at the follow-up visit.

5. A five-year-old is being treated for an acute attack of asthma using racemic epinephrine (epineph-rine hydrochloride) nebulizer stat. Which finding indicates an adverse effect of this medication?

   ○ **A.** Excitability

   ○ **B.** Tremors

   ○ **C.** Heart rate 150

   ○ **D.** Nausea

6. The client is being treated with intravenous Vancomycin for MRSA when the nurse notes redness on the client's neck and chest. Place in ordered sequence the actions to be taken by the nurse:

   ○ **A.** Call the doctor.

   ○ **B.** Stop the IV infusion of Vancomycin.

   ○ **C.** Administer Benadryl as ordered.

   ○ **D.** Take the vital signs.

7. A client with leukemia is receiving oral prednisolone (Prednisone). An expected side effect of the prolonged use of prednisoline is which of the following?

   ○ **A.** Weight loss

   ○ **B.** Decreased appetite

   ○ **C.** Hirsutism

   ○ **D.** Integumentary bronzing

8. Which laboratory result would concern the nurse caring for a client who is receiving furosemide (Lasix)?

   ○ **A.** Potassium level of 2.5

   ○ **B.** Sodium level of 140

   ○ **C.** Glucose level of 110

   ○ **D.** Calcium level of 8

9. Which instruction should be given to a client taking Lugol's solution prior to a thyroidectomy?

   ○ **A.** Take at bedtime.

   ○ **B.** Take the medication with juice.

   ○ **C.** Report changes in appetite.

   ○ **D.** Avoid sunshine while taking the medication.

10. A client is admitted to the recovery room following an exploratory laparotomy. Which medication should be kept nearby?

 ○ **A.** Nitroprusside (Nipride)

 ○ **B.** Naloxone hydrochloride (Narcan)

 ○ **C.** Flumazenil (Romazicon)

 ○ **D.** Diphenhydramine (Benadryl)

11. A client with renal failure has an order for erythropoietin (Epogen) to be given subcutaneously. The nurse should teach the client to report which of the following?

 ○ **A.** Severe headache

 ○ **B.** Slight nausea

 ○ **C.** Decreased urination

 ○ **D.** Itching

Answer Rationales

1. Answer C is correct. Alendronate sodium is a drug used to treat osteoporosis. Let's use testing strategies for this question. Look at answers A and C; these are opposites. When you are in bed, you are lying down. The drug should not be given while lying down, nor should it be taken with medication or with estrogen. In answer C, you are upright. This drug causes gastric reflux, so you should remain upright and take it with only water. Notice the clue in the name of the drug: *fosa*, as in fossils. All the drugs in this category contain the syllable *dronate*.

2. Answer B is correct. This drug is in the same category as the chemotherapeutic agent tamoxifen (Nolvadex) used for breast cancer. In the case of Evista, this drug is used to treat osteoporosis. Notice that the *E* stands for estrogen. This drug has an agonist effect, so it binds with estrogen and can cause hot flashes. This drug does not cause leg cramps, urinary frequency, or cold extremities, so answers A, C, and D are incorrect.

3. Answer C is correct. Glucophage can cause renal problems. The dye used in cardiac catheterizations is also detrimental to the kidneys. The client may be placed on sliding scale insulin for 48 hours after the dye procedure or until renal function returns. Note the syllable *phage*, as seen in the syllable *phagia*, which means eating. Also note that answers A and C are opposites. Answer A is incorrect because the medication should be withheld; answer B is incorrect because limiting the amount of protein in the diet prior to the exam has no correlation to the medication. Taking the medication with water is not necessary, so answer D is incorrect.

4. Answer C is correct. *SR* means sustained release. These medications cannot be altered. In answers A and B, crushing or opening the capsule is not allowed. In answer D, the doctor should be notified immediately.

5. Answer C is correct. Adverse effects of epinephrine include hypertension and tachycardia. Answers A, B, and D are expected side effects of racemic epinephrine.

6. The correct order is B, D, A, C.

7. Answer C is correct. Notice that the testing strategy "odd item out" can be used in this question. Answers A, B, and D are symptoms of Addison's disease. Answer C is the answer that is different from the rest. Hirsutism, or facial hair, is a side effect of cortisone therapy.

8. Answer A is correct. Furosemide (Lasix) is a loop diuretic. Note that most of the loop diuretics end in *ide*. In answers B, C, and D, the findings are all within normal limits.

9. Answer B is correct. Lugol's solution is a soluble solution of potassium iodine and should be given with juice because it is bitter to taste. In answer A the medication can be taken at another time, so it is incorrect. Reporting changes in appetite is unnecessary, so answer C is incorrect. Answer D is incorrect because it is also unnecessary.

10. Answer B is correct. During the postoperative period, narcotics are given. Narcan is the antidote to narcotics, so answer B is correct. Nipride is utilized to lower blood pressure, so answer A is incorrect. Romazicon is the antidote for the benzodiazepines, so answer C is incorrect. Benadryl is an antihistamine, so answer D is incorrect.

11. Answer A is correct. Severe headache can indicate impending seizure activity. Slight nausea is expected when beginning the therapy, so answer B is incorrect. A client with renal failure already has itching and decreased urination, so answers C and D are incorrect.

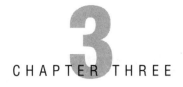

CHAPTER THREE

Caring for the Client with Disorders of the Respiratory System

---

Terms you'll need to understand

- ✓ Acute respiratory failure
- ✓ Apnea
- ✓ Asthma
- ✓ Atelectasis
- ✓ Bronchitis
- ✓ Continuous positive airway pressure (CPAP)
- ✓ Cor pulmonale
- ✓ Cyanosis
- ✓ Dyspnea

- ✓ Emphysema
- ✓ Empyema
- ✓ Hemoptysis
- ✓ Hypoxemia
- ✓ Hypoxia
- ✓ Pleural effusion
- ✓ Pleurisy
- ✓ Pneumonia
- ✓ Pulmonary embolus
- ✓ Tachypnea

Nursing skills you'll need to master

- ✓ Assessing breath sounds
- ✓ Providing tracheostomy care
- ✓ Collecting sputum
- ✓ Teaching proper use of an inhaler (MDI and DPI)
- ✓ Performing chest physiotherapy
- ✓ Assisting with thoracentesis

- ✓ Obtaining a throat culture
- ✓ Performing venipuncture
- ✓ Administering medication
- ✓ Managing chest drainage system
- ✓ Maintaining oxygen therapy
- ✓ Maintaining assisted ventilation

Chronic Obstructive Pulmonary Disease

Chronic obstructive pulmonary disease (COPD) exists when prolonged disease or injury has made the lungs less capable of meeting the body's oxygen needs. Examples of COPD include chronic bronchitis, emphysema, and asthma.

Chronic Bronchitis

Chronic bronchitis, an inflammation of the bronchi and bronchioles, is caused by continuous exposure to infection and non-infectious irritants, such as cigarette smoke. The condition is most common in those ages 40 to 55. Chronic bronchitis may be reversed with the removal of noxious irritants, although it is often complicated by chronic lung infections. These infections, which are characterized by a productive cough and dyspnea, can progress to right-sided heart failure and pulmonary hypertension. Chronic bronchitis and emphysema have similar symptoms that require similar interventions.

Emphysema

Emphysema is the irreversible overdistention of the airspaces of the lungs, which results in destruction of the alveolar walls. Clients with emphysema are classified as *pink puffers* or *blue bloaters*. Pink puffers may complain of exertional dyspnea without cyanosis. Blue bloaters develop chronic hypoxia, cyanosis, polycythemia, cor pulmonale, pulmonary edema, and eventually respiratory failure.

Physical assessment reveals the presence of a barrel chest, use of accessory muscles, coughing with the production of thick mucoid sputum, prolonged expiratory phase with grunting respirations, peripheral cyanosis, and digital clubbing.

In identifying emphysema, a chest x-ray reveals hyperinflation of the lungs with flattened diaphragm. Pulmonary studies show that the residual volume is increased while vital capacity is decreased. Arterial blood gases reveal hypoxemia.

Many symptoms of chronic bronchitis and emphysema are the same; therefore, medications for the client with chronic bronchitis and emphysema include bronchodilators, steroids, antibiotics, and expectorants. Oxygen should be administered via nasal cannula at 2–3 liters/minute. Close attention should be given to correcting acid-base imbalances, meeting the client's nutritional needs, avoidance of respiratory irritants, prevention of respiratory infections, providing oral hygiene, and client teaching regarding medications.

CAUTION

When administering antibiotics, a separate IV line should be established for the administration of amino-phylline—a bronchodilator—because incompatibilities can exist with some antibiotics and the administration of a bronchodilator. If only one access is established, the SAS (saline, administer drug, saline) procedure should be used.

The client receiving aminophylline should be placed on cardiorespiratory monitoring because amino-phylline affects heart rate, respiratory rate, and blood pressure. In this scenario, toxicity can occur rapidly. Toxic symptoms include nausea, vomiting, tachycardia, palpitations, hypotension, shock, coma, and death.

The therapeutic range for aminophylline is as follows: 10–20 mcg/mL.

Asthma

Asthma is the most common respiratory condition of childhood. *Intrinsic (nonallergenic) asthma* is precipitated by exposure to cold temperatures or infection. *Extrinsic (allergenic or atopic) asthma* is often associated with childhood eczema. Both asthma and eczema are triggered by allergies to certain foods or food additives. Introducing new foods to the infant one at a time helps decrease the development of these allergic responses. Easily digested, hypoallergenic foods and juices should be introduced first, including rice cereal and apple juice, which may be given at six months of age. Cow's milk should not be given to the infant before one year of age. Symptoms of asthma include expiratory wheeze; shortness of breath; and a dry, hacking cough, which eventually produces thick, white, tenacious sputum. In some instances an attack may progress to status asthmaticus, leading to respiratory collapse and death.

Management of the client with asthma includes maintenance therapy with mast cell stabilizers and leukotriene modifiers. Treatment of acute asthmatic attacks includes the administration of oral or inhaled short-term or long-term B2 agonist and anti-inflammatories as well as supplemental oxygen. Methylxanthines, such as aminophylline, are rarely used for the treatment of asthma. These drugs, which can cause tachycardia and dysrhythmias, are administered as a last resort. Antibiotics are frequently ordered when a respiratory infection is present.

Acute Respiratory Infections

Acute respiratory infections, such as pneumonia, are among the most common causes of death from infectious diseases in the United States. Pneumonia is the fifth major cause of death in persons over age 65.

Pneumonia

Pneumonia is an inflammation of the parenchyma of the lungs. Causative organisms include bacteria, viruses, and fungi. Some of these organisms are listed here:

▶ Pneumococcus

▶ Group A beta hemolytic streptococcus

▶ Staphylococcus

▶ Pseudomonas

▶ Influenza types A and B

▶ Cytomegalovirus

▶ Aspergillus fungiatus

▶ Pneumocystis carinii

Presenting symptoms depend on the causative organism. The client with viral pneumonia tends to have milder symptoms, whereas the client with bacterial pneumonia might have chills and fever as high as 103°. Clients with cytomegalovirus, pneumocystis carinii, or aspergillus will be acutely ill. General symptoms of pneumonia include

▶ Hypoxia

▶ Tachypnea

▶ Tachycardia

▶ Chest pain

▶ Malaise

▶ Fever

▶ Confusion (especially in the elderly client)

Care of the client with pneumonia depends on the causative organism. The management of bacterial pneumonias includes antibiotics, antitussives, antipyretics, and oxygen. Antibiotics that may be ordered include penicillin G, tetracycline, garamycin, and erythromycin. Viral pneumonias do not respond to antimicrobial therapy, but are treated with antiviral medication such as Symmetrel (amantadine). Fungal pneumonias are treated with antifungal medication such as Nizoral (ketoconazole). Additional therapies for the client with pneumonia include providing for fluid and nutritional needs, obtaining frequent vital signs, and providing oral hygiene. Supplemental oxygen and chest percussion and drainage should be performed as ordered by the physician

> **CAUTION**
>
> Some medications used in the treatment of pneumonia require special attention:
>
> ▶ **Tetracycline**—Should not be given to women who are pregnant or to small children because of the damage it can cause to developing teeth and bones.
>
> ▶ **Garamycin**—An aminoglycoside, it is both ototoxic and nephrotoxic. It is important to monitor the client for signs of toxicity. Serum peak and trough levels are obtained according to hospital protocol.
>
> Peak levels for aminoglycosides are drawn 30 minutes after the third or fourth IV infusion . Trough levels for aminoglycosides are drawn 30 minutes before the third or fourth IV infusion. The therapeutic range for garamycin is 4–10 mcg/mL.

Pleurisy

Pleurisy, an inflammation of the pleural sac, can be associated with upper respiratory infection, pulmonary embolus, thoracotomy, chest trauma, or cancer. Symptoms include

- ▶ Sharp pain on inspiration

- ▶ Chills

- ▶ Fever

- ▶ Cough

- ▶ Dyspnea

Chest x-ray reveals the presence of air or fluid in the pleural sac. Management of the client with pleurisy includes the administration of analgesics, antitussives, antibiotics, and oxygen therapy. The presence of pleural effusion can require the client to have a thoracentesis. It is the nurse's responsibility to position the client for the procedure and to monitor for signs of complications related to the procedure. The nurse should assess the client's vital signs, particularly changes in respirations and blood pressure, which can reflect impending shock from fluid loss or bleeding. The nurse should also observe the client for signs of a pneumothorax.

Nursing Skill: Positioning the client for a thoracentesis

- ▶ Sitting on the edge of the bed with feet supported and with the head and arms resting on a padded over bed table)

- ▶ Sitting astride a chair with the arms and head resting on the back of the chair

- ▶ Lying on the unaffected side with the head of the bed elevated 30 to 45 degrees (for clients unable to sit upright)

Tuberculosis

Tuberculosis (TB) is a highly contagious respiratory infection caused by the mycobacterium tuberculosis. It is transmitted by droplets from the respiratory tract. Airborne precautions, as outlined by the Centers for Disease Control (CDC), should be used when caring for the client with tuberculosis.

> **NOTE**
>
> Standard precautions and transmission-based precautions are provided in Appendix A, "Things You Forgot," which is on the CD.

Diagnosis includes the administration of the Mantoux skin test, sometimes referred to as the Purified Protein Derivative (PPD), which is read in 48–72 hours. The presence of a positive Mantoux test indicates exposure to TB but not active infection. A chest x-ray should be ordered for those with a prior positive skin test. A definite diagnosis of TB is made if the sputum specimen is positive for the tubercle bacillus. Factors that can cause a false positive TB skin test include nontuberculous mycobacterium and inoculation with BCG vaccine. Factors that can cause a false negative TB skin test include anergy (a weakened immune system), recent TB infection, age, vaccination with live viruses, overwhelming TB, and poor testing technique. Management of the client with TB includes the use of ultraviolet light therapy and the administration of antimycobacterial drugs. Medication regimens can consist of several drugs including Myambutol (ethambutol), INH (isoniazid), Rifadin (rifampin), and PZA (pyrazinamide). The use of multiple drug therapy has reduced treatment time from two years to as little as six months; however, drug resistant forms may require longer treatment periods. Clients are no longer considered infectious after three negative sputum samples have been obtained. Surgical management may include a wedge resection or lobectomy.

Influenza

Influenza is an acute highly contagious infection that primarily affects the upper respiratory tract. Symptoms of influenza include the following:

▶ Chills and fever greater than 102° F.

▶ Sore throat and laryngitis

▶ Runny nose

▶ Muscle aches and headache

Complications of influenza include pneumonia, exacerbations of Chronic Obstructive Pulmonary Disease (COPD), and myositis. More serious complications include pericarditis and encephalitis. Children, the elderly, and those with chronic illness are more likely to develop severe complications; therefore, it is recommended that these clients receive annual immunization. The vaccine is given in the fall, prior to the onset of annual outbreaks, which occur in the winter months. The vaccine is produced in eggs; therefore, it should not be given to anyone who is allergic to egg protein. Children age two and older can receive the nasal vaccine as well as adults.

Treatment of influenza is aimed at controlling symptoms and preventing complications. Interventions for the client with influenza include bed rest, increased fluid intake, decongestant nasal sprays, antitussives with codeine, and antipyretics. Antibiotics are indicated if the client develops bacterial pneumonia. Antiviral medication such as Relenza (zanamivir) and Tamiflu (oseltamivir) are used for the prevention as well as the treatment of influenza A and B and can be used to reduce the duration and severity of symptoms. Symmetrel (amantadine) or Flumadine (rimantadine) are also used to prevent or decrease symptoms of the flu.

Acute Respiratory Failure

Acute respiratory failure can be defined as the lungs' failure to meet the body's oxygen requirements. One acute respiratory condition you need to be familiar with is acute respiratory distress syndrome, commonly known as ARDS.

Acute Respiratory Distress Syndrome

Acute respiratory distress syndrome, commonly known as *ARDS* or *noncardiogenic pulmonary edema*, occurs mostly in otherwise healthy persons. ARDS can be the result of anaphylaxis, aspiration, pulmonary emboli, inhalation burn injury, or complications from abdominal or thoracic surgery. ARDS may be diagnosed by a chest x-ray that will reveal emphysematous changes and infiltrates that give the lungs a characteristic appearance described as ground glass. Assessment of the client with ARDS reveals

- ▶ Hypoxia
- ▶ Sternal and costal retractions
- ▶ Presence of rales or rhonchi
- ▶ Diminished breath sounds
- ▶ Refractory hypoxemia

Care of the client with ARDS involves

- ▶ Use of assisted ventilation
- ▶ Monitoring of arterial blood gases

▶ Attention to nutritional needs

▶ Frequent change in position, placement in high Fowler's position, prone position, or use of specialized beds to minimize consolidation of infiltrates in large airways

▶ Investigational therapies, including the use of vitamins C and E, aspirin, interleukin, and surfactant replacements

Pulmonary Embolus

Pulmonary embolus refers to the obstruction of the pulmonary artery or one of its branches by a clot or some other undissolved matter, such as fat or a gaseous substance. Clots can originate anywhere in the body but are most likely to migrate from a vein deep in the legs, pelvis, kidney, or arms. *Fat emboli* are associated with fractures of the long bones, particularly the femur. *Air emboli*, which are less common, can occur during the insertion or removal of a central line. Common risk factors for the development of pulmonary embolus include immobilization, fractures, trauma, cigarette smoking, use of oral contraceptives, and history of clot formation.

TIP

Remember the three Fs associated with fat emboli:

▶ Fat

▶ Femur

▶ Football player

Fat emboli are associated with fracture of long bones (such as a fractured femur); most fractured femurs occur in young men 18–25, the age of most football players.

Symptoms of a pulmonary embolus depend on the size and location of the clot or undissolved matter. Symptoms include

▶ Chest pain

▶ Dyspnea

▶ Syncope

▶ Hemoptysis

▶ Tachycardia

▶ Hypotension

▶ Sense of apprehension

- Petechiae over the chest and axilla

- Distended neck veins

Diagnostic tests to confirm the presence of pulmonary embolus include chest x-ray, pulmonary angiography, lung scan, and ECG to rule out myocardial infarction. Management of the client with a pulmonary embolus includes

- Placing the client in high Fowler's position

- Administering oxygen via mask

- Giving medication for chest pain

- Using thrombolytics/anticoagulants

Antibiotics are indicated for those with septic emboli. Surgical management using umbrella-type filters is indicated for those who cannot take anticoagulants as well as for the client who has recurrent emboli while taking anticoagulants. Clients receiving anticoagulant therapy should be observed for signs of bleeding. PT, INR, and PTT are three tests used to track the client's clotting time. You can refer to Chapter 13, "Caring for the Client with Disorders of the Cardiovascular System," for a more complete discussion of these tests.

> **CAUTION**
>
> Streptokinase is made from beta strep; therefore, clients with a history of strep infections may respond poorly to anticoagulant therapy with streptokinase because they might have formed antibodies.
>
> Streptokinase is not clot specific; therefore, the client may develop a tendency to bleed from incision or injection sites.

Emerging Infections

The CDC (1994) defines *emerging infections* as diseases of infectious origin with human incidences occurring within the past two decades. Emerging illnesses are likely to increase in incidence in the near future. Two respiratory conditions listed as emerging infections are Severe Acute Respiratory Syndrome (SARS) and Legionnaire's disease.

Severe Acute Respiratory Syndrome

Severe Acute Respiratory Syndrome (SARS) is caused by a coronavirus. Symptoms include

- Fever

- Dry cough

- Hypoxemia
- Pneumonia

In identifying SARS, a chest x-ray reveals "ground glass" infiltrates with bilateral consolidation occurring sometimes within 24–48 hours, thus suggesting the rapid development of acute respiratory failure. SARS has occurred with greater frequency in Asia, although cases have also been confirmed in Canada, Switzerland, and Germany; therefore, a history of recent travel is significant

The SARS virus can be found in nasopharyngeal and oropharyngeal secretions, blood, and stool. Diagnostic tests for SARS include

- Sputum cultures for Influenza A, B, and RSV
- Serum tests to detect antibodies IgM and IgG
- Reverse transcriptase polymerase chain reaction tests performed to detect RNA of SARS CoV

Two tests on two different specimens must be positive to confirm the diagnosis. Test results are considered negative if no SARS CoV antibodies are found 28 days after the onset of symptoms.

The client suspected of having SARS should be cared for using airborne and contact precautions. Management includes the use of antibiotics to treat secondary or atypical pneumonia. Antivirals or retrovirals can be used to inhibit replication. Respiratory support, closed system for suctioning, and the use of surfactant replacement may be ordered.

Legionnaire's Disease

Legionnaire's disease is caused by gram negative bacteria found in both natural and manmade water sources. Bacterial growth is greater in stored water maintained at temperatures ranging from 77° to 107° F. Risk factors include

- Immunosuppression
- Diabetes
- Pulmonary disease

Legionnaire's involves the lungs and other organs. The symptoms include

- Productive cough
- Dyspnea

- Chest pain

- Diarrhea

- Fever

Diagnostic tests include a urinary antigen test that remains positive after initial antibiotic therapy. Management includes the use of antibiotics, oxygen, provision of nutrition, and hydration. The drug of choice for treating Legionnaire's disease is Zithromax (azithromycin). Transmission-based precautions are not necessary when caring for the client with Legionnaire's disease because there is no indication of human-to-human transmission.

Diagnostic Tests for Review

These are simply some of the tests that are useful in diagnosing pulmonary disorders. You should review the normal lab values as well as any special preparations for the client undergoing those tests. In addition, think about the care given to clients after the procedures have been completed. For instance, the client who has undergone a bronchoscopy will have a depressed gag reflex, which increases the chance of aspiration. No food or fluid should be given until the gag reflex returns. The tests for diagnosing pulmonary disorders are as follows:

- CBC

- Chest x-ray

- Pulmonary function tests

- Lung scan

- Bronchoscopy

Pharmacology Categories for Review

The client with a respiratory disorder should be managed with several categories of medications. The client with an acute respiratory condition, such as bacterial pneumonia, is given an antibiotic to fight the infection, antipyretic medication for fever and body aches, and an antitussive for relief of cough. The client with a chronic respiratory condition may receive many of the same medications, with the addition of a steroid or bronchodilator. The following list contains the most commonly prescribed categories of medications used to treat clients with respiratory conditions:

- Antibiotics

- Antivirals

- ▶ Antituberculars
- ▶ Antitussives
- ▶ Antipyretics
- ▶ Bronchodilators
- ▶ Expectorants
- ▶ Leukotriene modifiers
- ▶ Mast-cell stabilizers
- ▶ Steroids

Exam Prep Questions

1. When performing an assessment on the client with emphysema, the nurse finds that the client has a barrel chest. The alteration in the client's chest is due to:

   ○ **A.** Collapse of distal alveoli

   ○ **B.** Hyperinflation of the lungs

   ○ **C.** Long-term chronic hypoxia

   ○ **D.** Use of accessory muscles

2. The nurse notes that a client with COPD demonstrates more dyspnea in certain positions. Which position is most likely to alleviate the client's dyspnea?

   ○ **A.** Lying supine with a single pillow

   ○ **B.** Standing or sitting upright

   ○ **C.** Side lying with the head elevated

   ○ **D.** Lying with head slightly lowered

3. When reviewing the chart of a client with long standing lung disease, the nurse should pay close attention to the results of which pulmonary function test?

   ○ **A.** Residual volume

   ○ **B.** Total lung capacity

   ○ **C.** FEV1/FVC ratio

   ○ **D.** Functional residual capacity

4. The physician has ordered O_2 at 3 liters/minute via nasal cannula. O_2 amounts greater than 3 liters / minute are contraindicated in the client with COPD because:

   ○ **A.** Higher concentrations result in severe headache.

   ○ **B.** Hypercapnic drive is necessary for breathing.

   ○ **C.** Higher levels will be required later to raise the pO_2.

   ○ **D.** Hypoxic drive is needed for breathing.

5. The client taking a bronchodilator tells the nurse that he is going to begin a smoking cessation program when he is discharged. The nurse should tell the client to notify the doctor if his smoking pattern changes because he will:

   ○ **A.** Need his medication dosage adjusted

   ○ **B.** Require an increase in antitussive medication

   ○ **C.** No longer need annual influenza immunization

   ○ **D.** Not derive as much benefit from inhaler use

6. Lab results indicate that the client's serum aminophylline level is 17mcg/mL. The nurse recognizes that the aminophylline level is:

   ○ **A.** Within therapeutic range

   ○ **B.** Too high and should be reported

   ○ **C.** Questionable and should be repeated

   ○ **D.** Too low to be therapeutic

7. The morning weight for a client with emphysema indicates that the client has gained 5 pounds in less than a week, even though his oral intake has been modest. The client's weight gain may reflect which associated complication of COPD?

   ○ **A.** Polycythemia

   ○ **B.** Cor pulmonale

   ○ **C.** Left ventricular failure

   ○ **D.** Compensated acidosis

8. The nurse is teaching the client the appropriate way to use a metered dose inhaler. Which action indicates the client needs additional teaching?

   ○ **A.** The client takes a deep breath while depressing the inhaler.

   ○ **B.** The client places the inhaler two fingers from the mouth.

   ○ **C.** The client waits 15 seconds before using the inhaler a second time.

   ○ **D.** The client exhales slowly using purse lipped breathing.

9. The client with COPD may lose weight despite having adequate caloric intake. When counseling the client in ways to maintain an optimal weight, the nurse should tell the client to:

   ○ **A.** Continue the same caloric intake and increase the amount of fat intake

   ○ **B.** Increase his activity level to stimulate his appetite

   ○ **C.** Increase the amount of complex carbohydrates and decrease the amount of fat intake

   ○ **D.** Decrease the amount of complex carbohydrates while increasing calories, protein, vitamins, and minerals

10. The client has been receiving garamycin 65 mg IVPB every 8 hours for the past 6 days. Which lab result indicates an adverse reaction to the medication?

    ○ **A.** WBC 7500

    ○ **B.** Serum glucose 92

    ○ **C.** Protein 3.5

    ○ **D.** Serum creatinine 2.0

Answer Rationales

1. Answer B is correct. Clients with emphysema develop a barrel chest due to the trapping of air in the lungs, causing them to hyperinflate. Answers C and D are common in those with emphysema but do not cause the chest to become barrel shaped. Answer A does not occur in emphysema.

2. Answer B is correct. The client with chronic obstructive pulmonary disease has increased difficulty breathing when lying down. His respiratory effort is improved by standing or sitting upright or by having the bed in high Fowler's position. Answers A, C, and D do not alleviate the client's dyspnea; therefore they are incorrect.

3. Answer C is correct. The FEV1/FVC ratio indicates disease progression. As COPD worsens, the ratio of FEV1 to FVC becomes smaller. Answers A and B reflect loss of elastic recoil due to narrowing and obstruction of the airway. Answer D is increased in clients with obstructive bronchitis.

4. Answer D is correct. In clients with COPD, respiratory effort is stimulated by hypoxemia. Answers A and C are incorrect because higher levels would rob the client of the drive to breathe. Answer B is an incorrect statement.

5. Answer A is correct. Changes in smoking patterns should be discussed with the physician because they have an impact on the amount of medication needed. Answer B is incorrect because clients with COPD are placed on expectorants, not antitussives. Answer C is incorrect because an annual influenza vaccine is recommended for all those with lung disease. Answer D is incorrect because benefits from inhaler use should be increased when the client stops smoking.

6. Answer A is correct. The therapeutic range for aminophylline is 10–20 mcg/ml. Answers B and D are incorrect. There are no indications that the results are questionable; therefore, repeating the test as offered by answer C is incorrect.

7. Answer B is correct. Cor pulmonale, or right sided heart failure, is a possible complication of emphysema. Answers A and D do not cause weight gain, so they're incorrect. Answer C would be reflected in pulmonary edema, so it's incorrect.

8. Answer C is correct. The client should wait 60 seconds before using the inhaler a second time. The client's wait time of 15 seconds indicates that the client needs further teaching. Answers A, B, and D indicate that the client understands the correct use of the inhaler.

9. Answer D. The client with COPD needs additional calories, protein, vitamins, and minerals. Answer A is incorrect because the client needs more calories but not more fat. Answer B is not feasible, will increase the O_2 demands, and will result in further weight loss. Answer C leads to excess acid production and an increased respiratory workload.

10. Answer D is correct. The serum creatinine is elevated, indicating renal impairment. Answers A, B, and C are within normal limits.

Suggested Readings and Resources

▶ Centers for Disease Control and Prevention: www.cdc.gov.

▶ American Lung Association: www.lungusa.org.

▶ The Pathology Guy: www.pathguy.com.

▶ Health24: www.health24.com.

▶ Ignatavicius, D., and Workman, S. *Medical Surgical Nursing: Critical Thinking for Collaborative Care*. 6th ed. Philadelphia: Elsevier, 2008.

▶ Brunner, L., and Suddarth, D. *Textbook of Medical Surgical Nursing*. 12th ed. Philadelphia: Lippincott Williams & Wilkins, 2009.

▶ LeMone, P., and Burke, K. in *Medical Surgical Nursing: Critical Thinking in Client Care*. 4th ed. Upper Saddle River, NJ: Pearson Prentice Hall, 2008.

▶ Lewis, S., Heitkemper, M., Dirksen, S., O'Brien, P,. and Bucher, L. *Medical Surgical Nursing: Assessment and Management of Clinical Problems*. 7th ed. Philadelphia: Elsevier, 2007.

▶ Lehne, R. *Pharmacology for Nursing Care*. 7th ed., Philadelphia: Elsevier, 2009.

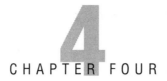

CHAPTER FOUR

Caring for the Client with Disorders of the Genitourinary System

---

Terms you'll need to understand

- ✓ Anuria
- ✓ Arteriovenous graft
- ✓ Cutaneous ureterostomy
- ✓ Cystectomy
- ✓ Cystitis
- ✓ Dialysis
- ✓ Dysuria
- ✓ End stage renal failure
- ✓ Fistula
- ✓ Glomerulonephritis
- ✓ Hematuria
- ✓ Ileal conduit
- ✓ Ileal reservoir
- ✓ Nephrectomy
- ✓ Nephrotic syndrome
- ✓ Oliguria
- ✓ Polyarteritis nodosa
- ✓ Scleroderma
- ✓ Systemic lupus erythematosus

Nursing skills you'll need to master

- ✓ Performing urinary catheterization (male and female)
- ✓ Administering medication
- ✓ Performing bladder irrigation
- ✓ Assessing and caring for AV shunt
- ✓ Performing peritoneal dialysis
- ✓ Performing stoma care
- ✓ Collecting urine specimen (clean catch, sterile, 24 hour)
- ✓ Assisting with renal biopsy
- ✓ Caring for central lines

The genitourinary system includes the kidneys, ureters, urinary bladder, prostate, and testes. Disorders of this system can be divided into conditions that affect the kidneys and urinary tract, which includes the ureters and bladder. Renal disorders are of particular significance because the kidneys contribute to our health in a number of ways. The kidneys play a primary role in maintaining fluid volume and electrolyte balance, filtering waste for elimination, maintaining blood pressure, synthesizing red blood cells, and metabolizing vitamin D. Disorders of the ureters and bladder affect the storage and elimination of urine. Male genitourinary disorders, such as prostatitis and epididymitis, can result from infection. Others, such as benign prostatic hypertrophy, can result from the physiologic changes associated with aging. Although these disorders are not as serious as renal disorders, those affected experience significant physical and emotional changes. In this chapter we review the most common conditions affecting the genitourinary system.

Acute Glomerulonephritis

Acute glomerulonephritis is an antigen-antibody response occurring from one to two weeks following infection with Group A β-hemolytic *Streptococcus*. Other causes include systemic lupus erythematosus, scleroderma, and polyarteritis nodosa.

Signs and symptoms include

- Dark, smoke-colored urine
- Hypertension
- Headache
- Nausea and vomiting
- Oliguria

Routine urinalysis typically reveals elevations in specific gravity, hematuria, and proteinuria. Blood studies reveal elevations in blood urea nitrogen (BUN), serum creatinine, and erythrocyte sedimentation rates. A positive antistreptolysin (ASO) titer indicates prior infection with Group A β-hemolytic *Streptococcus*. Two additional studies may be ordered to determine the extent of kidney damage. These studies are a 24-hour urine to check for creatinine clearance and a renal biopsy, which shows cellular changes in the glomerular tissue.

CAUTION

Know the normal ranges for urine specific gravity, BUN, and serum creatinine.

The management of the client with acute glomerulonephritis includes the use of

- ▶ Antibiotics
- ▶ Antihypertensives
- ▶ Diuretics
- ▶ Steroids
- ▶ Bed rest
- ▶ Strict monitoring of fluid intake and output
- ▶ Limited intake of sodium and protein
- ▶ Limited intake of potassium during periods of oliguria
- ▶ Assess for signs of edema and circulatory overload

Chronic Glomerulonephritis

Chronic glomerulonephritis refers to a long-term inflammation of the glomerular capillaries. The condition may follow an episode of acute glomerulonephritis or a milder antigen-antibody reaction.

Signs and symptoms include

- ▶ Proteinuria
- ▶ Pedal edema
- ▶ Weight loss
- ▶ Nocturia
- ▶ Gastrointestinal complaints
- ▶ Anemia
- ▶ Peripheral neuropathy
- ▶ Gout
- ▶ Hypertension
- ▶ Increased serum creatinine
- ▶ Increased BUN
- ▶ Normal or below normal urine specific gravity

Management of the client with chronic glomerulonephritis is largely symptomatic. Medications include diuretics, antihypertensives, and antianemics. Hyperkalemia is treated with Kayexelate (sodium polystyrene sulfonate), which can be given alone or with sorbitol. Strict monitoring of fluid intake and output and restriction of dietary protein and sodium are essential in the prevention of fluid overload.

End Stage Renal Disease

End stage renal disease (ESRD) is a progressive, irreversible deterioration in renal function in which the kidneys are no longer able to maintain metabolic as well as fluid and electrolyte balance. Urea and other nitrogenous wastes are retained in the blood stream, necessitating management by peritoneal dialysis, hemodialysis, or renal transplant.

Peritoneal Dialysis

Peritoneal dialysis involves the instillation of dialysate via a flexible catheter implanted into the peritoneal cavity. Osmotic pressure allows waste products to be returned with the dialysate. Strict adherence to sterile technique is essential to prevent infection and peritonitis.

Symptoms of peritonitis include

▶ Fever

▶ Abdominal discomfort

▶ Return of cloudy dialysate

Hemodialysis

Hemodialysis is accomplished by using a dialyzer, which serves as a synthetic semipermeable membrane. Vascular access is obtained through the use of a subclavian, jugular, or femoral catheter as well as the placement of a fistula or arteriovenous graft.

Complications associated with hemodialysis include viral infection, hypotension, cramps, febrile reactions, nausea and vomiting, and disequilibrium syndrome. The client with disequilibrium syndrome experiences symptoms of cerebral edema, including confusion and irritability. Disequilibrium syndrome is managed by slowing or discontinuing the dialysis session and administering Osmitrol (mannitol).

> **CAUTION**
>
> Do not check blood pressure or perform venous sticks in the extremity with a vascular access because damage can occur to the access site. The presence of a bruit indicates the access site is patent.
>
> Do not administer rapid-acting antihypertensives prior to hemodialysis because some are not removed by dialysis and the client is more likely to experience shock. Check with the physician to see which medications can be given to the client scheduled for hemodialysis.

Renal Transplantation

Renal transplant can be obtained from a cadaver or living, compatible donor. The transplanted kidney is placed within the pelvis to provide greater protection against traumatic injury. Following transplantation, the client is placed on lifetime therapy with immunosuppressives, biologic response modifiers, and monoclonal antibodies. Commonly used medications administered after renal transplant include

- Azathioprine (Imuran)
- Corticosteroids (Prednisone)
- Cyclosporine (Sandimmune, Neoral)
- Tacrolimus (Prograf)
- Sirolimus (Rapimmune)

Mycophenolate (CellCept) has been approved by the FDA solely for the prevention of renal transplant rejection.

> **NOTE**
>
> Neoral (cyclosporine) should be mixed with orange juice, milk, or chocolate milk before administration. The medication should be given in a glass container or in the special container that comes with the medication.

Nephrotic Syndrome

Nephrotic syndrome can be caused by glomerulonephritis, systemic illness, or an acute allergic response. Diagnosis is based on the client's symptoms, renal function tests, and 24-hour urine test for creatinine clearance.

Nephrotic syndrome involves a collection of symptoms that include

▸ Marked proteinuria

▸ Generalized edema (anasarca)

▸ Hypoalbuminemia

▸ Hypercholesterolemia

Management of the client with nephrotic syndrome includes

▸ Bed rest

▸ Prevention of skin breakdown

▸ Daily weight

▸ Strict intake and output

▸ Moderate protein intake with sodium restrictions

▸ Medications, including steroids and immunosuppressives

Urinary Calculi

Urinary calculi (urolithiasis, kidney stones) can result from immobility, cancer, increased intake of vitamin D, or overactivity of the parathyroids. Urinary calculi are more common in men, particularly in those 30–50 years of age, and occur in all age groups with greater frequency in the spring and summer months. Kidney stones are more commonly made up of calcium, magnesium, phosphorus, or oxalate.

Symptoms associated with kidney stones include

▸ Flank pain

▸ Fever

▸ Nausea and vomiting

▸ Changes in urinary output

Diagnostic measures include x-ray with contrast media, CBC, and a 24-hour urine test. The helical CT is the most diagnostic tool for locating kidney stones.

Management of the client with kidney stones includes

▸ Use of IV fluids

▸ Pain management

- ▶ Extracorporeal shock wave lithotripsy (ECSWL)

- ▶ Straining the urine to detect passage of the stone

- ▶ Surgical management

- ▶ Dietary alterations for those with recurring calcium, uric acid, or oxalate stones

Urinary Tract Infections

Urinary tract infections (UTIs) are caused by pathologic microorganisms of the urinary tract. UTIs represent 40% of hospital-acquired infections, with most of those being due to contamination during catheterization or instrumentation. Ascending infection with fecal material (E. coli) accounts for over one half of all UTIs. Symptoms of UTIs depend on whether the infection affects the bladder (cystitis) or the kidney (pyelonephritis). Symptoms of UTI include

- ▶ Pain and burning on urination

- ▶ Urinary frequency and urgency

- ▶ Flank pain

- ▶ Fever

- ▶ Nausea and vomiting

Management of the client with a UTI includes the use of specific antibiotics, urinary antispasmodics, and increased fluids.

Genitourinary Disorders

Two of the most common genitourinary disorders affecting men are prostatitis and benign prostatic hyperplasia. Inflammation of the prostate can occur after a viral illness or infection with a sexually transmitted disease. Benign prostatic hypertrophy is associated with injury and with aging.

Prostatitis

Prostatitis is classified as either bacterial or nonbacterial. Bacterial prostatitis is associated with infection of the urethra or lower urinary tract. Although there is no identifiable organism, nonbacterial prostatitis can result in a chronic infection.

Signs and symptoms of acute bacterial prostatitis include:

▶ Chills and fever

▶ Dysuria

▶ Urethral discharge

▶ Erectile dysfunction

▶ Perineal pain that radiates to the sacral area

Diagnosis is based on the client's symptoms and urine culture. Management of the client with prostatitis includes the use of antibiotics, such as Bactrim (trimethoprim-sulfamethoxazole), bed rest, and sitz baths.

Benign Prostatic Hyperplasia

One of the most common pathological conditions in men over age 50 is benign prostatic hyperplasia (BPH). Enlargement of the prostate can obstruct the vesicle neck or prostatic urethra, leading to incomplete emptying of the bladder and urinary retention. Retention of urine causes dilation of the ureters and kidneys and contributes to the development of urinary tract infections.

Signs and symptoms of BPH include

▶ Increased frequency of urination

▶ Nocturia

▶ Urinary urgency

▶ Hesitancy in starting urination

▶ Decrease in the volume and force of urinary stream

▶ Feeling of bladder fullness

▶ Recurrent urinary tract infections

Diagnostic tests include urinalysis, renal function tests, digital rectal exam, and complete blood studies.

Medical management of BPH includes the use of alpha-adrenergic receptor blockers, such as tamsulosin (Flomax) and antiandrogens, such as finasteride (Proscar). Saw palmetto has been used to treat mild to moderate BPH, although its effectiveness has not been established.

> **CAUTION**
>
> Women who are pregnant or who might become pregnant should avoid handling crushed or broken antiandrogen medication because of the risk to birth defects in the male fetus.

Surgical management of BPH includes removal of the prostate. The most common surgical procedure for BPH is a transurethral prostatectomy (TURP). The most common complication following a TURP is hemorrhage; therefore, it is imperative that the urinary output is assessed for amount and color.

> **CAUTION**
>
> The use of saw palmetto may result in a false lowering of the PSA level thus delaying diagnosis and treatment of prostate cancer.
>
> The presence of bright red urine with increased viscosity and clots following a TURP indicates arterial bleeding and should be reported to the doctor immediately.
>
> The presence of dark red urine with less viscosity and few clots following a TURP indicates venous bleeding, which can be managed by applying traction to the urethral catheter.

Bladder Cancer

Malignancies of the bladder are the fourth leading cause of cancer in the United States. Risk factors in bladder cancer include

- ▶ Recurrent bacterial UTI
- ▶ High cholesterol intake
- ▶ Pelvic radiation
- ▶ Environmental carcinogens, including certain dyes
- ▶ Smoking (primary cause)

Symptoms of bladder cancer include visible painless hematuria, infection, dysuria, and frequency of urination. Pelvic and back pain are common with metastasis.

Diagnostic tests include cystoscopy, CT scan, biopsy, and ultrasonography. Management of the client with bladder cancer depends on the grade, the degree of local invasion, and the client's age as well as physical and mental status. Surgical management includes cystectomy with the creation of a urinary diversion.

> **CAUTION**
>
> Types of urinary diversions that may be performed following a cystectomy are ileal conduit, ileal reservoir, ureterostomy, and ureterosigmoidostomy. It is important for the nurse to review these because some require the client to wear an external appliance and some do not.

Chemotherapeutic management includes a combination of Folex (methotrexate), Adrucil (5 florourouracil), Velblane (vinblastine), and Adriamycin (doxorubicin). In cases where cystectomy is not performed, the client may be treated by intravesicle therapy with BCG vaccine (TheraCyst). Clients receiving intravesicle therapy can continue to eat and drink before therapy but should avoid urinating for at least two hours after instillation of the medication. This allows sufficient exposure time to the medication. During dwell time, the client should be reminded to change positions every 20 minutes so that the entire surface of the bladder is exposed to the medication. Afterward, the client is encouraged to drink additional fluids to remove drug residue.

Diagnostic Tests for Review

Routine diagnostic tests, including CBC and urinalysis, are ordered for the client with disorders of the renal and urinary system. Specific tests such as intravenous pyelogram and CT scan are ordered to detect structural abnormalities. The complete metabolic panel reflects changes in electrolytes that result from renal disease. The tests are as follows

▶ CBC

▶ Complete metabolic panel

▶ Urinalysis

▶ Intravenous pyelogram

▶ CT scan

Pharmacology Categories for Review

Renal disorders affect many other organ systems including the cardiovascular system and hematopoietic system. Clients with renal disease will receive medication from a number of different categories depending on their condition. These medications include:

▶ Antibiotics

▶ Antihypertensives

- ▶ Antineoplastics
- ▶ Antispasmodics
- ▶ Diuretics
- ▶ Immunosuppressives

Exam Prep Questions

1. A client hospitalized with acute glomerulonephritis has a positive ASO titer. The nurse understands that the client's current illness is due to a:

   ○ **A.** History of uncontrolled hypertension

   ○ **B.** Prior bacterial infection

   ○ **C.** Prolonged elevation in blood glucose

   ○ **D.** Drug reaction that led to muscle breakdown

2. The physician has prescribed hydralazine (Apresoline) for a client with acute glomerulonephritis. Which finding indicates that the drug is having the desired effect?

   ○ **A.** The client's appetite has improved.

   ○ **B.** Creatinine levels have returned to normal.

   ○ **C.** The client's blood pressure has decreased.

   ○ **D.** Urinary output is amber in color.

3. A client with acute glomerulonephritis requests a snack. Which snack is most therapeutic?

   ○ **A.** Orange juice

   ○ **B.** Banana

   ○ **C.** Applesauce

   ○ **D.** Warm broth

4. The physician has ordered Prednisone 50 mg daily to promote diuresis in a client with nephrotic syndrome. The nurse should administer the medication:

   ○ **A.** In a single dose at bedtime

   ○ **B.** With a snack or glass of milk

   ○ **C.** With water to promote absorption

   ○ **D.** Prior to arising in the morning

5. A client receiving Gentamycin (garamycin) IVPB has a morning peak level of 12 micrograms/mL. The nurse should:

   ○ **A.** Notify the physician because the level is too high.

   ○ **B.** Administer the medication at the scheduled time.

   ○ **C.** Request an order to administer the medication IM.

   ○ **D.** Repeat the level 30 minutes before the next dose.

6. The nurse is teaching the client with an ileal conduit regarding skin care to prevent excoriation. The nurse should tell the client to empty the collection bag:

   ○ **A.** Every hour

   ○ **B.** When it is half full

   ○ **C.** Once daily

   ○ **D.** When it is one-third full

7. A client with end stage renal disease has been managed by peritoneal dialysis. Which finding should be reported to the doctor immediately?

   ○ **A.** The amount of dialysate return is less than that instilled.

   ○ **B.** The client complains of abdominal pain and nausea.

   ○ **C.** The dialysate return is colorless in appearance.

   ○ **D.** The client has lost two pounds in the last week.

8. The nurse notes dark red bleeding and a few clots in the catheter of a client two days after a TURP. The nurse should first:

   ○ **A.** Prepare the client for a return to surgery.

   ○ **B.** Apply traction to the urethral catheter.

   ○ **C.** Document the findings as normal.

   ○ **D.** Decrease the client's IV rate.

9. A client is admitted with a tentative diagnosis of bladder cancer. Which finding most likely contributed to the development of bladder cancer?

   ○ **A.** Two PPD cigarette use for 25 years

   ○ **B.** Frequent urinary tract infections

   ○ **C.** Employment in the textile industry

   ○ **D.** A history of renal calculi

10. The nurse is providing dietary instructions to a client with oxylate renal calculi. The nurse should tell the client to avoid which of the following snacks:

    ○ **A.** Strawberries

    ○ **B.** Cheese

    ○ **C.** Chicken nuggets

    ○ **D.** Banana

Answer Rationales

1. Answer B is correct. A positive antistreptolysin titer indicates infection with Group A β-hemolytic *Streptococcus*, a bacteria. Answers A and C are not associated with acute glomerulonephritis so they are incorrect. Answer D, rhabdomyolysis, is not associated with infection making it incorrect.

2. Answer C is correct. Apresoline (hydralazine) is an antihypertensive. A decrease in BP indicates the medication is working. Answers A, B, and D indicate that the overall condition of the client is improving, but they are not the result of therapy with hydralazine.

3. Answer C is correct. Applesauce would provide vitamins and carbohydrates. Answers A and B are high in potassium, and answer D is a liquid that is high in sodium. Clients with AGN have elevated levels of potassium and sodium that require dietary restrictions, so answers A, B, and D are incorrect.

4. Answer B is correct. Prednisone, a steroid, should be given with a snack or meal to prevent gastric irritation. Answer C would cause pain and gastric upset, making it incorrect. Answers A and D do not include providing food with the medication, so they are incorrect.

5. Answer A is correct. The therapeutic range for Garamycin is 4–10 micrograms/mL. Because the drug is both ototoxic and nephrotoxic, the physician should be notified. Answers B and C are incorrect choices because they would increase the peak level. Answer D refers to the time for drawing a trough level, making it incorrect.

6. Answer D is correct. Emptying the collection when it is one-third full prevents the likelihood of the urine leaking. Answer A isn't necessary or feasible, so it is incorrect. Waiting until it is half full or more as suggested in answers B and C increases the likelihood that the collection bag will lose contact with the skin, allow for soiling and contributing to excoriation; therefore B and C are incorrect.

7. Answer B is correct. Abdominal pain, nausea, fever, and return of cloudy dialysate are indications of peritonitis, which requires immediate antibiotic therapy. Diminished or slow return of dialysate, as mentioned in answer A, is managed by having the client turn from side to side to facilitate return flow, so it is incorrect. Answers C and D reflect good management, making them incorrect.

8. Answer B is correct. The appearance of dark red blood with a few clots indicates a venous bleed. Traction to the uretheral catheter and increasing the client's fluid intake should be tried first before calling the doctor. Answer A would be indicated for the client with an arterial bleed, which is characterized by bright red bleeding and many clots, so it is incorrect. Answer C is not the best because documentation should reflect exactly what was assessed and the nurse's action, so it's incorrect. Answer D is incorrect because increasing fluids will help keep the catheter free of clots.

9. Answer A is correct. Cigarette smoking is the most significant factor in the development of bladder cancer. Answers B and C might have contributed but are not as likely as answer A; therefore, they are incorrect. Answer D involves the kidneys, not the bladder, so it is incorrect.

10. Answer A is correct. Strawberries, peanuts, rhubarb, and spinach are food sources high in oxylate. Answers B, C, and D are suitable snacks for the client with oxylate renal calculi, so they are incorrect.

Suggested Reading and Resources

▶ Ignatavicius, D., and Workman, S. *Medical Surgical Nursing: Critical Thinking for Collaborative Care.* 6th ed. Philadelphia: Elsevier, 2008.

▶ Brunner, L., and Suddarth, D. *Textbook of Medical Surgical Nursing.* 12th ed. Philadelphia: Lippincott Williams & Wilkins, 2009.

▶ LeMone, P., and Burke, K. *Medical Surgical Nursing: Critical Thinking in Client Care.* 4th ed. Upper Saddle River, NJ: Pearson Prentice Hall, 2008.

▶ Lewis, S., Heitkemper, M., Dirksen, S., O'Brien, P., and Bucher, L. *Medical Surgical Nursing: Assessment and Management of Clinical Problems.* 7th ed. Philadelphia: Elsevier, 2007.

▶ Lehne, R. *Pharmacology for Nursing Care,* 7th ed. Philadelphia: Elsevier, 2009.

▶ National Institute of Diabetes & Digestive & Kidney Diseases: www.niddk.nih.gov.

▶ University of Utah Health Sciences Center: www-medlib.med.utah.edu.

▶ National Kidney Foundation: www.kidney.org.

▶ Nephropathy Support Network: www.igansupport.org.

▶ American Urological Association: www.afud.org.

▶ National Kidney and Urologic Diseases Information Clearinghouse: www.kidney.niddk.nih.gov.

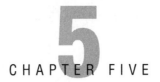

CHAPTER FIVE

Caring for the Client with Disorders of the Hematopoietic System

---

Terms you'll need to understand

- ✓ Dyspnea
- ✓ Fatigue
- ✓ Hemarthrosis
- ✓ Hemolysis
- ✓ Jaundice
- ✓ Leukopenia
- ✓ Otitis media
- ✓ Pallor
- ✓ Paresthesia
- ✓ Pruritis
- ✓ Tachypnea
- ✓ Thrombocytopenia
- ✓ Tinnitus
- ✓ Upper respiratory infections

Nursing skills you'll need to master

- ✓ Performing a blood transfusion
- ✓ Administering platelets
- ✓ Performing Z track IM technique

Anemia

When anemia occurs, people have a decrease in the number of red blood cells or a decrease in the ability of these red blood cells to carry oxygen. The causes and symptoms of anemia are listed here:

▶ Increased red blood cell destruction

▶ Blood loss

▶ Poor dietary iron intake

▶ Poor absorption

▶ Parasites

Symptoms of anemia:

▶ Fatigue

▶ Pallor

▶ Tachypnea

▶ Cardiac changes

▶ Dyspnea

▶ Headaches

▶ Dizziness

▶ Growth retardation

▶ Depression

▶ Late sexual maturation

CAUTION

Children with persistent anemia may experience frequent bouts of otitis media and upper respiratory infections.

Pernicious Anemia

In pernicious anemia, the intrinsic factor is missing, resulting in an inability to absorb cyanocobalamin (Vitamin B12). Pernicious anemia is common in the elderly and clients who have had a gastric resection. It can also occur from poor dietary intake of foods containing B12, especially in people on vegetarian diets or those lacking dairy products.

Symptoms of pernicious anemia include

- ▶ Pallor
- ▶ Jaundice
- ▶ Smooth, beefy red tongue
- ▶ Fatigue
- ▶ Weight loss
- ▶ Paresthesia
- ▶ Reduced vibratory and position senses
- ▶ Ataxia

The treatment for this is the administration of injections of cyanocobalamin (Vitamin B12). The injections are given weekly until adequate levels are reached, and then monthly for maintenance.

Aplastic Anemia

This type of anemia occurs when there is depression of the blood-forming elements of the bone marrow. The cells are replaced with fat. The symptoms of aplastic anemia are as follows:

- ▶ Decreased erythrocytes
- ▶ Leukopenia
- ▶ Thrombocytopenia

Some of the causes of aplastic anemia are

- ▶ Drug toxicity
- ▶ Radiation exposure
- ▶ Multiple blood transfusions
- ▶ Autoimmune states
- ▶ Hepatitis B

Treatments of aplastic anemia include

- ▶ Identifying and removing the offending agent
- ▶ Performing a bone marrow transplant
- ▶ Immunosuppressive therapies

Sickle Cell Anemia

A client with sickle cell anemia has red blood cells that have an abnormal crescent shape, causing an impairment in tissue perfusion. Low oxygen levels can cause the client's cells to sickle. Due to this, these cells cannot properly circulate through the system. The most common crisis these clients have is vasocclusive crisis, in which the client has a lack of oxygen to a specific area, causing hypoxia and necrosis to that area. Because bone marrow transplant is the only potential cure for sickle cell anemia, treatments are usually aimed at avoiding crises and preventing complications. Some treatments for sickle cell anemia are listed here:

▶ Short-term blood transfusion administration (for example, during aplastic crises or before major surgeries)

▶ Teach client to avoid contact sports and take frequent rest periods

EXAM ALERT

An easy way to remember major treatment therapies is to remember the letters H H O P:

▶ H—Heat

▶ H—Hydration

▶ O—Oxygen

▶ P—Pain relief

NOTE

The vasocclusive crisis is the only crisis type that causes the client to have pain.

Sickle cell crises might be preceded by recent infection, stressors, dehydration, extrenous activity, or exposure to high altitudes.

Iron Deficiency Anemia

There is a simple lack of iron in this disorder. The cause may be the result of poor dietary intake of iron sources. The symptoms of iron deficiency anemia are the same as general anemia. There are a few for severe, prolonged anemia that are different (included here):

▶ Brittle nails

▶ Cheilosis (corner of the mouth ulcers)

▶ Pica (craving to eat unusual substances such as clay or starch)

▶ Koilonchyia (concave or spoon-shaped fingernails)

▶ Sore tongue

The treatment for iron deficiency anemia is as follows:

- Increasing dietary intake of iron (good sources of iron include egg yolk; green, leafy vegetables; dried fruit; iron-fortified cereals; peanut butter; raisins; and liver)
- Administering iron supplements by mouth or intramuscularly

> **CAUTION**
>
> Intramuscular iron (Imferon) is given through the IM Z track method.
>
> Iron elixir should be administered through a straw to prevent staining the teeth.

Cooley's Anemia (Thalassemia Major)

This disorder is inherited as an autosomal recessive disorder. This client's red blood cells are destroyed prematurely. Note that this disease is mainly found by lab results. The treatment for Cooley's anemia includes frequent blood transfusions. When multiple blood transfusions are given, reduce iron overload and hemosiderosis with subcutaneous chelating injections of deferoxamine (Desferal).

Hemophilia

In this disorder an abnormal clotting pattern occurs, resulting in an ineffective clot. Hemophilia is inherited as a sex-linked disorder. The mother passes this disorder to her male children. Clients lacking factor VIII have hemophilia A; clients lacking factor IX have hemophilia B. The symptoms of hemophilia include

- Bleeding and bruising easily
- Hemorrhaging from minor cuts
- Joint hemorrhages
- Post-operative hemorrhaging
- Nose bleeds
- Hematuria

The complications are as follows:

- Internal bleeding
- Intracranial bleeding
- Hemarthrosis

Cryoprecipitates are no longer used because HIV and hepatitis cannot be removed. Treatment of hemophilia includes the following: DDAVP for mild hemophilia and Von Willebrand disease, purified factor VIII concentrate (monoclonal), and recombinant factor VIII concentrate (which is sold as a drug, not as a drug product). These three products are the only recommended treatments for controlling the bleeding associated with hemophilia.

Polycythemia Vera

This disorder is characterized by thicker than normal blood. With polycythemia vera, there is an increase in the client's hemoglobin of 18g/dl, RBC of 6 million/mm, or hematocrit at 55% or greater and increased platelets. The following are some symptoms of polycythemia vera:

▶ Enlarged spleen

▶ Dizziness

▶ Ruddy or flushed (plethoric) complexion

▶ Tinnitus

▶ Fatigue

▶ Paresthesia

▶ Dyspnea

▶ Pruritis

▶ Burning sensation in fingers and toes (erythromelagia)

Treatments of polycythemia vera include

▶ Phlebotomy

▶ Hydroxyurea (Droxia) administration

▶ Hydration

▶ Anticoagulant therapy

CAUTION

With polycythemia, the client is at risk for cerebrovascular accident (CVA), myocardial infarction (MI), and bleeding due to dysfunctional platelets.

Diagnostic Tests for Review

The diagnostic tests for the client with hematopoietic disorders are the same as any other routine hospitalization of a client (CBC, urinalysis, and chest x-ray). Specific tests, such as the Schilling test for B12 deficiency, are used to evaluate certain disorders. These tests need to be reviewed prior to taking an exam for a better understanding of the disease process:

- ▶ Schilling test
- ▶ CBC with differential
- ▶ Hemoglobin electrophoresis

Pharmacology for Review

The client with a hematopoietic disorder will receive a number of medications to stimulate red blood cell production and replace needed vitamins or nutrients. Analgesics are also a requirement for the pain associated with some diseases. You'll need to review certain drug classifications prior to the test for knowledge of their effects, side effects, and adverse reactions:

- ▶ Antianemics
- ▶ Analgesics
- ▶ Vitamins

Exam Prep Questions

1. A 50-year-old client with sickle cell disease is admitted with a diagnosis of pneumonia. Which nursing intervention would be most helpful to prevent a vasocclusive crisis?

   ○ **A.** Obtaining blood pressures every 2 hours

   ○ **B.** Administering pain medication every 3–4 hours as ordered

   ○ **C.** Monitoring arterial blood gas results

   ○ **D.** Administering IV fluids at an ordered rate of 200ml/hr

2. Which clinical manifestation, noted in a client with pernicious anemia, would indicate that the client has been noncompliant with B12 injections?

   ○ **A.** Hyperactivity in the evening hours

   ○ **B.** Weight gain of 5 pounds in one week

   ○ **C.** Paresthesia of hands and feet

   ○ **D.** Diarrhea stools several times a day

3. The nurse is caring for a 70-year-old client with anemia who is receiving a blood transfusion. Assessment findings reveal crackles on chest auscultation and distended neck veins. What is the nurse's initial action?

   ○ **A.** Slow the transfusion.

   ○ **B.** Document the finding as the only action.

   ○ **C.** Stop the blood transfusion and turn on the normal saline.

   ○ **D.** Assess the client's temperature.

4. The nurse caring for a client with iron deficiency has performed dietary teaching of foods high in iron. The nurse recognizes that teaching has been effective when the client selects which meal plan?

   ○ **A.** Hamburger, French fries, and orange juice

   ○ **B.** Sliced veal, spinach salad, whole-wheat roll

   ○ **C.** Vegetable lasagna, Caesar salad, toast

   ○ **D.** Bacon, lettuce, and tomato sandwich, potato chips, and tea

5. The nurse is administering iron by the Z track method. Which technique would the nurse utilize to prevent tracking of the medication?

   ○   **A.** Inject the medication in the deltoid muscle.

   ○   **B.** Use a 22-gauge needle.

   ○   **C.** Omit aspirating for blood prior to injecting.

   ○   **D.** Draw up 0.2 ml of air after the proper medication dose.

6. The nurse caring for a client with anemia recognizes which clinical manifestation as one specific for a hemolytic type of anemia?

   ○   **A.** Jaundice

   ○   **B.** Anorexia

   ○   **C.** Tachycardia

   ○   **D.** Fatigue

7. A client with leukemia has been receiving injections of Neulasta (pegfilgrastim). Which laboratory value reveals that the drug is producing the desired effect?

   ○   **A.** Hemoglobin of 13.5g/dl

   ○   **B.** White blood cell count of 6,000/mm

   ○   **C.** Platelet count of 300,000/mm

   ○   **D.** Iron level of 75ug/dl

8. The nurse is performing discharge teaching on a client with polycythemia vera. Which would be included in the teaching plan?

   ○   **A.** Avoid large crowds.

   ○   **B.** Keep the head of the bed elevated at night.

   ○   **C.** Wear socks and gloves when going outside.

   ○   **D.** Know the signs and symptoms of thrombosis.

9. A 15-year-old client with iron deficiency anemia and a ruptured ectopic pregnancy needs a blood transfusion prior to surgery. The client's mother is a Jehovah's Witness and refuses to sign the blood permit. Which nursing action is most appropriate?

   ○   **A.** Give the blood without the mother's permission.

   ○   **B.** Coax the mother to change her mind.

   ○   **C.** Allow the client to sign the permit.

   ○   **D.** Notify the physician of the mother's refusal.

10. The physician has ordered a minimal bacteria diet on a client with neutropenia. Which seasoning is not permitted for this client?

   ○ **A.** Salt

   ○ **B.** Lemon juice

   ○ **C.** Pepper

   ○ **D.** Ketchup

Answer Rationales

1. Answer D is correct. Hydration is needed to prevent slowing of blood flow and occlusion. It is important to perform the assessments in answers A, B, and C, but D is the best intervention for the prevention of the crisis.

2. Answer C is correct. B12 is an essential component for proper functioning of the peripheral nervous system. Clients without proper B12 will have symptoms such as paresthesia due to the deficiency. Answers A and D don't occur with pernicious anemia. The client would have weight loss rather than weight gain as in answer B.

3. Answer A is correct. The client is exhibiting symptoms of fluid volume excess and slowing the rate would be the proper action. The nurse would not stop the infusion of blood as in answer C. Answers B and D would not help.

4. Answer B is correct. This selection is the one with the highest iron content. Other foods high in iron include Cream of Wheat, oatmeal, liver, collard greens, mustard greens, clams, chili with beans, brown rice, and dried apricots. Answers A, C, and D are not high in iron.

5. Answer D is correct. The 0.2 ml of air that would be administered after the medication with an intramuscular injection would allow the medication to be dispersed into the muscle. In answer A, the muscle is small. Answer C is an incorrect procedure, and answer B doesn't help with prevention of tracking.

6. Answer A is correct. The destruction of red blood cells causes the release of bilirubin, leading to the yellow hue of the skin. Answers C and D occur with anemia but are not specific to hemolytic. Answer B does not relate.

7. Answer B is correct. Neulasta is given to increase the white blood cell count in patients with leukopenia. This white blood cell count is within the normal range, showing an improvement. Answers A, C, and D are not specific to the drug's desired effect.

8. Answer D is correct. Patients with polycythemia have an increased risk for thrombosis and must be aware of the symptoms. Answers A, B, and C do not relate to this disorder.

9. Answer D is correct. This is the only option that is appropriate for the nurse to legally use at this point. The doctor is performing the surgery and must be notified of the mother's refusal. Answers A and C are not legal options, and answer B is inappropriate.

10. Answer C is correct. Ground pepper is an unprocessed food and will not be allowed due to the possible bacteria. Answers A, B, and D would be processed.

Suggested Reading and Resources

▶ Kee, J. *Laboratory and Diagnostic Tests with Nursing Implications*. New York: Prentice Hall, 2010.

▶ Brunner, L. and Suddarth, D. *Textbook of Medical-Surgical Nursing*. 12th ed. Philadelphia: Lippincott Williams & Wilkins, 2009.

▶ Hogan, M. *Child Health Nursing Reviews and Rationales*. 2nd ed. NJ: Prentice Hall, 2007.

▶ Ignatavicius, D., and Workman, S. *Medical-Surgical Nursing: Critical Thinking for Collaborative Care*. 6th ed. Philadelphia: Elsevier, 2007.

▶ Deglin, J., and Vallerand, A., *Davis Drug Guide for Nurses*. Philadelphia: F.A. Davis, 2009.

▶ Lewis, S., Heitkemper, M., Dirkson, S., O'Brien, P., and Bucher, L. *Medical Surgical Nursing: Assessment and Management of Clinical Problems*. 7th ed. Philadelphia: Elsevier, 2007.

▶ Rinehart, W., Sloan, D., and Hurd, C., *NCLEX Exam Cram*. Indianapolis: Que Publishing, 2007.

▶ Horkenberry, M., and Wilson, D. *Wong's Nursing Care of Infants and Children*. 8th ed. St. Louis: Mosby, 2007.

▶ Epocrates: www.epocrates.com.

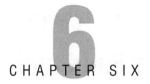

CHAPTER SIX

Caring for the Client with Disorders of Fluid and Electrolyte Balance and Acid/Base Balance

Terms you'll need to understand

✓ Acidosis

✓ Active transport

✓ Alkalosis

✓ Diffusion

✓ Electrolyte

✓ Filtration

✓ pH

Nursing skills you'll need to master

✓ Evaluating pH in clients

Basic Knowledge of Fluid and Electrolyte Balance

Although fluid and electrolyte balance and acid/base balance are separate entities, they are directly related to one another. For example, dehydration results in a decrease in the pH or metabolic acidosis, whereas overhydration results in an increase in the pH or metabolic alkalosis. To understand how this happens, let's review the basics of fluid movement across the cell membrane.

Fluid constantly moves in and out of the cell through a process known as *osmosis*. This fluid is compartmentalized into *intracellular* fluid (fluid that is within the cell) and *extracellular* fluid (fluid that is outside the cell). Two thirds of the body's fluid is intracellular. The remaining one third, or extracellular fluid, is divided between the intravascular and interstitial spaces.

Diffusion is the process whereby molecules move from an area of higher concentration to an area of lower concentration. Diffusion is affected by the amount and type of molecular particles. These molecular particles are removed from body fluid as they pass through semipermeable membranes in a process known as *filtration*.

Molecular particles can also pass from an area of lower concentration to one of higher concentration by a process known as *active transport*. Diffusion and active transport allow positively charged particles, called *cations*, and negatively charged particles, called *anions*, to pass in and out of the cell. These particles are also known as *electrolytes* because they are positively or negatively charged. As these cations and anions concentrate, they result in changes in the pH. Some examples of anions are bicarb (HCO_3-), chloride ($Cl-$), proteins, phosphates, and sulfates. Examples of cations are sodium ($Na+$), potassium ($K+$), magnesium ($Mg++$), and calcium ($Ca++$).

An *acid* is a substance that releases a hydrogen ($H+$) ion when dissolved in water, and a *base* is a substance that binds with a hydrogen ion when released in water. Therefore, when there is a decrease in bicarbonate hydrogen ions (HCO_3-) or an accumulation of carbonic acid, acidosis exists; when there is an increase in bicarbonate hydrogen ions (HCO_3-) or a loss of carbonic acid, alkalosis exists.

Within this chapter we will discuss how these factors affect acid/base balance (pH) and the regulation of electrolytes. You will also discover the disease processes that contribute to these alterations.

Regulation of pH and Its Effect on Fluid and Electrolytes

The body maintains its pH by keeping the ratio of HCO_3 (bicarb) to H_2CO_3 (carbonic acid) at a proportion of 20:1. HCO_3 or bicarbonate is base, whereas carbonic acid is acidic. This relationship constantly changes and is compensated for by the kidneys and lungs. The normal pH is 7.35–7.45, with the ideal pH being 7.40. If the carbonic acid concentration increases, acidosis occurs and the client's pH falls below 7.40. A pH below 7.35 is considered *uncompensated acidosis*. If the HCO_3 concentration increases, alkalosis occurs and the client's pH is above 7.40. A pH above 7.45 is considered *uncompensated alkalosis*.

How the Body Regulates pH

Two buffer systems in the body assist in regulating pH:

▸ **Kidneys**—By retaining or excreting $NaHCO_3$ (sodium bicarb) or by excreting acidic urine or alkaline urine. They also help by reabsorbing $NaHCO_3$– and secreting free H+ ions.

▸ **Lungs**—By retaining carbonic acid in the form of CO_2 (carbon dioxide) or by rapid respirations excreting CO_2.

When there is a problem with either the lungs' or kidneys' capability to compensate, an alteration in this balance results.

Let's discuss the alteration in acid/base balance as it affects electrolytes and pH.

Metabolic Acidosis

Metabolic acidosis results from a primary gain of carbonic acid or a loss of bicarbonate HCO_3 with a pH below 7.40.

Causes of Metabolic Acidosis

The following are some causes of metabolic acidosis:

▸ **Certain disease states**—Disease states that create excessive metabolism of fats in the absence of usable carbohydrates, leading to the accumulation of ketoacids.

▸ **Diabetes mellitus**—Lack of usable insulin, leading to hyperglycemia and ketoacidosis.

▸ **Anorexia**—Leading to cell starvation.

▶ **Lactic acidosis**—Due to muscle and cell trauma, such as myocardial infarction.

▶ **Renal failure**—Leading to waste accumulation in the body and elevated levels of creatinine, BUN, uric acid, and ammonia. All these substances are acidic.

▶ **Diarrhea**—With a loss of HCO_3. This loss of HCO_3 and fluid leads to dehydration. When the client is dehydrated, acidosis is likely.

▶ **Excessive ingestion**—Ingestion of aspirin or other acids.

▶ **Overuse of diuretics**—Particularly nonpotassium-sparing diuretics.

▶ **Overwhelming systemic infections**—Also called *sepsis*. Overwhelming infections lead to cell death and nitrogenous waste accumulation.

▶ **Terminal stages of Addison's disease**—Adrenal insufficiency results in a loss of sodium and water. This leads to a decrease in blood pressure and hypovolemic shock.

Symptoms of Metabolic Acidosis

The following list highlights symptoms of metabolic acidosis that a nurse needs to be aware of for both the exam and for on-the-job observations:

▶ **Neurological**—Headache, lethargy, drowsiness, loss of consciousness, coma, death

▶ **Gastrointestinal**—Anorexia, nausea, vomiting, diarrhea, fruity breath

▶ **Respiratory**—Hyperventilation (due to stimulation of the hypothalamus)

▶ **Renal**—Polyuria and increased acid in the urine

▶ **Lab values**—Decreased pH, decreased $PaCO_2$, decreased serum CO_2, often increased potassium

Care of the Client with Metabolic Acidosis

Metabolic acidosis is rarely present without an underlying disease process. Treatment involves early diagnosis and treatment of the causative factors:

▶ **Monitor the potassium level (K+) and treat accordingly**—Because potassium (K+) is an intracellular cation, changes in potassium levels commonly occur with metabolic acidosis. The symptoms of hyperkalemia are malaise, generalized weakness, muscle irritability, flaccid paralysis, nausea, and diarrhea. If the potassium is excreted through the kidneys, hypokalemia can result. The symptoms of hypokalemia are diminished reflexes, weak pulse, depressed U waves on the ECG, shallow respirations, shortness of breath, and vomiting.

CAUTION

If administering potassium, always check renal function prior to administration. The kidney assists in regulating potassium. If the client has renal disease, a life-threatening hyperkalemia can result. Because potassium is bitter to taste, it should be administered with a juice such as orange juice, grape juice, tomato juice, or apple juice. Ascorbic acid also helps with absorption of the potassium. If administering an IV, always control infusion by using an IV pump or controller. An infusion that is too rapid can result in cardiac arryhythmias. If giving IV, dilute the potassium with IV fluids to prevent hyperkalemia and burning of the vein.

▶ **Treat diabetes**—Treat with insulin for hyperglycemia; treat with glucose for hypoglycemia.

▶ **Treat hypovolemia**—Treat with a volume expander and blood transfusions and treat shock.

▶ **Treat renal failure**—Treatment includes dialysis or transplant and dietary modification. The diet for renal failure clients should control protein, sodium, and fluid. Supplemental calories and carbohydrates are suggested.

▶ **Treat lactic acidosis**—Treatment includes oxygen and $NaHCO_3$.

▶ **Treat Addison's disease**—Treatment includes cortisone preparations, a high sodium diet, and fluids for shock.

Nursing care of the client with metabolic acidosis includes frequent monitoring of vital signs and attention to the quality of pulses, and intake and output. Those with diabetes should be taught the importance of frequent blood glucose checks.

Respiratory Acidosis

Respiratory acidosis occurs when there is a decrease in the rate of ventilation to the amount of carbonic acid production. Hypoventilation leads to CO_2 accumulation and a pH value less than 7.35. Loss of the lungs as a buffer system causes the kidneys to compensate. In chronic respiratory acidosis, the kidneys attempt to compensate by retaining HCO_3.

Causes of Respiratory Acidosis

The following list highlights causes of respiratory acidosis you need to know. All these involve accumulation of carbonic acid (CO_2) and/or a lack of oxygenation:

▶ Over sedation or anesthesia.

▶ Head injury (particularly those affecting the respiratory center). This type of head injury leads to an increase in intracranial pressure and suppression of the respirations.

▶ Paralysis of the respiratory muscles (for example, Guillian-Barré, myasthenia gravis, or spinal cord injury).

▶ Upper airway obstruction.

▶ Acute lung conditions (such as pulmonary emboli, pulmonary edema, pneumonia, or atelectasis).

▶ Chronic obstructive lung disease.

▶ Prolonged overbreathing of CO_2.

> **CAUTION**
>
> When the client has been given general anesthesia followed by narcotic administration, there is a risk of narcotic overdose. The nurse should keep naloxone hydrochloride (Narcan) available as the antidote for narcotic overdose. Flumazenil (Romazicon) is the antidote for the client who is admitted with an overdose of benzodiazepines such as diazepam (Valium).

Symptoms of Respiratory Acidosis

The following list gives the symptoms of respiratory acidosis you need to know:

▶ **Neurological**—Dull sensorium, restlessness, apprehension, hypersomnolence, coma

▶ **Respiratory**—Initially increased respiratory rate, perspiration, increased heart rate; later, slow respirations and periods of apnea or Cheyne-Stokes respirations (breathing marked by periods of apnea lasting 10–60 seconds followed gradually by hyperventilation) with resulting cyanosis

> **CAUTION**
>
> Cyanosis is a late sign of hypoxia. Early signs are tachycardia and tachypnea.

Caring for the Client with Respiratory Acidosis

Care of the client with respiratory acidosis includes attention to signs of respiratory distress, maintaining a patent airway, encouraging fluids to thin secretions, and chest physiotherapy.

CAUTION

Percussion, vibration, and drainage should be done on arising, before meals, and prior to bedtime. Mouth care should be offered after percussion, vibration, and drainage. Cupped hands should be used to prevent trauma to the skin and bruising.

Effective toys for children with asthma or cystic fibrosis are toys such as horns, pinwheels, and whistles. These toys prolong the expiratory phase of respirations and help with CO_2 exhalation. The best sport is swimming.

Metabolic Alkalosis

Metabolic alkalosis results from a primary gain in HCO_3 or a loss of acid that results in a pH level above 7.45.

Causes of Metabolic Alkalosis

The following list highlights causes of metabolic alkalosis that you need to be aware of:

▶ Vomiting or nasogastric suction that may lead to loss of hydrochloric acid

▶ Fistulas high in the gastrointestinal tract that may lead to a loss of hydrochloric acid

▶ Steroid therapy or Cushing's syndrome (hypersecretion of cortisol) that may lead to sodium, hydrogen (H+) ions, and fluid retention

▶ Ingestion or retention of a base (for example, calcium antacids or $NaHCO_3$)

Symptoms of Metabolic Alkalosis

Symptoms of metabolic alkalosis include

▶ **Neurological**—Fidgeting and twitching tremors related to hypokalemia or hyperkalemia

▶ **Respiratory**—Slow, shallow respirations in an attempt to retain CO_2

▶ **Cardiac**—Atrial tachycardia and depressed T waves related to hypokalemia

▶ **Gastrointestinal**—Nausea, vomiting, and diarrhea causing loss of hydrochloric acid

▶ **Lab changes**—pH levels above 7.45, normal or increased CO_2, increased $NaHCO_3$

Caring for the Client with Metabolic Alkalosis

The following items are necessary care items a nurse should know for treating clients with metabolic alkalosis:

▶ Administering potassium replacements

▶ Observing for dysrhythmias

▶ Observing intake and output

▶ Assessing for neurological changes

CAUTION

A positive Trousseau's sign indicates hypocalcemia and is done by applying a blood pressure cuff to the arm and observing for carpo-pedal spasms. Another assessment tool is the Chvostek's sign, which is done by tapping the facial nerve (C7) and observing for facial twitching. This test also indicates hypocalcemia.

Respiratory Alkalosis

Respiratory alkalosis is related primarily to the excessive blowing off of CO_2 through hyperventilation. Causes of respiratory alkalosis include

▶ Hypoxia

▶ Anxiety

▶ High altitudes

Symptoms of Respiratory Alkalosis

The following list details symptoms of respiratory alkalosis that you will need to know as a nurse and for the exam:

▶ **Neurological**—Numbness and tingling of hands and feet, tetany, seizures, and fainting

▶ **Respiratory**—Deep, rapid respirations

▶ **Psychological**—Anxiety, fear, and hysteria

▶ **Lab changes**—Increased pH, decreased $PaCO_2$, decreased K+ levels, and normal or decreased CO_2 levels

Care of the Client with Respiratory Alkalosis

The following list includes steps for caring for clients suffering from respiratory alkalosis:

▶ To correct respiratory alkalosis, the nurse must determine the cause for hyperventilation. Some causes for hyperventilation are stress and high altitudes. Treatments include

   ▶ Stress reduction

   ▶ Sedation

   ▶ Breathing in a paper bag to facilitate retaining CO_2 or using a re-breathing bag

   ▶ Decreasing the tidal volume and rate of ventilator settings

---

CAUTION

Use the following acronym to help you with respiratory and metabolic questions on the exam:

ROME: Respiratory Opposite, Metabolic Equal

This means, in respiratory disorders the pH is opposite to the CO_2 and HCO_3, and in metabolic disorders the pH is equal to or moves in the same direction as the CO_2 and HCO_3. Here's an explanation:

▶ Respiratory acidosis—pH down, CO_2 up, HCO_3 up

▶ Metabolic acidosis—pH down, CO_2 down, HCO_3 down

▶ Respiratory alkalosis—pH up, CO_2 down, HCO_3 down

▶ Metabolic alkalosis—pH up, CO_2 up, HCO_3 up

Normal Electrolyte Values

It is important for you to know these normal electrolyte values. You need to be aware of these so that you can associate alterations in them with the acid/base balance. Note that you are likely to encounter questions on the exam that use these values:

▶ **Sodium (Na+) 135–145 meq/L**—Maintains acid/base balance, maintains extracellular volume, and maintains urine concentration

▶ **Potassium (K+) 3.5–5.5 meq/L**—Regulates protein synthesis, glycolysis, and glycogen synthesis

▶ **Calcium (Ca++) 4.5–5.5 meq/L or 8.5–10.5 mg/L**—Helps with the strength and density of bones and teeth, normal clotting, and muscle contractility

▶ **Chloride (Cl–) 95–105 meq/L**—Assists the formation of hydrochloric acid, maintenance of acid/base balances, and maintaining osmotic pressure

- **Phosphorus (Ph+) 2.5–4.5 mg/dL**—Assists with activation of B complex, cell development, CHO, fat and protein metabolism, and formation and activation of ATP (adenosine triphosphate—creb cycle)

- **Magnesium (Mg++) 1.5–2.5 meq/L**—Helps with muscle contraction, DNA synthesis, and activation of ATP and B complex

EXAM ALERT

A quick way to remember the normal electrolyte ranges is an acronym:

Miss—Magnesium (Mg+)

Piggy—Phosphorus (Phos+)

And

Kermit—Potassium (K+)

Came—Calcium (Ca+)

Home—HCO3 (bicarbonate)

On—oxygen saturation

Cloud—Chloride (Cl-)

Nine—Sodium (Na+)

Changes Associated with Aging

The following list gives you factors related to fluid and electrolyte balance and acid/base balance with aging clients:

- Presence of chronic health problems such as:

    - Diabetes mellitus

    - Renal failure

    - Osteoporosis

    - Liver disease

- Poor appetite

- Medications that can change electrolytes such as:

    - Diuretics

    - Laxatives

- ▶ Antacids
- ▶ Aspirin and NSAIDS
- ▶ Skin breakdown
- ▶ Osteoporosis
- ▶ Constipation
- ▶ Lack of muscle mass

Exam Prep Questions

1. The client is admitted to the unit with a potassium level of 2.4 meq/L. The client with a potassium level of 2.4 meq/L would exhibit symptoms of:

   ○ **A.** Peaked T waves

   ○ **B.** U waves

   ○ **C.** Muscle rigidity

   ○ **D.** Rapid respirations

2. The client is admitted with hypokalemia. An IV of normal saline is infusing at 80 ml/hour with 10 meq of KCl/hour. Prior to beginning the infusion, the nurse should:

   ○ **A.** Check the sodium level.

   ○ **B.** Check the magnesium level.

   ○ **C.** Check the creatinine level.

   ○ **D.** Check the calcium level.

3. The client is admitted to the labor and delivery unit with preeclampsia. An IV of magnesium sulfate is begun per pump. Which finding would indicate hypermagnesemia?

   ○ **A.** Urinary output of 60 ml per hour

   ○ **B.** Respirations of 30 per minute

   ○ **C.** Absence of the knee-jerk reflex

   ○ **D.** Blood pressure of 150/80

4. The client presents to the unit with complaints of shortness of breath. A tentative diagnosis of respiratory acidosis related to pneumonia is made. Which finding would support this diagnosis?

   ○ **A.** pH of 7.45, CO_2 of 45, HCO_3 of 26

   ○ **B.** pH of 7.35, CO_2 of 46, HCO_3 of 27

   ○ **C.** pH of 7.34, CO_2 of 30, HCO_3 of 22

   ○ **D.** pH of 7.44, CO_2 of 32, HCO_3 of 25

5. The client with Cushing's disease will most likely exhibit signs of:

   ○ **A.** Hypokalemia

   ○ **B.** Hypernatremia

   ○ **C.** Hypocalcaemia

   ○ **D.** Hypermagnesemia

6. The nurse is responsible for teaching the client regarding dietary choices to provide needed magnesium. Which food is a good source of magnesium?

   ○ **A.** Apple

   ○ **B.** Spinach

   ○ **C.** Liver

   ○ **D.** Squash

7. The client with hyperparathyroidism will exhibit signs of:

   ○ **A.** Hypokalemia

   ○ **B.** Hyponatremia

   ○ **C.** Hypercalcemia

   ○ **D.** Hyperphosphatemia

8. A client with metabolic acidosis associated with diabetes mellitus is admitted to the unit. A blood glucose of 250 mg/dl is present. Which symptom will most likely accompany ketoacidosis?

   ○ **A.** Oliguria

   ○ **B.** Polydipsia

   ○ **C.** Perspiration

   ○ **D.** Tremors

9. An elderly client is admitted to the unit with a temperature of 100.2°, urinary specific gravity of 1.032, and a dry tongue. The nurse should anticipate an order for:

   ○ **A.** An antibiotic

   ○ **B.** An analgesic

   ○ **C.** A diuretic

   ○ **D.** An IV of normal saline

10. Which diet selection contains the most potassium and should be removed from the tray of the client with renal failure?

   ○ **A.** Peach

   ○ **B.** Baked potato

   ○ **C.** Marshmallows

   ○ **D.** Bread

Answer Rationales

1. Answer B is correct. The normal potassium level is 3.5–5.5 meq/dl. Answer A is incorrect because it indicates an elevated potassium level. Answer C is incorrect because the muscles will be flaccid with hypokalemia. Answer D is incorrect because the respirations will be shallow not rapid.

2. Answer C is correct. The client receiving potassium needs to be evaluated for renal function because regulation of potassium is primarily done within the kidneys. It is not necessary to check the sodium, magnesium, or calcium level prior to beginning potassium, so answers A, B, and D are incorrect.

3. Answer C is correct. The signs of toxicity to magnesium are oliguria (less than 30 ml/hour urinary output), respirations less than 12 per minute, and absence of the deep tendon reflexes. In answer A the urinary output is within normal limits. If it falls below 30, you should further evaluate for toxicity. In answer B if the respirations fall below 12, the infusion should be discontinued and oxygen support maintained. The blood pressure is within normal limits in answer D.

4. Answer B is correct. The client with respiratory acidosis will have a pH that is decreased and CO_2 excretion will be inhibited due to the respiratory problems. The HCO_3 will also be increased because the kidneys are the compensating organ. Answer A is alkalosis, answer C is metabolic acidosis, and answer D is compensated alkalosis.

5. Answer B is correct. The client with Cushing's has hyperadrenal function. These clients retain sodium and water. They do not typically lose potassium or calcium or retain magnesium.

6. Answer B is correct. Dark green vegetables and legumes contain large amounts of magnesium. The other food choices do not provide significant sources of magnesium.

7. Answer C is correct. The client with hyperparathyroidism will have elevated calcium levels. Calcium is pulled from the bone into the serum. These clients frequently have renal calculi and osteoporosis. They do not have hypokalemia, hyponatremia, or hyperphosphatemia. They will have hypercalcemia and hypophosphatemia.

8. Answer B is correct. A blood glucose level of 250 mg/dl is elevated. Symptoms of hyperglycemia are polyuria, polydipsia, and polyphagia. The client will also have a decreased sensorium and tachypnea. Answers A, C, and D are all symptoms of hypoglycemia (testing technique: odd man out).

9. Answer D is correct. The client is hypovolemic and hyponatremic. The slight elevation in the temperature might be related to the dehydration. The normal specific gravity is 1.010–1.020; therefore, this finding shows urinary concentration. There is not enough data to support a need for an antibiotic, as in answer A, an analgesic as in B, or a diuretic as in C.

10. Answer B is correct. The skin of the potato contains large amounts of potassium, and potassium should be limited in the client with renal failure. A peach contains some potassium, but not as much as the baked potato, so answer A is incorrect. The marshmallows and bread contain minimal amounts of potassium, so answers C and D are incorrect.

Suggested Reading and Resources

▶ Hogan, M., and Wane, D. *Fluid, Electrolytes, and Acid-Base Balance*. Upper Saddle River, NJ: Pearson, 2003.

▶ Paradiso, C. *Lippincott's Review Series: Fluid and Electrolytes*. Philadelphia: Lippincott, 1998.

▶ Rinehart, W., Sloan, D., and Hurd, C., *Exam Cram NCLEX-RN*. Indianapolis: Que, 2005.

CHAPTER SEVEN

Caring for the Client with Burns

Terms you'll need to understand

- ✓ Allograft
- ✓ Autograft
- ✓ Biosynthetic graft
- ✓ Burn shock
- ✓ Consensus formula
- ✓ Contracture
- ✓ Debridement
- ✓ Donor site
- ✓ Emergent phase of burn injury
- ✓ Eschar

- ✓ Heterograft
- ✓ Homograft
- ✓ Intermediate phase of burn injury
- ✓ Jobst garment
- ✓ Lund and Browder method
- ✓ Palm method
- ✓ Parkland formula
- ✓ Rehabilitative phase of burn injury
- ✓ Rule of Nines
- ✓ Total body surface area (TBSA)

Nursing skills you'll need to master:

- ✓ Performing sterile dressing change
- ✓ Administering medications
- ✓ Transfusing blood and blood products
- ✓ Performing tracheostomy suction and care
- ✓ Monitoring central venous pressure

- ✓ Caring for central lines
- ✓ Assessing a burn injury using the Rule of Nines
- ✓ Calculation of IV fluid requirements using the Parkland formula and the Consensus formula

Although the incidence of burn injury has declined, burns still account for about 2,000,000 injuries each year in the United States. According to the American Burn Association (2000), more than 51,000 persons require hospital care each year for treatment of their injuries. Those with burns greater than 25% total body surface area (TBSA) are at risk of dying from smoke inhalation and other complications associated with burns. Young children and the elderly are particularly vulnerable to local and systemic effects of burns because their skin is naturally thinner. Burns are the third leading cause of death in children under age 14 and are in the top 10 of causes of death for all age groups.

Burns generally occur from one of three major sources:

▶ Thermal injuries (hot liquid, open flame)

▶ Electrical injuries (household current, lightning)

▶ Chemical injuries (alkaline or acid liquids or powders)

Radiation injuries are most likely to occur with industrial accidents where radioactive energy is produced or in situations where radioactive isotopes are used as is the case with cancer treatment. More discussion on radiation injuries can be found in Chapter 18, "Emergency Nursing."

Most burns are thermal injuries that occur in the home. Cooking accidents from hot grease or stove fires result in a significant number of injuries, as do scalds from bath water that is too hot.

CAUTION

To prevent scalds, hot water heaters should be set no higher than 120° Fahrenheit.

Carbon monoxide, sulfur oxides, cyanide, chlorine, and other toxins are released from household contents during a fire. Inhalation of these gases damages the lower airway, resulting in the collapse of the alveoli and increasing the possibility of acute respiratory distress syndrome.

Burn Classifications

Before discussing caring for the client with burns, we must first look at how burns are classified. Treatment of the client with burns is dictated by whether the injury is classified as a *minor burn*, *moderate burn*, or *major burn*. These classifications are dependent on the degree of tissue involved and the total body surface area affected by the injury. Burns are further classified in terms of the depth of tissue destroyed or the *thickness* of the burn injury. The following list gives you an idea of the different degrees of burns, the symptoms experienced with the injury, and the expected time of healing:

▶ **Superficial partial thickness (first degree)**—Tissue damage is confined to the epidermis and possibly a portion of the dermis. This is the type of injury produced by sunburn or a low-intensity flash. The skin appears red but blanches with pressure. Blisters may or may not be present. The client usually complains of tingling, increased skin sensitivity, and pain that is relieved by the application of cool water or lotions containing aloe. The injury heals within a week. Although the skin peels, there is no scarring.

▶ **Deep partial thickness (second degree)**—Tissue damage involves the epidermis, upper dermis, and portions of the deeper dermis. Deep partial thickness injury is common in scalds and flash flames. The area involved appears blistered with weeping and edema. The client experiences pain and increased skin sensitivity, which increases with exposure to air. The use of sterile sheets and overbed cradles minimizes contact with the air and makes the client more comfortable. Morphine sulfate or other opiate analgesics are given intravenously to control pain.

CAUTION

Pain medication is given intravenously to provide quick, optimal relief and to prevent overmedication as edema subsides and fluid shift is resolving.

Deep partial thickness injury generally heals in two to four weeks, although infection can delay healing. Infection can also take a deep partial thickness injury to a full thickness injury.

▶ **Full thickness (third degree)**—Tissue damage involves the epidermis and entire dermis. The damage usually extends into subcutaneous tissue, including connective tissue, muscle, and bone. Full thickness burns result from prolonged exposure to hot liquids or open flame, electrical current, or exposure to chemical agents. Depending on the source of the injury, the affected area can appear dry, pale white, edematous, leathery, or charred. Destruction of nerve endings leaves the affected areas relatively pain free. Complicating the care of the client with full thickness injury is the development of hypovolemic burn shock, hyperkalemia, and anemia. Electrical injuries, which appear as whitish areas at the points of entry and exit, can result in changes in heart rhythm or complete cardiac standstill.

> **CAUTION**
>
> The cardiac status of a client with electrical burns should be closely monitored for at least 24 hours following the injury to detect changes in electrical conduction of the heart.
>
> Full thickness burns can damage muscles, leading to the development of myoglobinuria, in which urinary output becomes burgundy in color. The client with myoglobinuria may require hemodialysis to prevent tubular necrosis and acute renal failure.

Burn Measurement with TBSA

A second means of classifying burns is based on the percentage of tissue injured. Three methods are used to determine the total body surface area injured in a burn:

- ▶ **The Rule of Nines**—The Rule of Nines assigns percentages of 9 to major body surfaces. The breakdown is as follows: head = 9%, anterior trunk = 18%, posterior trunk = 18%, arms = 9% each, legs = 18% each, and perineum = 1%. The rule is demonstrated in Figure 7.1.

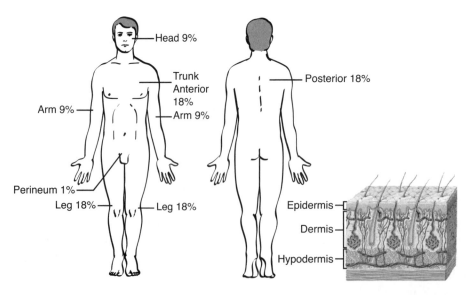

FIGURE 7.1
The Rule of Nines.

- ▶ **Lund and Browder method**—The Lund and Browder method of determining TBSA is more precise because it takes into account that anatomic parts, especially the head and legs, change with growth. Special charts divide the body into very small parts and provide for an estimate of the proportion of TBSA burned. The Lund and Browder method is used to estimate TBSA in children.

▶ **The palm method**—The percentage affected by scattered burns may best be calculated using the palm method. The size of the client's palm represents approximately 1% of the TBSA.

Minor burn injury involves a second degree burn or less than 15% of TBSA in adults and less than 10% in children. Or, it can involve a third degree burn of less than 2% TBSA but not involving areas requiring special care (face, eyes, ears, perineum, and joints of hands and feet). Minor burns do not include electrical burn injury, inhalation injury, those clients with concurrent illness or trauma, or age-related considerations.

Moderate burn injury involves second degree burns of 15%–20% TBSA in adults, 10%–20% in children, or third degree burns less than 10% TBSA that do not involve special care areas. Moderate burns, like minor burns, do not include electrical or inhalation injury, nor those with concurrent illness, trauma, or age-related considerations.

Major burn injury involves second degree burns greater than 25% TBSA in adults, 20% in children, or all third degree burns greater than 10% TBSA. Major burns include all burns involving the structures of the head and face, hands, feet, and perineum as well as electrical and inhalation injury, concurrent illness, and trauma regardless of age.

CAUTION

It will be beneficial to review your nursing textbooks for local and systemic reactions to burns because these injuries affect all body systems and cardiovascular and renal function in particular.

Nursing Care for Burn Victims

Caring for a burned client represents a unique challenge to even the most experienced nursing staff because few injuries pose a greater threat to the client's physical and emotional well-being. There are three phases of burn injury, each requiring various levels of client care. The three phases are

▶ Emergent

▶ Intermediate

▶ Rehabilitative

Psychological Care of a Burn Patient

Although interventions are focused on meeting the client's physiological needs during the emergent period, the nurse should keep in mind that the nature of the injury represents a time of extreme crisis for both the client and his family. Every effort should be made to provide emotional support by providing understandable explanations of procedures and making sure that the client is kept as comfortable as possible. When necessary, appropriate referrals should be made to clergy and other professionals. Interventions directed at stabilizing the client's condition as well as the type of emotional support will change as the client moves through the emergent, intermediate, and rehabilitative phases of injury.

The Emergent Phase

The emergent phase begins with the onset of burn injury and lasts until the completion of fluid resuscitation or a period of about the first 24 hours. During the emergent phase, the priority of client care involves maintaining an adequate airway and treating the client for burn shock.

Emergency care of burns at the site of injury includes

- Extinguishing the burn source

- Soaking the burn with cool water to relieve pain and to limit local tissue edema

- Removing jewelry and nonadherent clothing

- Covering the wound with a sterile (or at least clean) dressing to minimize bacterial contamination

- Brushing off chemical contaminants, removing contaminated clothing, and flushing the area with running water

CAUTION

The eyes should be irrigated with water immediately if a chemical burn occurs. Follow-up care with an ophthalmologist is important because burns of the eyes can result in corneal ulceration and blindness.

Major Burns in the Emergent Phase

If the injury is determined to be a major burn injury, the following additional interventions will be taken during the emergent phase of burn care. Assessment of the following needs to take place during this phase:

- Airway

- Breathing

- Circulation

> **CAUTION**
>
> Important steps in treating a burn client include
>
> ▶ **Treat airway and breathing**—Traces of carbon around the mouth or nose, blisters in the roof of the mouth, or the presence of respiratory stridor indicate the client has respiratory damage. Endotracheal intubation with assisted ventilation might be required to achieve adequate oxygenation.
>
> ▶ **Ensure proper circulation**—Compromised circulation is evident by slowed capillary refill, a drop in normal blood pressure, and decreased urinary output. These symptoms signal impending burn shock.

These interventions come next:

▶ Insertion of a large bore catheter for administering IV fluids

▶ Calculation of TBSA involved

▶ Calculation of fluid needs according to one of the fluid resuscitation formulas

> **CAUTION**
>
> It is important to remember that the actual burns might not be the biggest survival issue facing burn clients. Carbon monoxide from inhaled smoke can develop into a critical problem as well. Carbon monoxide combines with hemoglobin to form carboxyhemoglobin, which binds to available hemoglobin 200 times more readily than with oxygen. Carbon monoxide poisoning causes a vasodilating effect, making the client have a characteristic cherry red appearance. Emergency interventions for the client with carbon monoxide poisoning focus on early intubation and mechanical ventilation with 100% oxygen.

In the hours immediately following a major burn injury, loss of capillary permeability allows intravascular fluid to flood into the extracellular space. During the emergent or resuscitative phase, efforts are directed at preventing or reversing burn shock using fluid replacement formulas. Although there are a number of acceptable formulas for calculating fluid requirements, the Parkland formula and Consensus formula are most often used.

The Parkland Formula   The Parkland formula provides a large volume of IV fluid in the first 24 hours to prevent deepening hypovolemic shock and further acidosis. After the first 24 hours, the amount of fluid infused should be titrated according to the urinary output, with the goal of maintaining the output between 30 mL and 50 mL per hour.

The following example steps you through a calculation of TBSA using the Rule of Nines and the fluid requirements using the Parkland formula:

A client receives full thickness burns of the arms, chest, back, and head at 0600 hours. The client weighs 180 pounds. Using the Parkland formula, how much fluid should the client receive by 1400?

Parkland formula:

Ringer's Lactate 4 mL× kg body weight × % TBSA

Half of the amount is to be infused in the first 8 hours.

The remainder is to be infused over the next 16 hours.

With this information, what steps should you follow? The steps given below will help you calculate this if you have difficulty:

1. Calculate the TBSA using the Rule of Nines:

   arms (9% each arm) = 18% + chest (18%) + back (18%) + head (9%) = 63%

2. Convert the client's weight from pounds to kilograms:

   180 pounds ÷ 2.2 pounds (2.2 pounds = 1 kg) = 81.8 kg (round to 82 kg)

3. Calculate using the Parkland formula for fluid resuscitation:

   4 mL × 82 kg × 63 = 20,664 mL in 24 hours

   According to the Parkland formula, half the calculated volume of Lactated Ringer's solution is to infuse in the first 8 hours; one fourth is to infuse in the second 8 hours; and one fourth is to infuse in the remaining 8 hours.

4. The injury occurred at 0600; the first 8 hours will end at 1400. Therefore, the client should receive one half the total amount or 10,332 mL.

The Consensus Formula   Here's how you use the Consensus formula (for comparison with use of the Parkland formula):

Consensus formula:

Ringer's Lactate or other balanced saline solution 2mL 4 mL× kg body weight × % TBSA

Half of the amount is to be infused over the first 8 hours.

The remainder of the amount is to be infused over the next 16 hours.

CAUTION

Fluid replacement formulas are calculated from the time of injury rather than from the time of arrival in the emergency room.

With this information, what steps should you follow? The steps given here will help you calculate this if you have difficulty:

1. Calculate the TBSA using the Rule of Nines:

   arms (9% each arm) = 18% + chest (18%) + back (18%) + head (9%) = 63%

2. Convert the client's weight from pounds to kilograms:

180 pounds ÷ 2.2 pounds (2.2 pounds = 1 kg) = 81.8 kg (rounded to 82 kg)

3. Calculate using the Consensus formula for fluid resuscitation:

2 mL × 82 × 63 = 10,332 mL

4 mL × 82 × 63 = 20,664 mL

On the low end (2 mL), the amount to infuse over 24 hours would be 10,332 mL, with half to be infused in the first 8 hours and the remainder to be infused over the next 16 hours.

On the high end (4 mL), the amount to infuse over 24 hours would be 20,664 mL, with half to be infused in the first 8 hours and the remainder to be infused over the next 16 hours.

Additional Interventions

These additional interventions are taken after assessment of airway and establishing IV access for fluid replacement. Airway and maintaining fluid volume take priority over all the other interventions:

▶ Administering a tetanus booster

▶ Inserting a urinary catheter for determining hourly output

▶ Inserting a nasogastric tube attached to low suction to minimize the risk of aspiration

---

NOTE

Enteral feedings are usually instituted within the first 24 hours to meet the client's increased caloric needs and maintain the integrity of the intestinal mucosa thereby minimizing systemic sepsis. The client with major burn injury might require as much as 5,000 kilocalories a day.

▶ Elevating burned extremities to lessen edema formation

The Intermediate Phase

The intermediate phase of burn care begins about 48–72 hours following the burn injury. Changes in capillary permeability and a return of osmotic pressure bring about diuresis or increased urinary output. If renal and cardiac functions do not return to normal, the added fluid volume, which prevented hypovolemic shock, might now produce symptoms of congestive heart failure. Assessment of central venous pressure provides information regarding the client's fluid status.

> **NOTE**
>
> The central venous pressure (CVP) is read with the client in a supine position with the manometer level with the fourth intercostal space midaxillary line (often referred to as the *phlebostatic axis*). The normal CVP varies; however, the general range is between 5–12 mm H₂0 or 2–6 mm Hg. Increased CVP indicates fluid volume overload; decreased CVP indicates fluid volume deficit.

Additional complications found during the intermediate phase include infections, the development of Curling's ulcer, paralytic ileus, anemia, disseminated intravascular coagulation, and acute respiratory failure.

> **NOTE**
>
> Infections represent a major threat to the post-burn client. Bacterial infections (*staphylococcus, proteus, pseudomonas, escherichia coli,* and *klebsiella*) are common due to optimal growth conditions posed by the burn wound; however, the primary source of infection appears to be the client's own intestinal tract. As a rule, systemic antibiotics are avoided unless an actual infection exists.

During the intermediate phase, attention is given to removing the eschar and other cellular debris from the burned area. *Debridement*, the process of removing damaged tissue (eschar) in order to improve healing, can be done by placing the client in a tub or shower and gently washing the burned tissue away with mild soap and water. Hydrotherapy should be limited to 20 to 30 minutes to reduce the risk of fluid shifts. Enzymes, substances that digest the burned tissue, such as Elase or Santyl (collagenase) are important debriding agents for burn wounds.

> **CAUTION**
>
> Enzymatic debridement should not be used for burns greater than 10% TBSA, for burns near the eyes, or for burns involving muscle.

Following debridement, the wound is treated with a topical antibiotic and a dressing is applied (more on dressings is covered in the next section). Commonly used topical antibiotics include silver sulfadiazine (Silvadene); mafenide acetate (Sulfamylon); and silver nitrate, which can be used in an aqueous solution of 0.5% or Acticoat, a prepared dressing impregnated with silver nitrate. Silver nitrate has bacteriostatic properties that inhibit bacterial growth. Mafenide acetate, although painful, is useful in preventing *Pseudomonas* infections. Silvadene cools and soothes the burn wound but does not prevent infection.

Dressings for Burns

Dressings for burns include standard wound dressings (sterile gauze) and biologic or biosynthetic dressings (grafts, amniotic membranes, cultured skin, and artificial skin).

Standard Wound Dressings

The use of standard wound dressings makes the client more comfortable by preventing exposure of the wound to air. These dressings are usually applied every shift or once a day.

Biologic or Biosynthetic Dressings

Biologic dressings are obtained from either human tissue (homograft or allograft) or animal tissue (heterograft). These dressings, which are temporary, are used for clients with partial thickness or granulating full thickness injuries. The type of biologic dressing used depends on the type of wound and availability of the graft.

Homografts or allografts are taken from cadaver donors and obtained through a skin bank. These grafts are expensive and there is a risk of blood-borne infection. Heterografts or xenografts are taken from animal sources. The most common heterograft is pigskin because of its compatibility with human skin.

> **CAUTION**
>
> Certain religious and ethnic groups would be offended if offered a porcine (pigskin) graft.

Amniotic membrane is used for full thickness burns because it adheres immediately to the wound. It is also an effective covering for partial thickness burns until reepithealization occurs. Amniotic membrane is low in cost, and its size allows for coverage of large wounds.

Cultured skin can be obtained by using a biopsy of epidermal cells taken from unburned portions of the client's body. The cells are grown in a laboratory and grafted to generate permanent skin. The process is long and costly, and extreme care is needed to prevent damage and loss of the graft.

Artificial skin (Integra) made of synthetic material and animal collagen becomes a part of the client's skin. The graft site is pliable, there is less hypertrophic scarring, and its use is helping to eliminate the need for compression dressings like the Jobst garment during the rehabilitative phase of care.

Permanent grafts include the autograft or skin transferred from an unburned area of the client's body to the burn wound. The client generally experiences more pain from the donor site than from the burn wound because the donor site has many pain receptors. The client should receive pain medication, and both the donor site and graft site should be carefully monitored for signs of infection.

The Rehabilitative Phase

The last stage in caring for a client with burn injury is the rehabilitative stage. Technically, this stage begins with closure of the burn and ends when the client has reached the optimal level of functioning. In actuality, it begins the day the client enters the hospital and can continue for a lifetime. In the emergent and intermediate phases, the focus is on establishing and maintaining physiological equilibrium. In the rehabilitative phase, the focus is on helping the client return to preinjury life. If that is not possible, the focus is on helping the client adjust to the changes the injury has imposed.

Diagnostic Tests for Review

The following are routine tests done on most all hospital admissions. For this client, it is a way of monitoring the hemodynamic changes (development of anemia and so on) as well as changes in renal function. The chest x-ray lets the nurse know whether there has been an inhalation injury, a development of pneumonia, changes associated with ARDS, and so on. The complete metabolic panel gives information on electrolyte status, guiding the type of IV fluid to use, as well as whether additional electrolytes are needed. Here are the tests that should be performed:

▶ CBC

▶ Complete metabolic panel

▶ Urinalysis

▶ Chest x-ray

Pharmacology Categories for Review

A client with burn injuries is particularly vulnerable to infection because he has lost the first line of defense, the skin. In fact, post-burn infection is a major cause of morbidity and mortality; therefore, it is helpful to review topical antibiotics used to treat those with burns. Other complications of burns include anemia and stress ulcers. A review of medications used to treat anemia as well as medications to prevent ulcers and the bleeding that can occur will be helpful. Narcotic analgesics—particularly opiate derivatives—are used in controlling pain and providing sedation during the emergent and intermediate phases of burn care. A review of these categories, as seen in the following list, will better prepare you to care for a client with burns:

▶ Topical antibiotics

▶ Antianemics

▶ Antacids

▶ Narcotic analgesics

Exam Prep Questions

1. The nurse is caring for a client with an electrical burn. Which structures have the greatest risk for soft tissue injury?

- ○ **A.** Fat, tendons, and bones
- ○ **B.** Skin and hair
- ○ **C.** Nerves, muscle, and blood vessels
- ○ **D.** Skin, fat, and muscle

2. Which laboratory result would be expected during the emergent phase of a burn injury?

- ○ **A.** Glucose 100 mg/dL
- ○ **B.** Potassium 3.5 mEq/L
- ○ **C.** Sodium 142 mEq/L
- ○ **D.** Albumin 4.2 gm/dL

3. An African American client is admitted with full thickness burns over 40% of his body. In addition to the CBC and complete metabolic panel, the physician is likely to request which additional blood-work?

- ○ **A.** Erythrocyte sedimentation rate
- ○ **B.** Indirect Coombs
- ○ **C.** C reactive protein
- ○ **D.** Sickledex

4. A client weighing 76 kg is admitted at 0600 with a TBSA burn of 40%. Using the Parkland formula, the client's 24-hour intravenous fluid replacement should be:

- ○ **A.** 6,080 mL
- ○ **B.** 9,120 mL
- ○ **C.** 12,160 mL
- ○ **D.** 15,180 mL

5. On the third post-burn day, the nurse finds that the client's hourly urine output is 26 ml. The nurse should continue to assess the client and notify the doctor for an order to:

   ○ **A.** Decrease the rate of the intravenous infusion.

   ○ **B.** Change the type of intravenous fluid being administered.

   ○ **C.** Change the urinary catheter.

   ○ **D.** Increase the rate of the intravenous infusion.

6. A Jewish client requires grafting to promote burn healing. Which graft is most likely to be unacceptable to the client?

   ○ **A.** Isograft

   ○ **B.** Autograft

   ○ **C.** Homograft

   ○ **D.** Xenograft

7. During the rehabilitative phase, the client's burns become infected with _pseudomonas_. The topical dressing most likely to be ordered for the client is:

   ○ **A.** Silver sulfadiazine (Silvadene)

   ○ **B.** Poviodine (Betadine)

   ○ **C.** Mafenide acetate (Sulfamylon)

   ○ **D.** Silver nitrate

8. The CVP reading of a client with partial thickness burns is 6 mm H_2O. The nurse recognizes that the client:

   ○ **A.** Needs additional fluids

   ○ **B.** Has a normal CVP reading

   ○ **C.** May show signs of congestive failure

   ○ **D.** Would benefit from a diuretic

9. The physician has prescribed Protonix (pantoprazole) for a client with burns. The nurse recognizes that the medication will help prevent the development of:

   ○ **A.** Curling's ulcer

   ○ **B.** Myoglobinuria

   ○ **C.** Hyperkalemia

   ○ **D.** Paralytic ileus

10. The nurse has just completed the dressing change for a client with burns to the lower legs and ankles. The nurse should place the client's ankles in which position?

- ○ **A.** Internal rotation
- ○ **B.** Abduction
- ○ **C.** Dorsiflexion
- ○ **D.** Hyperextension

Answer Rationales

1. Answer A is correct. Fat, tendon, and bone have the most resistance. The higher the resistance, the greater the heat generated by the current, thereby increasing the risk for soft tissue injury. Answer B has intermediate resistance, so it is incorrect. Answer C is incorrect because it has very low resistance. Answer D has low to intermediate resistance, so it is incorrect.

2. Answer A is correct. Glucose levels rise as a result of the stress response during the emergent phase. Answers B, C, and D are within normal range. K+ and Na+ would be elevated, whereas albumin would be lowered during the emergent period due to increased permeability.

3. Answer D is correct. Sickle cell anemia and sickle cell trait are more prevalent in African American clients. The Sickledex test detects the presence of sickle cell anemia and sickle cell trait. Trauma can trigger a sickle cell crisis, which would complicate the treatment of the client. Answers A and C indicate inflammation, so they are incorrect. Answer B is incorrect because it detects circulating antibodies against RBCs.

4. Answer C is correct. The Parkland formula is 4 ml × kg × TBSA = 24-hr. fluid requirement, or 4 × 76 × 40 = 12,160 mL. Answer A is the fluid requirement for the first 8 hours after burn injury, so it's incorrect. Answer B is incorrect because it's the fluid requirement for 16 hours after burn injury. Answer D is an excessive amount given the client's weight and TBSA, so it's incorrect.

5. Answer D is correct. The urinary output should be maintained between 30 mL and 50 mL per hour. The first action should be to increase the IV rate to prevent increased acidosis. Answer A would lead to diminished output, so it is incorrect. There is no indication that the type of IV fluid is not appropriate as is suggested by answer B, making it incorrect. Answer C would not increase the client's output and would place the client at greater risk for infection, so it is incorrect.

6. Answer D is correct. Xenografts are taken from nonhuman sources. The most common sources are porcine, or pigskin, which would be offensive to both Jews and Muslims. Answer A refers to a graft taken from an identical twin, making it incorrect. Answer B is incorrect because it refers to a graft taken from the client's own skin. Answer C refers to a graft taken from a cadaver, making it incorrect.

7. Answer C is correct. Sulfamylon is effective in treating wounds infected with *pseudomonas*. The client should receive pain medication prior to dressing changes because the medication produces a burning sensation when applied to the wound. Answers A, B, and D are incorrect because they are used in the treatment of burns but are not effective against *pseudomonas* infections.

8. Answer B is correct. The normal CVP reading is 5–12 mm H_2O. Answer A is incorrect because the client does not need additional fluids. Answers C and D would be appropriate only if the CVP reading were greater than 12 mm H_2O.

9. Answer A is correct. Curling's ulcer, a stress ulcer, is a common occurrence in clients with burns. Protonix, a proton pump inhibitor, is effective in preventing ulcer formation. Answers B, C, and D are common in clients with burns but are not prevented by the use of Protonix, so they are incorrect.

10. Answer C is correct. Placing the ankles in dorsiflexed position helps prevent contractures. Answers A, B, and D will lead to contractures that may require surgical intervention, so they are incorrect.

Suggested Reading and Resources

▶ Ignatavicius, D., and Workman, S. *Medical Surgical Nursing: Critical Thinking for Collaborative Care.* 6th ed. Philadelphia: Elsevier, 2008.

▶ Brunner, L., and Suddarth, D. *Textbook of Medical Surgical Nursing.* 12th ed. Philadelphia: Lippincott Williams & Wilkins, 2009.

▶ LeMone, P., and Burke, K. in *Medical Surgical Nursing: Critical Thinking in Client Care.* 4th ed. Upper Saddle River, NJ: Pearson Prentice Hall, 2008.

▶ Lewis, S., Heitkemper, M., Dirksen, S., O'Brien, P., and Bucher, L. *Medical Surgical Nursing: Assessment and Management of Clinical Problems.* 7th ed. Philadelphia: Elsevier, 2007.

▶ Lehne, R. *Pharmacology for Nursing Care.* 7th ed. Philadelphia: Elsevier, 2009.

▶ Burn Recovery Center: www.burn-recovery.org.

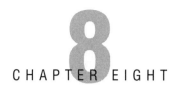

CHAPTER EIGHT

Caring for the Client with Sensorineural Disorders

Terms you'll need to understand:

- ✓ Aqueous humor
- ✓ Astigmatism
- ✓ Canal of Schlemm
- ✓ Cataract
- ✓ Conductive hearing loss
- ✓ Conjunctiva
- ✓ Cornea
- ✓ Decibel
- ✓ Glaucoma
- ✓ Hyperopia
- ✓ Intraocular pressure
- ✓ Legally blind
- ✓ Lens
- ✓ Macular degeneration
- ✓ Meniere's disease
- ✓ Mydriatic
- ✓ Myopia
- ✓ Myotic
- ✓ Otitis media
- ✓ Otosclerosis
- ✓ Ototoxic
- ✓ Presbycusis
- ✓ Presbyopia
- ✓ Retinal detachment
- ✓ Sensorineural hearing loss

Nursing skills you'll need to master:

- ✓ Performing sterile dressing change
- ✓ Administering eye drops, eye ointments, and ear drops
- ✓ Use of an ear wick
- ✓ Inserting and removing eye prosthesis
- ✓ Performing eye and ear irrigations
- ✓ Caring for hearing aids

Most of us will agree that the abilities to see, hear, taste, perceive touch, and smell are pretty important. Without the ability to smell, food would have little, if any, taste. The sense of touch lets us know when we experience something pleasurable or have been injured. No one would argue that this is unimportant. But of all the senses, the abilities to see and hear are considered most important, for they keep us informed about the world around us. In this chapter, we review problems affecting vision and hearing.

Disorders of the Eyes

Disorders of the eyes can be divided into the following categories:

▶ **Intraocular disorders**—Examples include cataracts and glaucoma.

▶ **Retinal disorders**—Examples of these are hypertensive retinopathy, diabetic retinopathy, and macular degeneration.

▶ **Refractive errors**—Examples include myopia, hyperopia, presbyopia, and astigmatism.

▶ **Traumatic injury**—Examples include hyphema, contusions, foreign bodies, lacerations, and penetrating injuries.

Intraocular Disorders

Intraocular disorders arise from within the eyeball. The primary intraocular disorders you need to understand are cataracts and glaucoma. These two diseases are discussed in the following sections.

Cataracts

Cataracts, opacities in the lens of the eye, result in the distortion of images projected onto the retina. Cataracts are associated with aging, trauma, disease of the eye, prolonged use of steroids, and exposure to sunlight or ultraviolet light. Congenital cataracts of the newborn are characterized by the absence of the red reflex.

CAUTION

An infant should be able to visually follow a moving object by three months of age. If unable to do so, the infant should have the vision evaluated by an ophthalmologist.

Symptoms of cataracts include

▶ Blurred, hazy vision

▶ Glare from bright lights

▶ Yellow, white, or gray discoloration of the pupil

▶ Gradual loss of vision

Cataract surgery is generally performed in an outpatient surgery center. The client is given a sedative to lessen anxiety. Medications such as Diamox (acetazolamide) are given to reduce intraocular pressure. Mydriatic eye drops such as Neo-Synephrine (phenylephrine) are used in combination with cycloplegics such as Cyclogyl (cyclophenolate HCl) to paralyze the muscles of accommodation. After the client is in the operative area, an intravenous injection of Versed (midazolam) can be given to induce light anesthesia followed by local anesthesia.

Removal of the affected lens is usually accomplished by an extracapsular cataract extraction (ECCE). The anterior portion of the lens is opened and removed along with the lens cortex and nucleus. The posterior lens capsule is left in place to provide support for the intraocular lens implant. Antibiotic steroid drops or ointments are instilled in the operative eye. In some instances a sterile patch and shield are applied to the operative eye.

Post-operatively the client is maintained in a semi-Fowler's position to prevent stress on the implant. Clients are usually discharged within 2–3 hours following surgery. Before discharging the client, the nurse should instruct the client.

▶ To avoid activities that would increase intraocular pressure, such as bending from the waist, blowing the nose, wearing tight shirt collars, closing the eyes tightly, and placing the head in a dependent position

▶ To report sharp, sudden pain in the operative eye

▶ To report bleeding, increased discharge, or lid swelling in the operative eye

▶ To report decreasing vision, flashes of light, or visual floaters

▶ To take a tub bath or to face away from the shower head when bathing

▶ In the proper way to administer eye medication

▶ To wear the protective shield when sleeping

Glaucoma

Glaucoma refers to a group of diseases that result in an increase in intraocular pressure. The three types of glaucoma and their characteristics are

▶ **Primary open-angle glaucoma (POAG)**—This is the most common form of glaucoma. POAG affects both eyes, is usually asymptomatic, and is caused by a decrease in the outflow of aqueous humor. The intraocular pressure in those with primary open-angle glaucoma averages between 22mm Hg and 32mm Hg. Symptoms of primary open angle glaucoma include

▶ Tired eyes

▶ Diminished peripheral vision

▶ Seeing halos around lights

▶ Hardening of the eyeball

▶ Increased intraocular pressure

▶ **Acute glaucoma**—This is sometimes called *narrow-angle glaucoma* and is less common. This is caused by a sudden increase in the production of aqueous humor. The onset of severe eye pain is sudden and without warning. Emergency treatment is necessary because rising intraocular pressure can exceed 30mm Hg resulting in loss of vision. Symptoms of acute glaucoma include the following:

▶ Sudden, excruciating pain around the eyes

▶ Headache or aching in the eyebrow

▶ Nausea and vomiting

▶ Cloudy vision

▶ Pupil dilation

▶ **Secondary glaucoma**—is related to ocular conditions that narrow the Canal of Schlemm or that alter eye structures involved in the production and circulation of aqueous humor.

NOTE

Normal intraocular pressure is 10–21mm Hg.

Management of a Client with Glaucoma

Conservative management of the client with glaucoma is aimed at reducing intraocular pressure with medications. Miotic eye drops such as Isopto Carpine (pilocarpine HCl) are instilled to constrict the pupil and increase the flow of aqueous humor. Beta blockers such as Timoptic (timolol) and carbonic anhydrase inhibitors like Diamox (acetazolamide) decrease the production of aqueous humor, thereby lowering the intraocular pressure. Osmotics like Osmitrol (mannitol) can be administered via IV to clients with acute glaucoma to rapidly reduce intraocular pressure and prevent permanent damage to the optic nerve.

Surgical management is indicated when medications fail to control the symptoms associated with open-angle glaucoma as well as for the client with acute glaucoma. A laser is used to create a hole, allowing the aqueous humor to drain more freely. Standard surgical therapy that creates a new drainage canal or destroys the structures responsible for the increase in intraocular pressure is reserved for the client whose condition does not respond to either medications or laser surgery.

Post-operatively the client is instructed to lie on the nonoperative side, to avoid taking aspirin, and to report severe eye or brow pain. Changes in vital signs, a decrease vision, and acute pain deep in the eye are symptoms of choroidal hemorrhage.

CAUTION

Clients with known or suspected glaucoma should avoid over-the-counter medications that can increase intraocular pressure. Medications such as Visine cause vasoconstriction, which is followed by rebound vasodilation. Rebound vasodilation can raise pressures within the eye.

Atropine is contraindicated in the client with glaucoma because it closes the Canal of Schlemm and raises intraocular pressure.

Retinal Disorders

Retinal disorders involve disorders of the innermost layer of the eye. The most common retinal disorders are hypertensive retinopathy, diabetic retinopathy, and macular degeneration. The following sections cover these retinal disorders in greater detail.

Hypertensive Retinopathy

Hypertensive retinopathy occurs in the client with a long history of uncontrolled hypertension. Elevations in diastolic blood pressure create a copper wire appearance in the retinal arterioles. If the blood pressure remains elevated, arterioles become occluded by the formation of soft exudates known as cotton wool spots. Treatment focuses on control of systemic hypertension. Left untreated, hypertensive retinopathy can result in retinal detachment and loss of vision.

Diabetic Retinopathy

Diabetic retinopathy is the result of vascular changes associated with uncontrolled diabetes mellitus. Vascular changes are inherent in all diabetics; however, good control of blood sugar helps reduce the severity of the disease. The two types of diabetic retinopathy are

> ▶ **Background diabetic retinopathy**—This leads to the development of microaneurysms and intraretinal hemorrhages.

> ▶ **Proliferative diabetic retinopathy**—This leads to the development of new, fragile blood vessels that leak blood and protein into the surrounding tissue.

The treatment of diabetic retinopathy depends on the type and the degree of tissue involvement. Laser surgery can be used to seal microaneurysms and prevent bleeding.

Macular Degeneration

Macular degeneration affects the portion of the eye involved with central vision. The two types of macular degeneration are

▶ **Atropic (dry)**—This form is characterized by sclerosing of retinal capillaries with loss of rod and cone receptors, decreased central vision, and complaints of mild blurred vision. The condition progresses faster in smokers than nonsmokers. The risk for macular degeneration can be reduced by eating a diet rich in antioxidants, lutein, and carotenoids.

▶ **Exudative (wet)**—This form is characterized by a sudden decrease in vision due to serous detachment of the pigmented epithelium of the macula. Blisters composed of fluid and blood form underneath the macula, resulting in scar formation and decreasing vision.

Treatment of macular degeneration is aimed at slowing the process. Laser therapy can be used to seal leaking blood vessels near the macula.

Retinal Detachment

Retinal detachment can result from a blow to the head, fluid accumulation in the subretinal space, or the aging process. Generally, the condition is pain-free; however, the client might complain of the following symptoms:

▶ Blurred vision

▶ Flashes of light

▶ Visual floaters

▶ Veil-like loss of vision

Management of Clients with Detached Retinas

Conservative management usually involves placing the client with the area of detachment in dependent position. The most common site for retinal detachment is the superior temporal area of the right eye. Sedatives and anxiolytics will make the client more comfortable. Spontaneous reattachment of the retina is rare, so surgical management is often required.

Surgical management includes the creation of a scar to seal the retina to the choroid or, by scleral buckling, to shorten the sclera and improve contact between the retina and choroid.

Post-op activity varies with the procedure used. If gas or oil has been instilled during the scleral buckling, the client is positioned on the abdomen with the head turned so that the operative eye is facing upward. This position is maintained for several days or until the gas or oil is absorbed. An alternative is to allow the client to sit on the bedside and place his head on an overbed table. Bathroom privileges are allowed, but the client must keep his head bowed. The following discharge instructions should be given to the client with a scleral buckling:

▶ Report any sudden increase in pain or pain accompanied by nausea.

▶ Avoid reading, writing, and close work for the first post-op week.

▶ Do not bend over so that the head is in a dependent position.

▶ Be careful not to bump the head.

Refractive Errors

Refractory errors refer to the capability of the eyes to focus images on the retina. Refractory errors are due to an abnormal length of the eyeball from front to back and the refractive power of the lens. Refractory errors include the following:

▶ **Myopia (nearsightedness)**—Images focus in front of rather than on the retina; this is corrected by a concave lens.

▶ **Hyperopia (farsightedness)**—Images focus behind rather than on the retina; this is corrected by a convex lens.

▶ **Presbyopia**—The crystalline lens loses elasticity and becomes unable to change shape to focus the eye for close work so that images fall behind the retina; this is age related.

▶ **Astigmatism**—An uneven curvature of the cornea causes light rays to be refracted unequally so that a focus point on the retina is not achieved.

Nonsurgical management of refractory errors includes the use of eyeglasses and contact lenses. Surgical management includes the following:

▶ **Radial keratotomy (RK)**—This treatment is used for mild to moderate myopia. Eight to sixteen cuts are made through 90% of the peripheral cornea. The incisions decrease the length of the eye by flattening the cornea. This allows the image to be focused nearer the retina.

▶ **Photorefractive keratotomy (PRK)**—This is used for the treatment of mild to moderate stable myopia and low astigmatism. An excimer laser is used to reshape the superficial cornea using powerful beams of ultraviolet light. One eye is treated at a time with a wait period of three months between surgeries. Complete healing can take up to six months.

▶ **Laser in-situ keratomileusis (LASIK)**—This is used for the treatment of nearsightedness, farsightedness, and astigmatism. An excimer laser is used to reshape the deeper corneal layers. Both eyes are treated at the same time. Complete healing can take up to four weeks. LASIK is thought to be better than PRK because the outer layer of the cornea is not damaged, there is less pain, and the healing time is reduced.

▶ **Intacs corneal ring**—This is the newest vision enhancement for nearsightedness. The shape of the cornea is changed by using a polymeric ring on the outer edges of the cornea. The surgery does not involve the use of a laser and is reversible. Healing to best vision is immediate, and replacement rings can be applied if the client's vision changes with aging.

Traumatic Injuries

Traumatic injuries to the eyes can occur from any activity. Traumatic injuries and their treatments include

▶ **Hyphema**—Hemorrhage in the anterior chamber as the result of a blow to the eye, Treatment includes bedrest in semi-Fowler's position, no sudden eye movement for 3–5 days, cycloplegic eyedrops, use of an eye patch and eye shield to protect the eye, and limited television viewing and reading.

▶ **Contusion**—Bruising of the eyeball and surrounding tissue. Treatment includes ice to the affected area and a thorough eye exam to rule out other eye injuries. Elevating the client's head 30 to 45 degrees will help to minimize edema and swelling.

▶ **Foreign bodies**—Objects that irritate or abrade the surface of the conjunctiva or cornea. Treatment includes transporting the client to the ER with both eyes covered by a cupped object, a visual assessment by a physician before treatment, and instillation of fluorescein followed by irrigation with normal saline to remove foreign particles.

▶ **Lacerations and penetrating injuries**—Corneal lacerations and penetrating injuries of the eye are considered emergencies because ocular contents can prolapse through the site of injury. Treatment can require the administration of IV antibiotics and surgery.

CAUTION

Objects protruding from the eye should never be removed by anyone except an ophthalmologist because greater damage can occur, including the displacement of ocular structures. Clients with penetrating eye injuries have the poorest prognosis for retaining vision.

Visual Tests for Review

Several tests are commonly used during a routine eye examination. These tests include the Snellen chart, which assesses visual acuity, and the Ishihara polychromatic chart, which assesses color vision. Some medications, such as antituberculars, can affect both visual acuity and color vision; therefore, the client should have a thorough eye exam before beginning therapy and every six months while taking the medication. The Ansler grid is used to detect changes caused by macular degeneration, whereas tonometry detects changes in intraocular pressure that are associated with glaucoma. These tests should be done at least once a year for clients over age 40.

Pharmacology Categories for Review

A number of medications are used to treat eye disorders. Mydriatics and cycloplegics are used for the client with cataracts. Miotics, beta blockers, and carbonic anhydrase inhibitors are ordered for the client with glaucoma to constrict the pupil and reduce pressure within the eye. It is important for you to review the side effects and contraindications for these medications:

- ▶ Cycloplegics
- ▶ Miotics
- ▶ Mydriatics
- ▶ Beta blockers
- ▶ Carbonic anhydrase inhibitors

Ear Disorders

Much of what we know about our world is gained through vision; however, a well-functioning auditory system is also important. Disorders of the ears and hearing loss create problems with everyday living. Some conditions, such as Meniere's disease, interfere with balance and coordination. Other conditions, such as otosclerosis and age-related presbycusis, affect our ability to receive and give information accurately. The client with a significant hearing loss often becomes confused, mistrustful, and socially isolated from family and friends. Disorders of the ears can be divided into the following conditions:

- ▶ Conditions affecting the external ear (otitis externa)
- ▶ Conditions affecting the middle ear (otitis media)

- ▶ Conditions affecting the inner ear (Meniere's disease, otosclerosis)

- ▶ Age-related hearing loss (presbycusis)

- ▶ Ear trauma

Otitis Externa

Otitis externa is often referred to as *swimmer's ear* because it occurs more often in hot, humid environments. The condition can result from an allergic response or inflammation. Allergic external otitis media is often the result of contact with hair spray, cosmetics, earrings, earphones, and hearing aids. It can occur from infectious organisms, including bacteria or fungi. Most infections are due to *pseudomonas aeruginosa*, *streptococcus*, *staphylococcus*, and *aspergillus*. In rare cases, a virulent form of otitis externa develops, spreading the infection into the adjacent structures of the brain and causing meningitis, brain abscess, and damage to cranial nerves.

The treatment of otitis externa is aimed at relieving pain, inflammation, and swelling. Topical antibiotics and steroids are used. Systemic antibiotics, either oral or intravenous, are used in severe cases.

Otitis Media

Otitis media is an infection of the middle ear that occurs more often in young children than adults because the eustachian tube of the child is shorter and wider than that of the adult. *H. influenza* is the most common cause of acute otitis media. Signs and symptoms of acute otitis media include pain, malaise, fever, vomiting, and anorexia.

Increased pressure can cause the tympanic membrane to rupture. Rupture of the tympanic membrane usually results in relief of pain and fever; however, repeated rupture can lead to scarring of the membrane with eventual loss of hearing.

Treatment of acute otitis media includes the use of systemic antibiotics, analgesics for pain, as well as antihistamines and decongestants to decrease fluid in the middle ear. Antibiotic therapy is continued for 7–10 days to ensure that the causative organism has been eliminated. If the tympanic membrane continues to bulge following antibiotic therapy, a small surgical incision is made in the tympanic membrane (myringotomy) and a PE (polyethelene tube) is inserted to allow continuous drainage of the middle ear.

Meniere's Disease

Meniere's disease is a disease of the inner ear characterized by a triad of symptoms: vertigo, tinnitus, and hearing loss of low tones. Symptoms can occur suddenly and can last from several hours to several days. The exact cause of Meniere's disease is unknown, but it is associated with allergies, as well as vascular and inflammatory responses that alter fluid balance.

Conservative management includes the use of antihistamines, antiemetics, and diuretics to control edema of the labyrinth and vasodilators to decrease vasospasm. Salt and fluid restrictions are recommended to decrease the amount of endolymphatic fluid produced. Cessation of smoking and limiting caffeine intake can also improve symptoms by helping to reduce vasoconstriction. Nicotinic acid has proven beneficial by producing a vasodilating effect.

Surgical management can involve an endolymphatic subarachnoid shunt or a labryinthectomy. Surgical management involving a labryinthectomy is controversial because hearing in the affected ear can be lost. Following surgery, the client will experience vertigo, nausea, and vomiting for several days.

Otosclerosis

Otosclerosis refers to the progressive hardening of the bony configuration known as the *stapes*, leaving them incapable of movement. Otosclerosis is the most common cause of conductive hearing loss. Symptoms of otosclerosis include tinnitus and conduction deafness.

Management of otosclerosis involves a stapedectomy. The diseased stapes is removed; then the oval window is sealed and rejoined to the incus using a metal or plastic prosthesis. Key points included in the care of the client who has had a stapedectomy are as follows:

▶ Tell the client that hearing might decrease after surgery due to swelling and accumulation of fluid but should improve as blood and fluid are absorbed.

▶ Instruct the client to avoid activities that increase pressure within the ear (such as blowing the nose, extreme head movement, drinking through a straw, and air travel). Avoiding crowds will lessen the chance of getting upper respiratory infections with symptoms such as coughing and sneezing. If the client must cough or sneeze, she should do it with an open mouth.

▶ Tell the client to report pain and changes in taste or facial sensation as well as drainage from the ear.

▶ Instruct the client to avoid getting water in the ears for at least six weeks after surgery. Tub baths are better than showers.

▶ Instruct the client to take medications (antibiotics and antiemetics) as prescribed.

Presbycusis

Presbycusis associated with aging is a common cause of sensorineural hearing loss. This type of hearing loss is the result of damage to the ganglion cells of the cochlea and decreased blood supply to the inner ear. Deficiencies in vitamins B9 and B12 also have been found to play a role in the development of presbycusis. Sensorineural hearing loss is also related to the use of oto-toxic drugs as well as exposure to loud noises.

> **NOTE**
>
> Hearing loss of 50 decibels affects the client's ability to distinguish parts of speech. Presbycusis affects the ability to hear high-frequency, soft consonant sounds (*t, s, th, ch, sh, b, f, p,* and *pa*).

Ear Trauma

Injury to the tympanic membrane can result in pain, infection, and hearing loss. Most ear trauma is the result of jabbing injuries that damage the eardrum and inner ear or blows to the ear that result in extreme changes in pressure. Children frequently use the ears (and the nose) as hiding places for foreign bodies that become lodged, interfering with hearing and creating a source of infection. Foreign bodies in the ear or nose should receive the attention of the physician who will remove them and provide appropriate follow-up treatment.

Assisting Clients with Hearing Loss

Devices to assist the client with a hearing loss include hearing aids and cochlear implants. If you are working with a client who is hearing impaired and he is not wearing a hearing aid, the following hints might prove helpful:

- ▶ Stand in front of the client when talking to him. Many hearing-impaired persons rely on lip reading and facial expression.

- ▶ Talk in a normal tone of voice. Raising your voice distorts the sound and can convey the wrong message.

- ▶ Keep the background noise to a minimum.

- ▶ Don't forget other means of communicating, such as writing, using pictures, and so on.

- ▶ Try to speak in lower tones. People hard of hearing can usually hear lower voices easier than a higher pitch. For example, they usually can hear a male easier than a female.

Diagnostic Tests for Review

Several diagnostic tests provide useful information in caring for the client with disorders of the ears. The CBC lets you know whether infection is present, and CAT scans and MRIs tell you of structural alterations. The Weber and Rinne tests are used to assess air and bone conduction.

Pharmacology Categories for Review

Several drug categories are used in the care of the client with disorders of the ears. These drug categories include antiinfectives for those with ear infections and decongestants and antihistamines for those with otitis media:

- ▶ Antiinfectives
- ▶ Antihistamines
- ▶ Decongestants
- ▶ Steroids

Exam Prep Questions

1. A client with retinal detachment of the right eye has a scleral buckling with instillation of silicone oil. Post-operatively the client should be positioned:

   ○ **A.** In semi-Fowler's position with the head in neutral position

   ○ **B.** Supine with the head turned to the right side

   ○ **C.** In low Trendelenburg position with the head in neutral position

   ○ **D.** Prone with the head turned to the left side

2. A client wearing corrective lenses has a visual acuity of 20/200. The nurse recognizes that the client:

   ○ **A.** Has proper correction for astigmatism

   ○ **B.** Is legally blind

   ○ **C.** Experiences age-related presbyopia

   ○ **D.** Has low night vision related to loss of rods

3. The physician has scheduled a client with hyperopia for LASIK surgery. Which statement describes the procedure?

   ○ **A.** Diagonal incisions are made in the cornea, but the central cornea is not incised.

   ○ **B.** The cornea is reshaped using pulsation of ultraviolet light on the central superficial tissues.

   ○ **C.** Superficial layers of the cornea are lifted while laser pulsation reshapes the deeper layers of tissue.

   ○ **D.** Vertical incisions are made in the central cornea followed by reshaping of the lens with pulsation of ultraviolet light.

4. A client admitted with glaucoma is being treated with miotic (pilocarpine) eye drops. Following administration of the medication, the nurse will note:

   ○ **A.** Dilation of the pupils

   ○ **B.** Diminished redness of the sclera

   ○ **C.** Decreased edema of the cornea

   ○ **D.** Constriction of the pupils

5. Following a stroke, an elderly client develops ptosis. When assessing the client, the nurse will note:

   ○ **A.** Drooping of the eyelid on the affected side

   ○ **B.** Inverted eyelid margins

   ○ **C.** Eversion of eyelid margins

   ○ **D.** Granulomatous inflammation of the eyelids

6. The physician has ordered an irrigation of the client's left ear for the removal of cerumen. To prevent vestibular stimulation, the fluid should be ___ degrees Fahrenheit:

   ○ **A.** 68

   ○ **B.** 76

   ○ **C.** 98

   ○ **D.** 120

7. The most suitable diet for the client with Meniere's disease is:

   ○ **A.** High in animal protein

   ○ **B.** Restricted in sodium

   ○ **C.** High in fat-soluble vitamins

   ○ **D.** Restricted in complex carbohydrates

8. A client with a diagnosis of acoustic neuroma asks the nurse to explain what is wrong with his hearing. The nurse's response is based on the knowledge that an acoustic neuroma is:

   ○ **A.** A malignant tumor of the inner ear with rapid metastasis

   ○ **B.** A malignant tumor of the fifth cranial nerve that affects hearing and chewing

   ○ **C.** A benign tumor of the auditory nerve that may cause destruction to the cerebellum

   ○ **D.** A highly vascular benign lesion of the middle ear that arises from the jugular vein

9. A pediatric client has been receiving Amoxicillin for acute otitis media. It is important the child receive all the medication. Which secondary disorder is associated with improper management of acute otitis media?

   ○ **A.** Cholesteatoma

   ○ **B.** Mastoiditis

   ○ **C.** Acoustic neuroma

   ○ **D.** Presbycusis

10. Following a tympanoplasty, the nurse should maintain the client in which position?

  ○ **A.** Semi-Fowler's with the operative ear facing down

  ○ **B.** Low Trendelenburg with the head in neutral position

  ○ **C.** Flat with the head turned to the side with the operative ear facing up

  ○ **D.** Supine with a small neck roll to allow for drainage

Answer Rationales

1. Answer D is correct. Following a scleral buckling with instillation of silicone oil or gas, the client should be positioned prone with the head turned so that the operative eye is facing upward. Answers A, B, and C would displace the oil and prevent it from enhancing a seal between the retina and choroid.

2. Answer B is correct. The client whose vision is corrected to 20/200 is by definition legally blind because he is able to see at 20 feet what the healthy eye can see at 200 feet. Answer A refers to a refractive error, which is corrected by eyeglasses or one of the laser procedures. Answer C is an inability to focus on near objects due to a loss of elasticity of the lens and is corrected by the use of bifocal eye glasses. Answer D does not apply because the client would experience difficulty with vision at night or in dim lighting. Answers A, C, and D are incorrect because they do not explain what is meant by a visual acuity of 20/200.

3. Answer C is correct. The LASIK procedure uses an excimer laser to correct nearsightedness, far-sightedness, and astigmatism. The superficial layers of the cornea are lifted, and laser impulses reshape the deeper corneal layers. Answer A refers to radial keratotomy, and answer B refers to photorefractive keratotomy, so they are incorrect. Answer D is an incorrect statement. Answers A, B, and D are incorrect because they do not describe LASIK surgery.

4. Answer D is correct. Miotics, such as pilocarpine, are administered to the client with glaucoma to cause pupillary constriction, thereby lowering intraocular pressure. Answer A is incorrect because miotics constrict the pupil. Answer B is incorrect because miotics do not diminish redness. Answer C is incorrect because miotics do not decrease edema of the cornea.

5. Answer A is correct. Ptosis or drooping of the eyelid can occur as the result of a stroke or Bell's palsy. Answer B refers to entropion, and answer C refers to ectropion, so they are incorrect. Answer D refers to chalazion, so it's incorrect. Answers B, C, and D are incorrect because they do not relate to ptosis.

6. Answer C is correct. Cerumen is removed using a mixture of water and hydrogen peroxide at body temperature. Answers A and B are incorrect because they are too cold. Answer D is incorrect because it is too hot.

7. Answer B is correct. A low sodium diet and nicotinic acid have been shown to be effective in reducing the symptoms of Meniere's disease. Answers A, C, and D are incorrect because they do not relieve the symptoms of Meniere's syndrome.

8. Answer C is correct. An acoustic neuroma is a benign tumor of the eighth cranial nerve. Because of its location it frequently involves the cerebellum. Damage to hearing, facial movement, and sensation are common. Answers A, B, and D are inaccurate statements therefore they are incorrect.

9. Answer B is correct. Mastoiditis is a secondary disorder that can result from untreated or inadequately treated acute or chronic otitis media. Answer A refers to a benign overgrowth of squamous cell epithelium, so it is incorrect. Answer C refers to a benign tumor, making it incorrect. Answer D is incorrect because it refers to sensorineural hearing loss associated with aging.

10. Answer C is correct. Following a tympanoplasty the client should be maintained flat with the head turned to the nonoperative side for at least 12 hours. Answers A, B, and D are incorrect positions following ear surgery.

Suggested Reading and Resources

▶ Ignatavicius, D., and Workman, S. *Medical Surgical Nursing: Critical Thinking for Collaborative Care.* 6th ed. Philadelphia: Elsevier, 2008.

▶ Brunner, L., and Suddarth, D. *Textbook of Medical Surgical Nursing.* 12th ed. Philadelphia: Lippincott Williams & Wilkins, 2009.

▶ LeMone, P., and Burke, K. in *Medical Surgical Nursing: Critical Thinking in Client Care.* 4th ed. Upper Saddle River, NJ: Pearson Prentice Hall, 2008.

▶ Lewis, S., Heitkemper, M., Dirksen, S., Obrien, P., and Bucher, L. *Medical Surgical Nursing: Assessment and Management of Clinical Problems.* 7th ed. Philadelphia: Elsevier, 2007.

▶ Lehne, R. *Pharmacology for Nursing Care.* 7th ed. Philadelphia: Elsevier, 2009.

▶ "Visual Impairment, Visual Disability and Legal Blindness": http://www.nlm.nih.gov/medlineplus/visionimpairmentandblindness.html

▶ emedicine from WebMD: www.emedicine.com

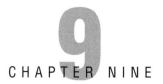

CHAPTER NINE

Caring for the Client with Cancer

Terms you'll need to understand

- ✓ Anovulation
- ✓ Cryptorchidism
- ✓ Dysphagia
- ✓ Dyspnea
- ✓ Emaciated
- ✓ Graft versus host disease
- ✓ Hyperthermia
- ✓ Nulliparity
- ✓ Postcoital
- ✓ Proliferation
- ✓ Pruritis
- ✓ Sepsis
- ✓ Spleenectomy

Nursing skills you'll need to master

- ✓ Knowing central line care
- ✓ Accessing a venous access device
- ✓ Safely working with radioactive materials
- ✓ Using patient control analgesia pumps
- ✓ Caring for the body after death

Cancer

Cancer occurs when an overproliferation of abnormal cells harms the host by growing into a body system or by robbing the body of nutrients.

Metastasis refers to the spread of cancer from a primary site to a secondary site.

> **NOTE**
>
> Common sites of metastasis are breast cancer (metastatic to the bone and brain) and lung cancer (to the liver and brain).

American Cancer Society's Seven Warning Signs of Cancer

Malignant, or cancer, cells are initiated by alterations in cell growth patterns. The American Cancer Society provides a list of warning signs to alert the public to occurrences that could indicate a problem. The following are the seven warnings you should know:

> **TIP**
>
> Remember the acronym CAUTION as a mnemonic to help you recall the seven warnings of cancer:
> - **C**hange in bowel or bladder habits
> - **A** sore that does not heal
> - **U**nusual bleeding or discharge
> - **T**hickening or lump in breast or elsewhere
> - **I**ndigestion or difficulty in swallowing
> - **O**bvious change in wart or mole
> - **N**agging cough or hoarseness

The Four Major Categories of Cancer

The different types of cancers are classified according to the tissue from which they originate. The following list identifies the major cancer groups:

- **Carcinoma**—Cancer arising from epithelial tissue (for example, basal cell carcinoma)
- **Sarcoma**—Cancer arising from connective tissue, muscle, or bone (for example, osteosarcoma)
- **Lymphoma**—Cancer arising from lymphoid tissue (for example, Burkitt's lymphoma)

▶ **Leukemia**—Cancer of the blood-forming cells in the bone marrow (for example, acute lymphocytic leukemia)

Risk Factors for Specific Cancers

Some environmental and intrinsic factors are associated with an increased incidence of certain cancers. Included here are risk factors associated with specific cancers:

▶ **Bladder**—Risk factors include smoking and environmental carcinogens such as dyes, paint, rubber, ink, and leather.

▶ **Breast**—Risk factors include a family history of first-degree relatives, the birth of the first child after age 30, menarche before age 12 and menopause after age 55, obesity, the use of birth control pills and hormonal replacement, alcohol intake, and a diet high in fat.

▶ **Cervical**—Risk factors include early sexual activity, early childbearing, multiple partners, human papillomavirus (HPV), human immunodeficiency (HIV) infection, smoking, the use of DES by the mother during pregnancy, and chronic cervical infections.

NOTE

The Gardasil vaccine is a medication that can be given for prevention of HPV. The American Cancer Society recommends routine HPV vaccination with Gardasil for females 11-12 years of age. The vaccine can be started as early as age nine. Gardasil is given in three doses over a six month time period. Caution should be used in administering to people with yeast or latex allergies.

▶ **Colon**—Risk factors include family history, polyps, chronic inflammatory bowel disease, alcohol use, smoking, and a diet high in fat and protein and low in fiber.

▶ **Esophagus**—Risk factors include use of tobacco, use of alcohol, and chronic irritation.

▶ **Hodgkin's lymphoma**—Risk factors include exposure to chemical agents and viral infections.

▶ **Larynx**—Risk factors include use of tobacco, nutritional deficiencies (riboflavin), chronic laryngitis, use of alcohol, and exposure to carcinogens.

▶ **Leukemia**—Risk factors include exposure to ionizing radiation, use of chemicals and drugs (for example, anticoagulants), genetics, people with Down syndrome, and people who are immunosuppressed.

▶ **Liver**—Risk factors include cirrhosis, hepatitis B, exposure to certain toxins, smoking, and alcohol use.

- **Lung**—Risk factors include smoking and secondhand smoke, air pollution, occupational exposure to radon, vitamin A deficiency, and heredity.

- **Multiple myeloma**—Risk factors include chemical and radiation exposure.

- **Ovarian**—Risk factors include a diet high in fat; alcohol use; a history of cancer of the breast, endometrium, or colon or a family history of ovarian or breast cancer; anovulation; nulliparity; and infertility.

- **Non-Hodgkin's lymphoma**—Risk factors include viral infections; exposure to chemical and/or ionizing radiation; autoimmune disorders.

- **Pancreas**—Risk factors include a diet high in fat, smoking, exposure to industrial chemicals, diabetes mellitus, and chronic pancreatitis.

- **Prostate**—Risk factors include race (African Americans), a history of prostate cancer in first degree relatives, high fat diet, and age (55 and older).

> **NOTE**
>
> Prostate specific antigen (PSA) is a laboratory test used to monitor response to treatment and to detect recurrence and progression of prostate cancer.

- **Renal**—Risk factors include tobacco use, exposure to industrial chemicals, obesity, hypertension, and dialysis.

- **Skin**—Risk factors include exposure to sun, exposure to various chemicals (arsenic and coal tar), scarring or chronic irritation of the skin, and ancestry (highest incidence in those of Celtic ancestry with red or blond hair, fair skin, and blue eyes).

> **CAUTION**
>
> Remember the alphabet A B C D when assessing skin lesions. If the answer is yes to any of the questions listed here, it could indicate a possible malignant lesion:
>
> - **A**—Is the lesion **a**symmetrical in shape?
> - **B**—Are the **b**orders of the lesion irregular?
> - **C**—Are there different **c**olors within the lesion?
> - **D**—Is the **d**iameter of the lesion more than 5mm?

- **Stomach**—Risk factors include a diet high in smoked foods and lacking in fruits and vegetables, gastric ulcers, Helicobacter pylori bacteria, heredity, pernicious anemia, and chronic gastritis.

- **Testes**—Risk factors include infections, genetic or endocrine factors, and cryptorchidism.

Cancer Prevention

An early diagnosis can mean a better cure rate for a patient with cancer. Certain cancers can even be prevented by interventions. The nurse can make a substantial impact by the use of education in preventive teaching and early detection techniques. One way the incidence of cancer can be decreased is by a change in eating habits. For example, with colon cancer the risk is decreased by the avoidance of fatty, fried foods and increasing the intake of fruits, vegetables, and whole grains. Another way to decrease incidence is by staying away from carcinogens such as smoking, alcohol, excessive sun exposure, and toxins. The nurse should also encourage the use of cancer screening, such as the prostate specific antigen test for males 50 or older and digital rectal exams for prostate cancer. Women should get a Papanicolaou (Pap) test for cervical cancer beginning three years after vaginal intercourse or after turning 21. Patients should get a colonoscopy (every 10 years beginning at age 50) and occult blood test for colon cancer. It is important for the nurse candidate to know the importance of patient education when studying for the NCLEX exam.

Patient Teaching

A part of the early detection process relies on the patient to perform regular exams to find any growths or abnormalities. The following gives information about the best time to perform these exams and the current recommendations by the American Cancer Society:

▶ Females should be instructed to perform breast self-exams monthly after menses.

▶ A baseline mammogram should be done at age 40 and yearly after age 40.

Clients should avoid the use of deodorant or body powder prior to the mammogram because these can produce areas that appear as calcifications.

> **CAUTION**
>
> Malignant breast masses appear most often in the upper outer quadrant of the breast. The most definitive diagnosis is made based on biopsy rather than lab or x-ray.

Management of the Client with Cancer

Treatments for cancer patients are focused on curing the cancer, prolonging survival time, or improving the quality of the patient's life. Clients with cancer usually die within weeks without treatment. The therapies included here can involve one treatment or a combination of all three:

▶ **Surgery**—This procedure is done to remove the tumor or the diseased tissue for a cure. Surgery can also be used to diagnose, as a preventive measure, as a palliative treatment, or for reconstruction. The care of the patient with surgery would be as any patient post-operatively with a focus on the body part involved or removed.

- **Radiation**—This is performed to shrink the tumor.

- **Chemotherapy**—This is undertaken to destroy cancer cells by interfering with mitosis or by destroying the cell wall.

Radiation

Radiation therapy is used to destroy cancer cells without destruction of the normal cells. The candidate for the NCLEX exam should review all aspects of nursing care dealing with radiation. This section focuses on the client with cervical cancer and the use of a sealed radiation source implanted inside the patient. In this case, the radiation is to the patient's cervix inserted through the vagina.

> **CAUTION**
>
> While the implant is in place, the client emits radiation but the client's body fluids are not radioactive.

Care of the client with radiation therapy implants requires that the nurse pay attention to time, distance, and shielding when caring for these clients. The nurse should

- Limit the amount of time spent in contact with the client.

- Maximize the distance by standing to the side of the bed and refraining from close contact.

- Shield herself by using a lead-lined apron during patient contact.

This type of radiation therapy is temporary. It is a contraindication for a nurse that is pregnant to care for these clients. Visitors should be limited to a 30-minute per day time span and instructions given to stay six feet from the radiation source. While the implant is in place, the nursing interventions focus on prevention of dislodgement. Accomplishment of this outcome is helped by instituting nursing measures, to include

- Bed rest

- Low residue diet (to decrease bowel contents)

- Foley catheter (to prevent collection of urine in the bladder)

The side effects and nursing care required for clients receiving radiation therapy depend on the specific area receiving the radiation. For example, uterine cancer radiation could cause damage to the colon and a client who has had radiation to the throat area could experience esophageal damage. General radiation side effects include fatigue, altered taste and anorexia, tissue fibrosis and scarring (can occur years after treatment), and skin problems. Radiation can result in drying, rashes, pruritis, and hyperpigmentation of the skin. Clients should be instructed to prevent drying by avoiding the following:

- ▶ Soaps

- ▶ Alcohol skin preparations

- ▶ Hot baths

CAUTION

Do not remove the markings placed on the skin by the radiologist.

NOTE

Clients who have received external radiation should avoid sun exposure to any radiated area during treatment and up to 12 months after treatment.

Chemotherapy

Chemotherapy has detrimental effects on the development of both normal and malignant cells. Chemotherapeutic agents include alkylating agents (which interfere with cell metabolism and growth), antitumor antibiotics (which interfere with the cell wall), cytoprotectants and colony-stimulating factors (which prevent problems associated with cancer treatments), topoisomerase inhibitors (break DNA and kills the cells), biological response modifiers (which charges the immune system), and hormones (which suppress hormonal-dependent tumors; an example is progesterone for ovarian cancer and estrogen for prostate or testicular cancer).

There are commonalities in the side effects of chemotherapeutic agents. You should become familiar with these side effects in preparation for the exam. Table 9.1 highlights the common side effects and some measures that are done to relieve them.

TABLE 9.1 Common Side Effects Associated with Chemotherapeutic Agents

Side Effect	Treatment
Anorexia, nausea, and vomiting	Antiemetics; small, frequent meals that are palatable and nourishing; avoidance of foods that are too hot or too spicy; a diet of soft bland foods.
Alopecia	Teach the client that hair loss will be immediate but not permanent; help the client select a wig before treatment begins. Note that the regrowth of hair is usually different from the hair that was lost. Cut long hair before therapy and avoid excessive combing of hair.
Bone marrow and platelet depression	Observe for petechiae and ecchymosis; use small-gauge needles; apply pressure over injection and venipuncture sites; avoid dental work; no aspirin; no enemas—use stool softeners to prevent straining; clients should avoid anal sex; use electric razors only. Teach to avoid crowds. Practice proper hand hygiene. Teach to not eat foods grown in or on the ground without cooking and peeling.
Mucosal membrane ulcerations	Rinse mouth with a solution of one-half strength peroxide and normal saline; xylocaine viscous (place on a cotton-tip applicator and apply to lesions); oral hygiene with a soft toothbrush.
Sterility	Sperm bank or egg deposits prior to chemotherapy administration.

Total Parenteral Nutrition

Clients with cancer often have inadequate nutrition due to the side effects of nausea, vomiting, and anorexia. These clients frequently require supplemental nutrition by the use of total parenteral nutrition (TPN).

> **NOTE**
>
> A central line is required for TPN administration.

Problems Associated with TPN

With TPN, the fluid is delivered directly into the venous system. This fluid has a high level of osmolarity, which can cause a fluid shift as well as electrolyte imbalances. The high dextrose content puts the client at risk for hyperglycemia and infection.

Dressing Changes for TPN

Because of the danger of infection, these clients are at a higher risk of developing sepsis. The following list gives the recommendations for the dressing change on the central line of a client receiving TPN:

▶ Sterile technique is utilized.

▶ Recommended dressing is a gauze dressing taped on all four sides or a transparent dressing.

Nursing Implementations

General nursing care for a client with TPN includes the following measures:

▶ Blood should not be drawn from the TPN port, but it can be drawn from the venous port.

▶ Avoid air entrance into the central line. If air embolism occurs, the nurse should clamp the catheter, place the client in the left Trendelenburg position, call the doctor, and administer ordered oxygen.

▶ TPN must be tapered to be discontinued.

NOTE

If the TPN is not immediately available and the infusion is empty, the nurse should hang D10W solution until the TPN is obtained.

▶ Monitor blood glucose levels and serum electrolytes

▶ Monitor weight

▶ TPN requires a pump or other type controller device system for administration

▶ Solution should be prepared under a laminar flow hood

▶ Any loose or soiled dressing should be changed immediately

Bone Marrow and Peripheral Stem Cell Transplantation (PSCT)

Bone marrow transplantation involves the destruction of the client's bone marrow (this is accomplished by high-dose chemotherapy administration and whole body irradiation). The client then receives a stem cell or bone marrow transplant infusion. Sources of stem cells include bone marrow, peripheral circulating blood, and umbilical cord.

Transplantation of bone marrow can be used to treat

▶ Aplastic anemia

▶ Thallassemia

▶ Sickle cell anemia

▶ Immunodeficiency disorders

▶ Certain cancers, such as acute leukemia, chronic myelogenous leukemia, Hodgkin's lymphoma, non-Hodgkin's lymphoma, and testicular cancer

Types of Transplants

The types of bone marrow transplants are based on the source of the donor cells. The three types of transplants available are

▶ **Autologous transplant**—Involves the harvesting, cryopreservation, and reinfusion of the client's own marrow to correct bone marrow hypoplasia resulting from chemotherapeutic drugs.

▶ **Allogenic transplant**—Involves the transplantation of bone marrow from a compatible donor. It has the following requirements:

  ▶ The prospective donor must be tissue and blood typed.

  ▶ The donor should be of the same racial and genetic type to be successful.

▶ **Syngeneic transplant**—Involves the transplantation of bone marrow from an identical twin; this type is rare.

Nursing Care After Transplantation

Until the new bone marrow takes, or *engrafts*, the client has no immunity or normal bone marrow function. This predisposes the client to infection and decreased thrombocytes. The candidate for the NCLEX exam must recognize the major risk of bleeding and infection in these clients. Interventions after a transplant focus on the assessment and prevention of complications of the transplant, including failure to engraft, graft versus host disease, and venocclusive disease. The nurse also institutes measures to reduce the risk of bleeding and infection, as well as treating these disorders if they occur. The nurse should

▶ Use sterile technique when performing care.

▶ Provide a private room.

▶ Allow no sick visitors.

▶ Assure no fresh flowers or plants are in the room.

▶ Place the client on a low bacteria diet that omits raw vegetables, pepper, and paprika, and includes only well-done meats.

▶ Assess for signs of complications or rejection of transplant, including jaundice, pain in right upper quadrant, weight gain, and hepatomegaly.

- ▶ Monitor for bleeding.

- ▶ Administer ordered blood transfusion.

- ▶ Administer ordered platelets.

- ▶ Institute bleeding precautions (please refer to depression of platelets for other bleeding precautions), including

  - ▶ Avoid IM injections

  - ▶ Avoid venipunctures

  - ▶ Avoid flossing of teeth

  - ▶ Avoid bending at the waist

  - ▶ No contact sports

- ▶ Monitor for infection.

CAUTION

An elevation of .5°F. could be significant in these clients.

- ▶ Pharmacological interventions include

  - ▶ Steroids

  - ▶ Immunosuppressants

  - ▶ Colony-stimulating factors

Hodgkin's Lymphoma

Hodgkin's lymphoma is a malignancy involving the lymph nodes. It is more prevalent in men and tends to peak in the early 20s and after age 50.

Clinical manifestations associated with Hodgkin's lymphoma include

- ▶ Coughing

- ▶ Dysphagia

- ▶ Dyspnea

- ▶ Enlargement of the cervical lymph node

- ▶ Fatigue

- Generalized pruritis

- Night sweats

- Pain in cervical lymph nodes when drinking (especially alcohol)

- Unexplained fever

- Weight loss

NOTE

A lymphoma client might first note this enlargement while shaving.

Diagnosis of Hodgkin's Lymphoma

Diagnosis of Hodgkin's lymphoma is made by assessment of previously mentioned clinical manifestations and by node biopsy results. The staging of involvement listed here becomes important in determining how far the disease has progressed:

- Biopsy confirms presence of Reed-Sternberg cells

- Staging of the disease by degree of involvement:

  - **1**—Single node or single site

  - **2**—More than one node, localized to a single organ on the same side of the diaphragm

  - **3**—Involvement of lymph nodes on both sides of the diaphragm

  - **4**—Diffuse involvement with disease disseminated in organs and tissues

Prognosis of Hodgkin's Lymphoma

Prognosis is dependent on the stage of the disease. If it's detected in the early stages, the prognosis for survival is good.

Treatment of Hodgkin's Lymphoma

Treatment of Hodgkin's depends on the stage of involvement. If the client is in stage 1 or 2, radiation is used alone; with more extensive involvement, though, chemotherapy is used with the radiation. The client might also undergo surgery to remove the spleen to help prevent the pooling of blood in this organ.

Diagnostic Tests for Review

Cancer clients require extensive diagnostic exams to determine the primary site of the cancer or tumor, as well as whether metastasis has occurred. The tests are also important in determining the treatment options: radiation, chemotherapy, and/or surgery. Laboratory exams such as carcinogenic embryonic acid (CEA) and prostate specific antigen (PSA) are important in determining the disease and its progression. Routine laboratory exams such as chest x-rays, urinalysis, and cell blood counts (CBCs) with differentials also need to be reviewed.

Particularly important when caring for the cancer client receiving chemotherapy is the CBC. This test monitors for the side effects and bone marrow depression that can result from antineoplastic drugs. These diagnostic tests include

- ▶ Biopsy
- ▶ Bone marrow aspiration
- ▶ Bronchoscopy
- ▶ CBC
- ▶ CEA
- ▶ CT scan
- ▶ Magnetic resonance imagery (MRI)
- ▶ Mammogram
- ▶ Mediastinoscopy
- ▶ PSA
- ▶ Radioactive scan

MRIs use a powerful magnet. Clients with metal in their body cannot take the exam. No metal can be in the room of the client receiving an MRI; therefore, tubings for equipment must be lengthened to accommodate the client on oxygen or other life support equipment. The candidate for the exam must consider the factors in the following list to determine whether an MRI would be contraindicated or whether special accommodations would need to be made for a client who is scheduled for an MRI:

- ▶ Pregnancy of client
- ▶ Client weight greater than 260 pounds (open MRI would be required due to client size)
- ▶ Clients with pacemakers or electronic implants

▸ Clients who have metal fragments, metal clamps, or aneurysm clips

▸ The ability of the client to communicate clearly

▸ Use of life support equipment

▸ Ability of the client to lie still in a supine position for 30 minutes

▸ Use of oxygen by the client

▸ Clients receiving an IV infusion

Pharmacology for Review

The nurse candidate writing for the NCLEX exam needs to be familiar with agents' side effects and adverse effects. Although most nurses who administer chemotherapeutic drugs have extensive training, these drugs can be tested on the NCLEX exam, and the candidate is expected to have knowledge of the drugs. The nurse must be aware of the impact of these drugs on the client's quality of life and recognize that some of these drugs have life-threatening, adverse effects. Nurses who administer chemotherapy must also keep in mind the importance of self-protection from the drug agents by wearing appropriate equipment when coming in contact with the agents. The following list contains the various kinds of chemotherapeutic agents:

▸ Alkylating agents

▸ Antiestrogens

▸ Antimetabolites

▸ Antineoplastics

▸ Antitumor antibiotics

▸ Biologic response modifiers

▸ Hormones

▸ Monoclonal antibodies

▸ Plant alkaloids

▸ Topoisomerase inhibitors

Drugs that treat the adverse effects of chemotherapeutic agents include

- ▶ Antianxiety
- ▶ Antibiotics
- ▶ Antiemetics
- ▶ Colony stimulating factors
- ▶ Erythropoietin
- ▶ Immunosuppressants
- ▶ Steroids

Exam Prep Questions

1. Which nursing intervention is most important when administering the chemotherapeutic drug Platinol (cisplatin)?

- ○ **A.** Administration of an IV bolus of fluid before and after the drug is given
- ○ **B.** Performing deep tendon reflex assessment every two hours after the infusion
- ○ **C.** Assessing the client's food intake
- ○ **D.** Auscultating breath sounds every four hours

2. A client diagnosed with metastatic cancer of the bone is exhibiting mental confusion and a BP of 160/100. Which laboratory value would correlate with the client's symptoms reflecting a common complication with this diagnosis?

- ○ **A.** Potassium 5.2 mEq/l
- ○ **B.** Calcium 13 mg/dl
- ○ **C.** Inorganic phosphorus 1.7 mEq/l
- ○ **D.** Sodium 138 mEq/l

3. A client with cancer has been placed on TPN. The nurse notes air entering the client via the central line. Which initial action is most appropriate?

- ○ **A.** Notify the physician.
- ○ **B.** Elevate the head of the bed.
- ○ **C.** Place the client in the left Trendelenburg position.
- ○ **D.** Stop the TPN and hang D51/2 NS.

4. The nurse is preparing a client for cervical uterine radiation implant insertion. Which will be included in the teaching plan?

- ○ **A.** TV or telephone use will not be allowed while the implant is in place.
- ○ **B.** A Foley catheter is usually inserted.
- ○ **C.** A high fiber diet is recommended.
- ○ **D.** Excretions will be considered radioactive.

5. The nurse is caring for a client with leukemia who is receiving the drug doxorubicin (Adriamycin). Which, if occurred, would be reported to the physician immediately due to the toxic effects of this drug?

  ○ **A.** Rales and distended neck veins

  ○ **B.** Red discoloration of the urine and an output of 75 ml the previous hour

  ○ **C.** Nausea and vomiting

  ○ **D.** Elevated BUN and dry, flaky skin

6. A client with cancer received platelet infusions 24 hours ago. Which of the following assessment findings would indicate the most therapeutic effect from the transfusions?

  ○ **A.** A Hgb level decrease from 8.9 to 8.7

  ○ **B.** A temperature reading of 99.4

  ○ **C.** A white blood cell count of 11,000

  ○ **D.** A decrease in oozing of blood from the IV site

7. The nurse is caring for a client receiving chemotherapy who is experiencing neutropenia. Which intervention would be most appropriate to include in the client's plan of care?

  ○ **A.** Assess the client's temperature every four hours due to risk of hypothermia.

  ○ **B.** Instruct the client to avoid large crowds and people who are sick.

  ○ **C.** Instruct the client in the use of a soft toothbrush.

  ○ **D.** Assess the client for hematuria.

8. A client with cancer becomes emaciated, requiring TPN to provide adequate nutrition. The nurse finds the TPN bag empty. Which fluid would the nurse select to hang until another bag is prepared in the pharmacy?

  ○ **A.** Lactated Ringer's

  ○ **B.** Normal saline

  ○ **C.** D10W

  ○ **D.** Normosol R

9. The nurse is caring for a client with possible cervical cancer. What clinical data would the nurse most expect to find in the client's history?

   ○ **A.** Postcoital vaginal bleeding

   ○ **B.** Nausea and vomiting

   ○ **C.** Foul-smelling vaginal discharge

   ○ **D.** Hyperthermia

10. A client is scheduled to undergo a bone marrow aspiration. Which position would the nurse assist the client into for this procedure?

   ○ **A.** Dorsal recumbent

   ○ **B.** Supine

   ○ **C.** High Fowler's

   ○ **D.** Lithotomy

Answer Rationales

1. Answer A is correct. Fluid administration is important to flush the drug through the renal system to prevent damage. Cisplatin can cause renal damage. Answers B, C, and D would not be important interventions with the drug administration, so they are incorrect.

2. Answer B is correct. Hypercalcemia is a common occurrence with cancer of the bone. The potassium level is elevated but does not relate to the diagnosis, so answer A is incorrect. Answers C and D are both normal levels, so they are incorrect.

3. Answer C is correct. The client is at risk for an air embolus. Placing the client in this position displaces air away from the right ventricle. Answers B and D would not help, so they are incorrect, and answer A would not be done first, so it's incorrect.

4. Answer B is correct. A catheter allows urine elimination without possible disruption of the implant. There is usually no restriction on TV or phone use, so answer A is incorrect. The client is placed on a low residue diet, so answer C is incorrect. The client's radiation is not internal; therefore, there are no special precautions with excretions, making answer D incorrect.

5. Answer A is correct. This drug can cause cardiotoxicity exhibited by changes in the ECG and congestive heart failure. Rales and distended neck veins are clinical manifestations of congestive heart failure, so answer A is correct. A reddish discoloration to the urine is a harmless side effect, so answer B is incorrect. An elevated BUN and dry, flaky skin are not specific to this drug, so answers C and D are incorrect.

6. Answer D is correct. Platelets deal with the clotting of blood. Lack of platelets can cause bleeding. Answers A, B, and C do not directly relate to platelets, so they are incorrect.

7. Answer B is correct. With neutropenia, the client is at risk for infection; therefore, he would need to avoid crowds and people who are ill. Answer A would not be appropriate. Answers C and D would correlate with a risk for bleeding, so they are incorrect.

8. Answer C is correct. D10W is the preferred solution to prevent complications from a sudden lack of glucose. Answers A, B, and D do not have glucose, so they are incorrect.

9. Answer A is correct. Vaginal bleeding or spotting is a common symptom of cervical cancer. Nausea and vomiting and foul-smelling discharge are not specific or common to cervical cancer, so B and C are incorrect. Hyperthermia does not relate to the diagnosis, so answer D is incorrect.

10. Answer C is correct. This procedure is usually done by the physician with specimens obtained from the sternum or the iliac crest. The high Fowler's position would be the best position of the ones listed to obtain a specimen from the client's sternum. Answers A, B, and D would be inappropriate positions for getting a biopsy from the sites indicated.

Suggested Reading and Resources

▶ American Cancer Society: www.cancer.org

▶ Epocrates: www.epocrates.com

▶ Kee, J. *Laboratory and Diagnostic Tests with Nursing Implications*. New York: Prentice Hall, 2010.

▶ Lacharity, L., Kumagai, C., and Bartz, B. *Prioritization, Delegation, & Assignment*. 2nd ed. St. Louis: Mosby Elsevier, 2006, 2011.

▶ Brunner, L., and Suddarth, D. *Textbook of Medical-Surgical Nursing*. 12th ed. Philadelphia: Lippincott Williams & Wilkins, 2009.

▶ Hogan, M. *Child Health Nursing Reviews and Rationales*. 2nd ed. Upper Saddle River, NJ: Pearson Prentice Hall, 2007.

▶ Ignatavicius, D., Workman, S. *Medical-Surgical Nursing: Critical Thinking for Collaborative Care*. 6th ed. Philadelphia: Elsevier, 2007.

▶ Deglin, J., and Vallerand, A., *Davis Drug Guide for Nurses*. Philadelphia: F.A. Davis, 2009.

▶ Lewis, S., Heitkemper, M., Dirkson, S., O Brien, P., and Bucher, L. *Medical Surgical Nursing: Assessment and Management of Clinical Problems*. 7th ed. Philadelphia: Elsevier, 2007.

▶ Rinehart, W., Sloan, D., and Hurd, C. *NCLEX Exam Cram*. Indianapolis: Que, 2007.

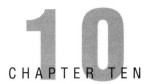

CHAPTER TEN

Caring for the Client with Disorders of the Gastrointestinal System

---

Terms you'll need to understand

✓ Ascites

✓ Gastrinoma

✓ Hepatomegaly

✓ Malaise

✓ Melena

✓ Odynophagia

✓ Splenomegaly

✓ String sign (see "Diagnosis of Crohn's")

✓ Tetany

✓ Steatorrhea

Nursing skills you'll need to master

✓ Performing ostomy care

✓ Assisting with a paracentesis

Ulcers

Ulcers are erosions that occur in the mucosal lining of the esophagus, stomach, or duodenum. Ulcers occur more frequently in men, post-menopausal women, those with a family history for ulcers, and those with type O blood.

Factors contributing to the development of ulcers include

▶ Irritants that increase the secretion of hydrochloric acid; nonsteroidal, anti-inflammatory drugs (NSAIDs) such as ibuprofen and Toradol; and steroids.

NOTE
NSAIDs and steroids should be administered with meals or food.

▶ Stress

▶ *H. Pylori* bacteria, which is treated with antibiotic therapy with doxycycline (tetracycline) or amoxicillin and metronidazole (Flagyl) and a bismuth compound or a proton pump inhibitor (PPI).

Types of Ulcers

An ulcer is referred to as *duodenal*, *gastric*, or *esophageal* depending on its location in the gastrointestinal system. The two most common locations for ulcers are the duodenum and gastric area. The clinical manifestations for these ulcers follow, with differentiating characteristics that you will need to know for the exam.

Duodenal

Duodenal ulcers are erosions that occur on the mucosa of the duodenum. These ulcers occur more frequently in people 30–60 years of age and occur more frequently than any other type of ulcer. The basic pathophysiology is a hypersecretion of stomach acid.

Unlike gastric ulcers, with duodenal ulcers, vomiting is uncommon. Clinical manifestations include

▶ Epigastric pain 2–3 hours after meals

▶ Pain that is relieved by food intake

▶ Melena

Gastric

When an erosion occurs in the gastric mucosa, the ulcer is classified as *gastric*. This type of ulcer usually occurs in people over 50. The pathophysiology of gastric ulcers involves a normal or hyposecretion of stomach acid.

Clinical manifestations include

- ▶ Midepigastric pain occurring from 1/2 to 1 hour after meals

- ▶ Discomfort that is increased by food consumption

- ▶ Vomiting (this is common and provides some relief of pain)

Diagnostic Tools for Ulcers

Ulcers are diagnosed by the patient history and a diagnostic test. The preferred diagnostic tool is the endoscopy exam because it allows direct visualization and biopsies of the area. The following are the major exams used to diagnose an ulcer:

- ▶ Upper gastrointestinal (GI) studies

- ▶ Barium swallow

- ▶ Endoscopy exam

- ▶ Gastric analysis

- ▶ H. Pylori bacteria (can be identified by a blood test, C13 urea breath test, or a stool exam)

- ▶ Biopsy

Treatment of Ulcers

The treatment of ulcers includes two potential paths. One path is the *conservative* path that includes treatment through dietary modifications and medications. Dietary modifications include avoiding highly seasoned or spicy foods, high fiber foods, caffeine, alcohol, smoking, and stress. The following highlights some medications used to treat ulcers:

- ▶ Antacids

- ▶ Antibiotics

- ▶ Histamine (H2 receptor) blockers

- ▶ Anticholinergics

- ▶ Antispasmodics

▶ Proton pump inhibitors

▶ Prostandin analogues such as misoprostol (Cytotec)

▶ Barrier drugs (for example, sucralfate [Carafate])

The second method of ulcer treatment involves surgery. The surgical procedure is a gastrectomy. Caring for a client who has had a gastrectomy includes assessment for

▶ Bleeding

▶ Shock

▶ Abdominal distention

> **CAUTION**
>
> In the first 12–24 hours, the nasogastric drainage should be small in amount but may be bright red in appearance. After 24 hours, the drainage should turn darker in color and decrease further in amount.
>
> Do not irrigate or move the NG tube after gastric surgery without a specific physician's order.

Dumping Syndrome

Post-gastrectomy problems can include the *dumping syndrome*. This syndrome is caused due to rapid emptying of food from the stomach into the jejunum. Symptoms of dumping syndrome include

▶ Dizziness

▶ Pallor

▶ Nausea

▶ Vomiting

▶ Palpitations

Treatment for clients with dumping syndrome include the following:

▶ Decreased fluids with meals

▶ Decreased carbohydrate intake

▶ Small, frequent meals

▶ Resting in recumbent position after meals

▶ Medications, including sedatives and antispasmodics, such as bentyl and pro-banthine and somastatin analogues, such as octreotide (sandostatin)

Inflammatory Bowel Disorders

There are two major inflammatory bowel diseases: Crohn's disease and ulcerative colitis. People 10–30 years of age have the greatest risk of developing these disorders. The causes are unknown, but these disorders can be triggered by agents such as pesticides, food additives, and radiation. A connection might also exist between a client's allergies or immune system.

Crohn's Disease (Regional Enteritis)

Crohn's disease is an inflammation of segments of the bowel, which leads to swelling, thickening, and abscess formation. The following lists symptoms associated with Crohn's disease:

▶ Abdominal pain

▶ Diarrhea

▶ Cramping

▶ Weight loss

▶ Anemia

▶ Ulcer formation

Diagnosis of Crohn's

In diagnosing Crohn's, you will see that barium studies reveal the presence of a string sign. A *string sign* is a narrowing of the lumen of the intestine that shows as such on the barium x-ray.

Treatment of Crohn's

Treating clients with Crohn's can involve several methods. Diet control, vitamins, medications, and surgery are possible treatments. The following highlights the treatment paths for Crohn's you should understand for the exam:

▶ Low-residue diet.

▶ Vitamin and iron supplements.

▶ Medications, including the following:

    ▶ Sedatives

    ▶ Antidiarrheals

    ▶ Steroids

- ▸ Antirheumatics

- ▸ Immunosuppressives

▸ Surgery for severe cases. A colectomy with a possible ileostomy may be performed.

> **NOTE**
>
> Prevention of skin problems is important after an ileostomy due to the liquid stool and high risk for excoriation of the skin.

Ulcerative Colitis

Ulcerative colitis is an inflammation of the colon and rectum. This disorder usually begins at the rectum and proceeds upward. This disease can result in systemic complications and a high mortality rate. The following highlights symptoms associated with ulcerative colitis that you should be aware of for the exam:

- ▸ Abdominal cramping

- ▸ Urgent defecation

- ▸ Vomiting

- ▸ Weight loss

- ▸ Fever

- ▸ Bloody diarrhea

- ▸ Decreased iron absorption

Diagnosis of Ulcerative Colitis

Ulcerative colitis is diagnosed by exams that visualize the distal portion of the intestines. The two diagnostic tools that follow are valuable in distinguishing this disease from other conditions that have similar symptoms:

- ▸ Barium enema

- ▸ Sigmoidoscopy

Treatment of Ulcerative Colitis

People with ulcerative colitis are treated with options similar to those that were discussed with Crohn's. Medications included in the following list emphasize additional drugs that the candidate needs to know for the exam:

▸ Anti-inflammatories

▸ Antibiotics

Diverticulitis

Diverticulosis occurs with the presence of sac-like outpouchings in the wall of the large intestine. Diverticulitis (the inflammation) results from the trapping of food and bacteria in the diverticula. This inflammation increases the risk of abscess formation and perforation.

Diverticulitis is more prevalent in elderly females who eat a diet containing seeds, nuts, and grains. The following list highlights symptoms of diverticulitis:

▸ Bowel irregularity

▸ Intervals of diarrhea

▸ Cramping pain in the left lower quadrant of the abdomen

▸ A low-grade fever

Diagnosis of Diverticulitis

Tools used to diagnose diverticulitis include a CBC that can reveal an elevation in white blood cells due to infection and sedimentation rate elevations that indicate inflammation. A CT scan can be a valuable tool if an abscess has occurred due to the diverticulitis. The following list highlights other exams that can demonstrate muscle thickness, narrowing of the colon, and direct visualization of the inflamed diverticulum:

▸ Barium studies

▸ Endoscopy exam

CAUTION

A barium enema would be contraindicated in clients with acute diverticulitis due to the possibility of perforation of the diverticulum.

Treatment of Diverticulitis

The paths used to treat diverticulitis depend on the severity of the problem. Conservative treatment includes diet and medications. If the client's symptoms do not improve or the client becomes acutely ill, surgery might be required. The following highlights the treatment options you need to be familiar with for the exam:

▶ Increased dietary intake of soft fiber foods (a low fiber diet is utilized during the acute episode)

▶ Increase in fluid intake (2–3 liters per day) within cardiac limits

▶ Medications, including

  ▶ Antispasmodics

  ▶ Fiber laxatives

  ▶ Analgesics

  ▶ Antibiotics

▶ Surgery (surgical intervention might be necessary due to hemorrhage, perforation, abscess formation, or bowel obstruction)

Gastroesophageal Reflux Disease (GERD)

GERD occurs when there is a problem, usually with the lower esophageal sphincter, that allows contents to reflux (back up) into the esophagus. The signs and symptoms include: dysphagia, odynophagia (painful swallowing), eructation, dyspepsia, and chest pain. Diagnosis is made by the use of PH monitoring (most accurate tool), endoscopic exam, and/or barium swallow.

Treatment of GERD is either conservative or surgical. Measures that might be used include the following:

▶ Avoid irritating foods (chocolate, fats, and acidic foods)

▶ Eliminate carbonated beverages and alcohol

▶ Serve frequent small meals

▶ Teach client to remain upright for 2–3 hours after eating and avoid eating within three hours of bedtime

▶ Medications: Antacids, histamine blockers, and proton pump inhibitors

▶ Endoscopic procedure: Stretta

▶ Surgery: Laparoscopic Nissen fundoplication (LNF)

> **NOTE**
>
> Long term reflux can lead to a condition called Barrett's esophagus, which can be a precursor to esophageal cancer. Monitoring and treatment of Barrett's esophagus includes periodic exams to identify and treat precancerous cells. Early treatment of these cells can prevent esophageal cancer development.

Diseases Associated with the Liver

The liver is a large internal organ. Liver function is complex and any dysfunction of this organ affects all body systems. Liver disorders are common and can result from substances that destroy the liver, such as alcohol (which causes pancreatitis and cirrhosis). These disorders can also result from a virus, such as hepatitis.

Hepatitis

Hepatitis is a viral infection of the liver. The five major types of hepatitis are known as hepatitis A, B, C, D, and E. Hepatitis A and E are similar in transmission: They have a fecal-oral route but are not chronic. Hepatitis B, C, and D have similar characteristics in that they are all transmitted by the same route: parenteral, perinatal, or sexual. Hepatitis G is one of the last types to be recognized and is transmitted by parenteral, sexual, and blood transfusions.

The following list gives you some important general management techniques for clients with all forms of hepatitis:

▶ Bed rest for those with prodromal or icteric symptoms

▶ Small and frequent increased calorie meals

▶ Increased fluid intake (3000 ml/day)

▶ Avoidance of drugs detoxified by the liver

▶ Cool baths and soothing lotions to treat pruritus

▶ Medications administered include steroids, anti-inflammatory drugs, and immunosuppressives

▶ The healthcare provider should practice standard precaution control measures while providing care for these clients

Hepatitis A

Hepatitis A is transmitted by the fecal-oral route. It can lead to an acute infection, but without the chronicity seen in other forms of the disease.

The symptoms of hepatitis A appear after an incubation period of 2–6 weeks. Hepatitis A is usually limited to 1–3 weeks of duration. The following list gives you the symptoms of hepatitis A:

► Malaise

► Fever

► Jaundice

► Nausea

► Vomiting

Diagnosis of Hepatitis A

Diagnosing hepatitis A requires a stool specimen. This specimen can reveal the hepatitis A antigen for 7–10 days before the illness and 2–3 weeks after symptoms appear. HAV antibodies are found in the serum after symptoms appear.

Treatment of Hepatitis A

Treatment of hepatitis A includes many parameters. First, prevention of the transmission of hepatitis A is a key element. Obtaining the two-dose hepatitis vaccine (Havrix) is recommended for adults 18 years or older and is highly recommended for the following groups: homosexuals; people traveling to unsanitary, poor-hygiene countries or locations; and healthcare workers.

The second dose of the vaccine should be given 6–12 months after the first dose. Protection begins a few weeks after the first dose and can last for up to 20 years. Administration of the immune globulin should be administered within 2 weeks of exposure to boost antibody protection and provide 6–8 weeks of passive immunity. The following three medications are important treatment options to remember for the exam:

► Hepatitis A vaccine (Havrix)

► Hepatitis A and hepatitis B combination drug (Twinrix) can be administered for persons over 18 years of age

► Serum immune globulin for exposure to the disease

CAUTION

Remember that hepatitis A has no long-term effects and is not chronic.

Hepatitis B

Hepatitis B is transmitted through parenteral, perinatal, or sexual routes. People at the greatest risk for hepatitis B include

- ▶ IV drug users
- ▶ Homosexual men
- ▶ Infants born to hepatitis B virus-infected mothers
- ▶ Healthcare workers
- ▶ Hemodialysis clients

Hepatitis B symptoms closely resemble hepatitis A's symptoms, but there is a much longer incubation period of 1–6 months. The following list gives you symptoms of hepatitis B that you will need to know for the exam:

- ▶ Malaise
- ▶ Fever
- ▶ Rash
- ▶ Jaundice
- ▶ Arthritis
- ▶ Abdominal pain
- ▶ Nausea

Diagnosis of Hepatitis B

In diagnosing hepatitis B, HBsAG can appear in the blood of infected clients for 1–10 weeks after exposure to the hepatitis B virus and for 2–8 weeks before the onset of symptoms. Clients who have HBsAg persist in serum for six or more months after an acute infection are considered to be carriers.

Treatment and Prevention of Hepatitis B

When it comes to treating this problem, there are a lot of unknowns for hepatitis B—and for all other forms of hepatitis as well. However, treatments are available for hepatitis B, and the following lists the treatments you should be familiar with:

- ▶ **Prevention by administration of the hepatitis B vaccine (HeptovaxRecombivax)—** The hepatitis B vaccine is administered IM in three doses. The second and third doses are given one month and six months, respectively, after the first dose. Doses are given in the deltoid muscle in adults.

▶ **Alpha interferon injections for chronic hepatitis B**—This medication can cause a flu-like reaction 3–6 hours after administration. Long-acting preparations (PEG-Intron, Pegasys) are given subcutaneously once weekly.

▶ **Hepatitis B immune globulin (HBIG)**—This gives passive immunity to hepatitis B for people who have been exposed to the hepatitis B virus but have never received the hepatitis vaccine. The drug should be administered within 24 hours of exposure to hepatitis B.

NOTE

The Centers for Disease Control recommends that the HBV vaccine be a part of routine child vaccination schedules.

▶ **Nucleoside analogs**: Lamivudine (Epivir), adefovir (Hepsera), entecavir (Baraclude), and telbivudine (Tyzeka) are a group of drugs that can be given orally. These drugs are administered for one year.

Hepatitis C

Hepatitis C is transmitted through the same routes as hepatitis B (parenteral, perinatal, or sexual). Cases of viral hepatitis not classified as A, B, or D are given the classification of hepatitis C. The age group with the highest incidence of hepatitis C is 40–59 years of age. Hepatitis B and C are similar, but a chronic carrier state exists more often with hepatitis C. More people with hepatitis C progress to chronic liver disease, including cirrhosis and liver cancer, than any other type of hepatitis.

Symptoms of hepatitis C are similar to those of hepatitis B. Some say the symptoms are mild and variable. The reason there are so many people predicted to have hepatitis C is because of the lack of symptoms and vagueness. Consequently, those infected often do not seek assistance. A great deal of people with hepatitis C are carriers of the disease but do not know they have it.

Diagnosis of Hepatitis C

Diagnosis of hepatitis C is confirmed by the presence of HCV (hepatitis C virus) in serum. A liver biopsy, to confirm the diagnosis and evaluate liver changes, might also be performed.

Treatment of Hepatitis C

The combination therapy used to treat hepatitis C (interferon and ribavirin) has been shown to produce positive results. Some clients experience complete remission from the drug regimen. These drugs are also used for relapses in the client's condition. The following are important to keep in mind for the exam:

▶ No vaccine is available for hepatitis C.

▶ Medications for treating hepatitis C include a combination of alpha interferon and ribavirin.

Hepatitis D

Hepatitis D is a delta hepatitis that requires the HBV surface antigen for replication. Only people with hepatitis B are at risk for hepatitis D. The virus is common among IV drug users, hemodialysis clients, and clients who have received multiple blood transfusions. Symptoms are similar to hepatitis B, except the incubation period is 3–20 weeks. These clients are also more likely to develop chronic active hepatitis and cirrhosis.

Diagnosis of Hepatitis D

Hepatitis D is diagnosed by a laboratory test. The presence of anti-delta antibodies in the presence of HBAg will be revealed in the test results.

Treatment of Hepatitis D

Treatment of hepatitis D includes alpha interferon.

Hepatitis E

Hepatitis E (HEV) is transmitted by the fecal-oral route. Like hepatitis A, it is not a chronic condition and has been found to develop mostly in persons living in underdeveloped countries. Many outbreaks have occurred in areas where flooding and heavy rains have occurred.

Symptoms are similar to hepatitis A, and the incubation period for this hepatitis is 15–64 days.

Diagnosis of Hepatitis E

Diagnosis is made by the presence of anti-HEV in serum.

Treatment of Hepatitis E

There is currently no known treatment for hepatitis E. Prevention is accomplished by practicing good hygiene and hand-washing techniques. Treatment with immune globulin after exposure has not been shown to be effective.

Hepatitis G

Hepatitis G virus (HGV) is one of the latest forms of hepatitis to be identified. It is spread parenterally, sexually, and by a blood transfusion. There is no known treatment at this time.

Prodromal Stage and Icteric Stage

Regardless of the type of hepatitis, clients experience symptoms associated with two stages: the *prodromal stage* and *icteric stage*. The prodromal stage of the hepatitis episode is the period of time when the client is exhibiting vague symptoms. This is the period when the patient's bile is not being excreted as it should (signified by dark urine and clay-colored stools) and is collecting in the bloodstream. When the bile has accumulated in the client's blood, the icteric stage begins and the client starts to exhibit symptoms such as jaundice, pruritus, and elevated liver enzymes.

Prodromal stage symptoms last from a few days to two weeks and include

▶ Fatigue

▶ Malaise

▶ Anorexia

▶ Nausea

▶ Vomiting

▶ Fever

▶ Dark urine

▶ Clay-colored stools

Icteric stage symptoms occur 5–10 days after the prodromal stage begins and include

▶ Jaundice

▶ Pruritus

▶ Tenderness in the right upper quadrant of the abdomen

▶ Hepatomegaly

▶ Elevated liver enzymes

Cirrhosis

Cirrhosis is the scarring or fibrosis of the liver, which results in the distortion of the liver structure and vessels. The most common causes of cirrhosis are alcoholism and hepatitis.

The following lists symptoms of cirrhosis you should know for the exam:

▶ Jaundice

▶ Spleenomegaly and hepatomegaly

▶ Chronic indigestion

▶ Constipation or diarrhea

- Weight loss

- Ascites

- Edema

- Petechiae

- Vitamin deficiencies of A, D, E, and K

- Changes in behavior, cognition, and speech

- Elevations in liver enzymes, BUN, and ammonia levels

Diagnosis of Cirrhosis

Liver functions are complex, requiring many diagnostic tests. These tests determine the extent of the cirrhosis, and the type of treatment depends on the condition of the liver. The candidate will need to know the following list of tests or exams important in diagnosing cirrhosis:

- Laboratory tests (liver enzymes, prothrombin time, and ammonia levels)

- Upper gastrointestinal x-ray

- CT scan

- Esophagogastroduodenoscopy (EGD)

- Liver biopsy

Treatment of Cirrhosis

The treatment regimen for clients with cirrhosis is based on the symptoms the client is exhibiting. For example, if the client is retaining fluids, diuretics are prescribed. Diet interventions include a diet to promote healing of liver tissue. The client would need increased calories, increased proteins, and low sodium food sources.

> **NOTE**
>
> If the client is in end-stage failure, protein sources are restricted.

Medications prescribed for clients with cirrhosis include antacids for gastric distress that could lead to bleeding, diuretics for fluid and ascites, and cathartics and enemas to correct the pH in the bowel and rid the body of ammonia. Other treatments the candidate should know for the exam include:

- Teach the client to avoid alcohol and medications detoxified by the liver

- Heme-test all stools and vomitus

- ▶ Record weight

- ▶ Intake and output

- ▶ Measure abdominal girth daily

- ▶ Use small needles for injections and maintain pressure for five minutes after injections due to bleeding tendencies

Pancreatitis

Pancreatitis is an acute inflammation of the pancreas associated with auto digestion. Enzymes secreted by the pancreas (lipase, amylase, trypsin, and so on) destroy the tissue of the pancreas. Consistent alcohol intake for 5–10 years is the common causative factor in middle-aged men with pancreatitis. The following list highlights some of the causes of pancreatitis:

- ▶ Biliary disease

- ▶ Alcoholism

- ▶ Bacterial or viral infections

- ▶ Blunt abdominal trauma

- ▶ Peptic ulcer disease

- ▶ Ischemic vascular disease

- ▶ Surgery on or near the pancreas

- ▶ Long-term use of steroids, thiazide diuretics, oral contraceptives, sulfonamides, or opiates

- ▶ Endoscopic retrograde cholangiopancreatography (ERCP) procedure

The symptoms of pancreatitis a client might exhibit include

- ▶ Epigastric pain radiating to the back

- ▶ Nausea and vomiting

- ▶ Abdominal distention

- ▶ Elevated blood and urine glucose levels

- ▶ Elevated serum lipase and amylase levels

- ▶ Decreased serum calcium levels

- ▶ Elevated white blood cells

- ▶ Steatorrhea (fatty stools)

Diagnosis of Pancreatitis

The nursing candidate should know that a diagnosis of acute pancreatitis is made by the clinical picture of the client and diagnostic tests. The major laboratory tests to diagnose this disorder are serum amylase and lipase. These tests will show an elevation with pancreatitis. More laboratory tests—for example, white blood cell counts and calcium, magnesium, and glucose levels—might also be done to determine a diagnosis. Other exams, x-rays, and endoscopic procedures that the candidate should know are included in the following list:

- CT scan
- MRI
- Endoscopic retrograde cholangiopancreatography (ERCP)

Treatment of Pancreatitis

The treatment modalities for the client with pancreatitis focus on relieving the client's symptoms and preventing or treating complications. The client is kept NPO, in the acute episode, with administration of IV fluids to inhibit stimulation and secretion of pancreatic enzymes. A nasogastric tube is usually inserted to decrease abdominal distention, prevent vomiting, and prevent hydrochloric acid from entering the duodenum. Other forms of therapy utilized to treat these clients include

- Observe for signs of bleeding. To prevent excessive bleeding, use small-gauge needles for IM, IV, or subcutaneous injections and maintain pressure for five minutes after any injections have been given.
- Medications, including the following:
    - Meperidine (Demerol)
    - Cimetadine (Tagamet)
    - Calcium gluconate
    - Viokase
    - Vitamins A, D, E, and K
    - Antibiotics
    - Insulin
- After oral feedings begin, the diet should be low fat and low protein and the client should avoid caffeine and alcohol
- ABGs to detect early complications
- Surgical intervention for gallstones that cannot be removed by ERCP or if complications such as pseudocysts and abscesses have formed

Cholecystitis/Cholelithiasis

Cholecystitis is inflammation of the gallbladder. Cholelithiasis occurs when gallstones are formed due to bile that is usually stored in the gallbladder hardening into stonelike material. Precipitates of cholesterol, bilirubin, and calcium produce gallstones.

Causes of gallbladder disease include a familial tendency for the development of this disease, but it can also be due to dietary habits. It is also associated with certain drugs, such as cholesterol-lowering agents. People with diabetes, hemolytic blood disorders, and Crohn's disease have a higher risk of development.

> **CAUTION**
>
> An easy way to remember who usually develops gallstones is to remember these four *F*s of gallbladder disease:
>
> ▶ Female (sex)
>
> ▶ Forty (usual age)
>
> ▶ Fat (usually obese)
>
> ▶ Fertile (usually have children)

Symptoms of Cholecystitis and Cholelithiasis

The symptoms that occur with cholecystitis (inflammation of the gallbladder) are usually associated with pain. The client might also exhibit jaundice of the skin, sclerae, and upper palate. With cholelithiasis (stones in the gallbladder), the stones might block the flow of bile from the gallbladder. Clinical manifestations include the following:

▶ Abdominal pain in RUQ, especially after a fatty meal. The pain can radiate to the right shoulder

▶ Abdominal distention

▶ Flatulence

▶ Steatorrhea

▶ Dyspepsia

▶ Clay colored stools and dark urine

▶ Nausea and vomiting

▶ Fever

Diagnosis of Cholecystitis/Cholethiasis

The following items are used to diagnose cholecystitis and cholethiasis:

▶ Abdominal x-ray

▶ Gallbladder ultrasound (the most frequently ordered test for diagnosis)

▶ Cholecystography using contrast media (telepaque, cholografin, or oragrafin):

  ▶ The client is held NPO for 10–12 hours before x-ray.

  ▶ A laxative or cleansing enema is ordered the evening prior to x-ray.

▶ Heptobiliary scan

▶ ERCP (used in clients who have an allergy to contrast media)

Treatment of Cholecystitis

Intervention for gallbladder inflammation and stones is supportive. Clients with cholecystitis might be treated conservatively or surgically. Conservative treatment is directed toward the relief of inflammation of the gallbladder and the elimination of pain. This goal is accomplished by placing the client NPO with IV fluids and NG suction. Anticholinergics may be given to help with the spasm of the smooth muscles.

Antibiotics are administered intravenously, especially if the client's WBC count is elevated. When the client has improved, diet intake is reinstituted with a gradual introduction of low-fat liquids and a high-protein, high-carbohydrate diet. Foods allowed and foods to avoid for clients recovering from a gallbladder attack are included here:

▶ **Foods allowed**—Skim milk, cooked fruits, rice, tapioca, lean meats, mashed potatoes, nongas-forming vegetables, bread, coffee, and tea

▶ **Foods to avoid**—Eggs, cream, pork, fried foods, cheese, rich dressings, gas-forming vegetables, and alcohol

Treatment of Cholethiasis

General treatments of cholethiasis include PO medication, lithotripsy procedures, and surgery. Small stones and radiolucent cholesterol stones can be treated with ursodeoxycholic acid (UDCA) or chenodeoxycholic acid (CDCA). These drugs are bile acids that can be used to dissolve the gallstones. It can take up to two years for the medication to work and is usually reserved for older clients who are not good surgical candidates. Approximately one half of people who take these drugs have a recurrence of the stones after the medication is stopped.

Another form of treatment that can be used for clients with gallstones is extracorporeal shock wave lithotripsy (ESWL). In this procedure, the client is placed in certain positions as repeated shock waves are directed at gallstones to cause them to fragment. After the stones are broken into small pieces, they can then pass through the common bile duct easily, be retrieved by endoscopy, or be dissolved by the bile acid drugs mentioned previously. This procedure is done on an outpatient basis, and the client resumes a regular routine within 48 hours.

The final type of treatment for gallstones is surgery. The surgeries that can be performed are laparoscopic and abdominal cholecystectomy. Laparoscopic surgery accounts for more than half of all cholecystectomies.

When this surgical procedure is used, a small incision or puncture wound is made through the abdominal wall. Other puncture wounds allow for the introduction of surgical instruments to remove the gallbladder and stones.

Laparoscopic surgery is usually performed as same-day surgery. Its advantages are less postoperative pain, decreased likelihood of paralytic ileus, and quicker resumption of preoperative activity.

The second type of procedure is the abdominal cholecystectomy. This procedure is reserved for those with large stones or with extensive involvement of the duct system. The surgical procedure involves ligation of the cystic duct and artery and removal of the gallbladder. Insertion of a penrose drain allows the drainage of serosanguinous fluid and bile into an absorbent dressing. If the common bile duct was manipulated, a T-tube is usually inserted in the duct to keep it open until swelling diminishes.

Clostridium Difficile

Clostridium difficile (C. difficile) is a serious bacterial infection that is a common cause of antibiotic associated diarrhea. The infection is highly associated with being in a healthcare setting. Risk factors for getting the bacteria include:

▶ Clients receiving antibiotic therapy

▶ Lengthy hospital stays

▶ Immunosuppressed clients

▶ Elderly clients

▶ Postoperative gastrointestinal surgery

Symptoms associated with C. difficile include:

▶ Watery diarrhea

▶ Fever

▶ Abdominal pain or cramping

The infection is diagnosed by a stool culture for the presence of C difficile. Management is accomplished by the administration of antibiotics (flagyl or vancomycin) and infection control. Infection control measures include:

▸ Placing clients with C. difficile in private rooms

▸ Contact precautions

▸ Strict hand hygiene

▸ Teaching family members infection-control measures

Food-Borne Illnesses

Food-borne illnesses commonly cause gastrointestinal problems in clients in the United States. These illnesses result when a person receives an infectious organism with the intake of food. The NCLEX candidate needs to be prepared to answer questions relating directly to these diagnoses. Table 10.1 discusses the most common types of illnesses and accentuates the major points of these disorders.

TABLE 10.1 Food-Borne Illnesses

Illness	Source of Infection	Symptoms	Treatment	Preventative Measures
Botulism (incubation time is 18–36 hours)	Improperly canned fruits and vegetables; it's less common in meats and fish	Nausea, vomiting, diarrhea, weakness, dysphagia, dysarthria, paralysis, respiratory failure	NPO, IV fluid replacement, trivalent botulism, antitoxin, and respiratory support	Home canning containers should be boiled for at least 20 minutes. Thoroughly cook meat.
E. coli (incubation time varies with specific strain)	Undercooked beef and shellfish; food contaminated with fecal material	Vomiting, diarrhea, abdominal cramping, fever; some cases have proven fatal due to rapid fluid loss and organ failure	IV fluid replacement and antibiotic administration	Thoroughly cook meat.
Salmonella (incubation time is 8–24 hours)	Contaminated food and drinks, raw eggs	Fever, nausea, vomiting, cramping, abdominal pain, diarrhea	NPO, IV fluid replacement	Good hand washing
Staphylococcal (incubation time is 2–4 hours)	Meat, dairy products, human carriers	Abrupt vomiting, abdominal cramping, diarrhea, weakness	Replacement of lost fluid volume and electrolytes	Properly prepare and store food.

Diagnostic Tests for Review

Most of the diagnostic exams for the gastrointestinal system are directly related to the anatomical area needing visualization. Along with the usual routine exams—for example, CBC, urinalysis, and chest x-ray—the NCLEX candidate should be knowledgeable of the preparation and care of clients receiving endoscopic exams. An example of special considerations for these exams is the need to assess the gag reflex before allowing oral intake after a gastroscopy procedure. The nurse candidate must also be aware of the risk of bleeding after a liver biopsy, as well as the possible breathing problems that can occur due to the sedation usually given for endoscopic exams. While reviewing these diagnostic exams, the candidate should be alert for information that would be an important part of nursing care:

- ▶ Barium enema

- ▶ Barium swallow

- ▶ Colonoscopy and sigmoidoscopy

- ▶ Endoscopic exams

- ▶ Gallbladder ultrasound

- ▶ Gastric analysis and biopsy

- ▶ H. Pylori

- ▶ Liver biopsy

- ▶ Liver panel blood tests

- ▶ pH motility studies

- ▶ Upper GI studies

Pharmacology for Review

An integral part of care to clients with gastrointestinal (GI) disorders is pharmacological intervention. These medications provide an improvement or cure of the clients' GI problems. The NCLEX candidate needs to focus on the classification of drugs in the following list. Most of these drugs are commonly given, which makes them more likely to be a part of the NCLEX exam. When reviewing these drug classifications, the candidate should think about the common side and adverse effects associated with the classification, such as the GI upset and bleeding associated with NSAIDs:

- ▶ Antacids

- ▶ Antispasmodics

- Antivirals
- Cathartics
- Corticosteroids
- Cytoprotective
- Fiber laxatives
- Hepatitis vaccines
- Histamine receptor blockers
- Immunosuppressives
- Interferons
- Nonsteroidal anti-inflammatory drugs
- Proton pump inhibitors

Exam Prep Questions

1. The physician is assessing renal function in a client with severe pancreatitis. Which laboratory finding would be the best indicator of a problem in this area?

   ○ **A.** Alkaline phosphatase 20U/L

   ○ **B.** Hemoglobin 14.6 g/dl

   ○ **C.** BUN 28 mg/dl

   ○ **D.** Creatinine 2.3 mg/dl

2. An 85-year-old client with diverticulitis has been vomiting and febrile for 12 hours. Where is the best location to assess skin turgor on this client?

   ○ **A.** Dorsal hand

   ○ **B.** Feet

   ○ **C.** Back of the arm

   ○ **D.** Sternum

3. The nurse is caring for a client with pancreatitis experiencing the process of lipolysis of the pancreas. Which assessment would be a priority because of the pathophysiology of lipolysis?

   ○ **A.** Checking for tetany-like movements

   ○ **B.** Assessing breath sounds

   ○ **C.** Obtaining vital signs

   ○ **D.** Palpating pedal pulses

4. A client scheduled for a Nissen repair for a hiatal hernia is being instructed preoperatively to use the incentive spirometer. Which statement indicates to the nurse that the client understands the teaching?

   ○ **A.** "These exercises will help to decrease my pain."

   ○ **B.** "I should use this device once a day."

   ○ **C.** "If I use this device, it will help in preventing pneumonia."

   ○ **D.** "I should do these breathing techniques while lying down flat in bed."

5. A nurse receives a report on a client three days postoperative abdominal surgery that includes four saturated dressing changes in eight hours. On assessment of this client, dehiscence and evisceration of the wound are noted. After applying a sterile, moistened 4-x-4, what is the nurse's next action?

○ **A.** Place the client in the dorsal recumbent position.

○ **B.** Notify the physician.

○ **C.** Wrap an Ace bandage around the abdomen.

○ **D.** Use a wheelchair to transport the client to the treatment room.

6. The nurse is caring for a client with a nasogastric tube in place. Assessment of the aspirate reveals a pH of 2.0. Which is the appropriate action?

○ **A.** Document the finding.

○ **B.** Notify the physician.

○ **C.** Remove the NG tube and replace it.

○ **D.** Turn the client side lying and reassess the aspirate.

7. A client diagnosed with an ulcer has been placed on tetracycline due to a positive helicobacter pyloric test result. Which food choice, when taken with the drug, could decrease its effectiveness?

○ **A.** Cabbage

○ **B.** Yogurt

○ **C.** Bran cereal

○ **D.** Bananas

8. A client with hepatitis C is scheduled for a liver biopsy. Which data, noted in the client's record, would receive priority?

○ **A.** Prothrombin time of 56 seconds

○ **B.** BUN of 22 mg/dl

○ **C.** Hematocrit 42%

○ **D.** Potassium 4.0 mEq/L

9. A client is being admitted with a diagnosis of possible pancreatitis. Which of the following is the best support for this diagnosis?

○ **A.** Pain is in the left upper quadrant of the abdomen

○ **B.** Client reports steatorrhea for the last three days

○ **C.** A serum amylase level of 366 U/L

○ **D.** Assessed diminished bowel sounds

10. A client with diverticulitis has received nutritional discharge instructions for a high-fiber diet. Which menu selection by the client would reinforce that the teaching was effective?

   ○ **A.** Spaghetti with meatballs and toast

   ○ **B.** Baked chicken and macaroni with cheese

   ○ **C.** Broccoli chicken stir fry and brown rice

   ○ **D.** Broiled liver and dinner roll

Answer Rationales

1. Answer D is correct. Creatinine is the most specific laboratory test for renal functioning; normal is 0.5–1.5mg/dl. Answers A and B do not relate to the kidney, so they are incorrect. Answer C can be abnormal with kidney function but is not as specific as the creatinine, so it's incorrect.

2. Answer D is correct. This is the best area to check in the elderly due to loss of skin elasticity that occurs with aging. Answers A, B, and C are all influenced by loss of elasticity more than the sternum, so they are incorrect.

3. Answer A is correct. Hypocalcemia is a specific manifestation of clients with pancreatitis and lipolysis, and tetany is a major characteristic of low calcium levels. Answers B, C, and D are all pertinent assessments but are not priorities with the pathophysiology of lipolysis, so they are incorrect.

4. Answer C is correct. Incentive spirometry's purpose is to prevent or treat atelectasis, which can lead to pneumonia. Answer A is a false statement, so it is incorrect. Answer B is incorrect because the timing is not as often as it should be. Answer D is wrong because it is best done sitting upright.

5. Answer B is correct. After the saline dressing is applied, the doctor should be notified for probable repair. Answer A is wrong because low Fowler's position should be used. Answer C will not help, so it's incorrect. Answer D is inappropriate at this time, so it's incorrect.

6. Answer A is correct. This finding is within normal range for gastric aspirate of 0–4. Answers B, C, and D would not be appropriate or necessary due to the normal reading, so they're incorrect.

7. Answer B is correct. Milk and dairy products can reduce the effectiveness of the drug when taken at the same time. Answers A, C, and D would not affect the drug, so they're incorrect.

8. Answer A is correct. An abnormal prothrombin time would receive priority due to the risk of hemorrhage with a liver biopsy. Answers B, C, and D are all normal values and don't relate to the procedure's risks, so they're incorrect.

9. Answer C is correct. The client's amylase level is elevated above the normal level of 200 U/L. This measurement is the most accurate indicator of pancreatitis and the most objective and specific. The answers in A, B, and D are also clinical manifestations of pancreatitis, but are not as specific as the laboratory value, so they are incorrect choices.

10. Answer C is correct. This diet has the highest amount of fiber. Answers A, B, and D have low amounts of fiber, so they're incorrect.

Suggested Reading and Resources

▶ Brunner, L., and Suddarth, D. *Textbook of Medical-Surgical Nursing*. 12th ed. Philadelphia: Lippincott Williams & Wilkins, 2009.

▶ Hogan, M. *Child Health Nursing Reviews and Rationales*. 2nd ed. Upper Saddle River, NJ: Pearson Prentice Hall, 2007.

▶ Ignatavicius, D., Workman, S. *Medical-Surgical Nursing: Critical Thinking for Collaborative Care*. 6th ed. Philadelphia: Elsevier, 2007.

▶ Deglin, J., and Vallerand, A., *Davis Drug Guide for Nurses*. Philadelphia: F.A. Davis, 2009.

▶ Lewis, S., Heitkemper, M., Dirkson, S., O Brien, P., and Bucher, L. *Medical Surgical Nursing: Assessment and Management of Clinical Problems*. 7th ed. Philadelphia: Elsevier, 2007.

▶ Rinehart, W., Sloan, D., and Hurd, C. *NCLEX Exam Cram*. Indianapolis: Que, 2007.

▶ Centers for Disease Control and Prevention: www.cdc.gov

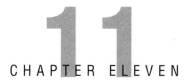

CHAPTER ELEVEN

Caring for the Client with Disorders of the Musculoskeletal System

---

Terms you'll need to understand

- ✓ Bone density
- ✓ Clostridium
- ✓ Crepitation
- ✓ Demineralize
- ✓ Dowager's hump
- ✓ Fasciotomy
- ✓ Isometric exercises
- ✓ Paresis
- ✓ Pathological fractures
- ✓ Purine
- ✓ TENS unit

Nursing skills you'll need to master

- ✓ Stump wrapping
- ✓ Caring for a client in traction
- ✓ Caring for a client with a cast
- ✓ Measuring and teaching crutch walking
- ✓ Measuring and teaching the use of canes
- ✓ Measuring and teaching the use of walkers

Fractures

A *fracture* is defined as simply a break in the continuity of the bone. Four major categories of bone fractures are classified according to the amount of tissue damage: simple or closed, compound, comminuted, and green stick. The first category is a *simple* or *closed fracture*. With a compound fracture, the skin surface is broken.

> **CAUTION**
>
> There is more danger of infection and osteomyelitis with compound fractures.

The third type of fracture is the *comminuted*, which causes damage to soft tissue nerves and blood vessels. The last major category is the *green stick*. This category occurs more often in children.

A fifth type of fracture is the *pathological fracture*. These fractures occur without major injury or trauma. The bones on these clients have been weakened by diseases such as osteoporosis, osteogenesis imperfecta, or metastatic cancer.

The nurse candidate must be aware of the need for early intervention in the care of clients with fractures. Symptoms indicating a fracture include

▶ Coolness and blanching distal to the break

▶ Crepitation

▶ Disalignment

▶ Shortness of the affected limb

▶ Swelling

▶ Pain

Treating Fractures

Treatment of fractures focuses on measures to limit movement, control pain, decrease edema, prevent complications, and promote healing. The following highlights the care you must know about for taking the exam. Treatment of a fracture includes

▶ Splinting the affected area

▶ Elevating the affected extremity

▶ Removing any jewelry from the extremity

- ▶ Administering medication, such as

  - ▶ Antibiotics for open fractures that are susceptible to gas-growing clostridium

  - ▶ Antithrombotics

  - ▶ Heparin

  - ▶ Enoxaparin (Lovenox)

  - ▶ Narcotics and muscle relaxers for pain

- ▶ Using traction

Traction

It is important to explore a little more on the traction treatment. Traction utilizes a pulling force to maintain proper alignment of the bone so that healing can occur. It can also reduce the fracture and decrease muscle spasms, which decreases pain. The following information outlines the types of traction and your role in the care of traction necessary for effectively taking the exam:

- ▶ **Manual traction**—Maintained by the caregiver's hand.

- ▶ **Skin traction**—Maintained by using straps or wraps applied to the skin (for example, Buck's traction [often used for fractured hips with 5–10 pounds of weight], which is shown in Figure 11.1).

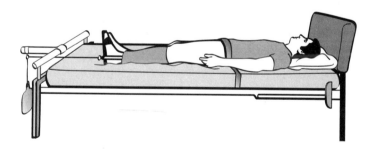

Figure 11.1 Example of Buck's traction.

- ▶ **Skeletal traction**—Maintained by using pins or wires inserted into the bone. This type of traction uses 15–30 pounds of weight (examples are 90-90, and Crutchfield tong traction, shown in Figure 11.2 and Figure 11.3, respectively).

- ▶ **Balanced suspension traction**—Maintained by using more than one force of pull to establish alignment (shown in Figure 11.4).

Here are some points to remember in maintaining traction:

▶ Weights must hang free.

▶ Linens should not lie on ropes.

▶ Ropes should remain within the pulley.

▶ Assess circulation, pulses, and movement of extremity.

▶ Except during an emergency, weights should not be removed on clients with skeletal traction in place.

▶ Skeletal traction requires specific assessment for signs of inflammation or infection at the entry sites of the pins or screws.

▶ Maintain proper body alignment.

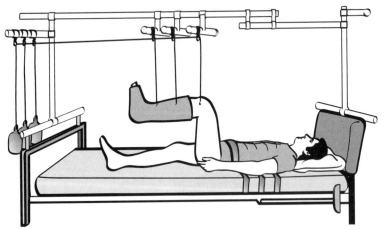

FIGURE 11.2 Example of 90-90 traction.

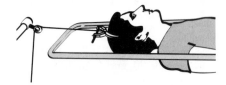

FIGURE 11.3 Example of the Crutchfield tong traction.

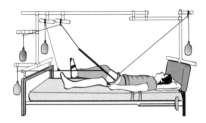

FIGURE 11.4 Example of balance suspension.

Casts

Related to traction is the use of casts for fracture healing. *Casts* are rigid devices used to keep a specific body part immobile. This allows the bone fragments to stay in place and heal. The following accentuates what you need to know about the management of the client with a cast:

▶ Allow the cast to dry from the inside out.

▶ Handle a wet cast with the palms of your hands.

▶ Place the extremity on a plastic-lined pillow.

▶ Note any drainage on the cast by circling it and noting the time of observation.

▶ Petal rough edges of the cast.

▶ Instruct the client not to scratch or place objects beneath the cast, such as hangers or toys.

▶ Evaluate any areas that feel hot (which might indicate that the client has an underlying infection).

▶ Relieve itching by blowing cool air from a blow dryer into the cast.

▶ Assess circulation, pulses, and movement of extremity.

Compartment Syndrome

A complication that can occur after a fracture is *compartment syndrome*. This is a serious condition resulting from pressure within different compartments (these separate the blood vessels, muscles, and nerves) that cause decreased circulation to the area—usually the leg and forearm. This disorder can lead to irreversible motor weakness, infection, and amputation of the limb.

A major element in compartment syndrome is prevention. The nurse candidate must be able to recognize the clinical manifestations of compartment syndrome, which include the following:

▶ Cyanosis

▶ Numbness

- Pain (especially pain that is unrelieved by medication)

- Pallor

- Paresis/paralysis

- Swelling

- Tingling

> **CAUTION**
>
> An easy way to remember the symptoms that should put you on alert for compartment syndrome is to remember the five *P*s:
> - Pain
> - Pallor
> - Pulselessness
> - Polar
> - Paresthesia

Treating Compartment Syndrome

Treatment of compartment syndrome requires a means to relieve the pressure. Two types of treatments can be used to accomplish this goal: bivalve treatment and fasciotomy. Bivalve treatment means cutting the cast on each side and is done if the cast is too tight, causing pressure and restricting blood flow. If symptoms persist, the client might require the second type of treatment—a surgical procedure called a *fasciotomy*. This is done by the surgeon making an incision through the skin and subcutaneous tissue into the fascia to relieve the pressure and improve circulation.

Osteomyelitis

Another complication that can occur with fractures is *osteomyelitis*. Osteomyelitis occurs when an infection has invaded the bone area. Clients at risk for osteomyelitis include the malnourished, the elderly, the overweight, and people who have a chronic illness (such as cardiovascular disease). The symptoms that can occur with osteomyelitis are

- Fever

- Malaise

- Swelling in the infected area

- Tenderness in the infected area

- Purulent drainage in the infected area

▶ Pain in the infected area

▶ Tachycardia

Treating Osteomyelitis

The treatment of osteomyelitis can involve several modalities. One course of treatment includes medications, which can include the use of antibiotics (the specific antibiotics used depend on the wound and blood culture results) and pain medication. Surgical debridement of the wound might also speed the elimination of infection in the bone. The following contains nursing interventions you need to know for the exam:

▶ Immobilize the body part.

▶ Administer pain medication.

▶ Perform neurovascular assessment.

▶ Perform sterile dressing changes.

▶ Teach the client how to use IV access devices for at-home antibiotic administration.

▶ Provide a diet high in protein and vitamin C.

Osteoporosis

Osteoporosis is a disease whereby bone demineralizes, resulting in bone density reduction. The wrist, hip, and vertebral column are most often affected. The density of bones decreases rapidly in postmenopausal women due to decreases in estrogen. It has been determined that almost one-half of women over age 65 have osteoporosis. The following highlights the risk factors associated with osteoporosis:

▶ Age (there's a greater incidence over age 60)

▶ Low body weight

▶ Race (it occurs more in Asian and Caucasian women)

▶ Sedentary lifestyle

▶ Low dietary calcium intake

▶ Smoking

▶ Alcohol consumption

▶ Decreased estrogen levels

▶ Excess caffeine intake

▶ Gender (more common in women)

▶ Family history of osteoporosis

Clinical manifestations of osteoporosis include

▶ Back pain

▶ Constipation

▶ Decrease in height

▶ Dowager's hump (humped back)

▶ Fractures

Treatment of Osteoporosis

Treatment of osteoporosis involves direct involvement of the client. Exercises to increase the muscles are recommended, including walking, swimming, and water aerobics. The client should also be taught to eat foods high in calcium, vitamin D, fiber, and protein. Foods high in calcium include molasses, apricots, breads, cereal, milk, dairy products (especially yogurt), beans, carrots, asparagus, and collard greens. They should also be taught to avoid alcohol and caffeine.

> **CAUTION**
>
> Excess caffeine can cause calcium to be excreted in the urine.

Another important aspect to teach clients with osteoporosis involves safety measures—for example, avoiding the use of throw rugs and teaching the clients to avoid falls.

Medications have been developed that are efficient in combating and preventing the disease, and some general medications are given for pain relief:

▶ Biphosphonates (examples are Fosamax, Boniva, and Didronel)

▶ Calcitonin

▶ Calcium supplements

▶ Estrogen for post-menopausal women

▶ Muscle relaxers

- NSAIDs

- Salmon calcitonin (Calcimar)

- Selective estrogen receptor modules, or SERMs (for example, Evista)

Gout

Gout is the formation of uric acid deposits in the joints, particularly the joint of the big toe. It is an arthritic condition resulting from the body's inability to metabolize purine foods. The buildup of uric acid, the end product of purines, causes inflammation in the joints involved. Symptoms of gout include painful joints and tophi (growths of urate crystals) that occur most often on the outer ear of the client with gout.

Treatment of the Client with Gout

Early attacks usually resolve themselves within a 10-day period without treatment, but most clients cannot tolerate the pain. The treatment regimen used for clients with gout follows two distinct paths: diet and drugs. Diet is the path directed toward decreasing purine in the diet. The following indicates foods that are low in purine and should be increased in the diet: cheese, eggs, fats, gelatin, milk, most vegetables, nuts, sugar, and cherries.

The client should avoid foods that are high in purine, including: dried beans, fish (especially sardines), liver, lobster, oatmeal, oysters, peas, poultry, spinach, mussels, and asparagus.

The second path of treatment for clients with gout is drugs, which are the primary element in the care of this client. Colchicine (Colsalide) with an NSAID is prescribed for the acute episode of gout. Allopurinol (Zyloprim) is used in chronic gout to both reduce the production of uric acid and promote the excretion of it. Other drugs that may be given include probenecid (Benemid) and losartan (Cozaar)

Rheumatoid Arthritis

Rheumatoid arthritis is a connective tissue disorder believed to be due to a C-reactive protein immune response. It is destructive to the joints and can cause deformities. The usual onset of the disease is between 30 and 50 years of age, and it affects women three times more often than men. The person with RA exhibits many symptoms. The following highlights the most common symptoms you need to be familiar with for the exam:

- Subcutaneous nodules (usually on the ulnar surface of the arm)

- Warmth, tenderness, and swelling in the affected joints

▶ Pericarditis

▶ Iritis of the eyes

▶ Weight loss

▶ Anorexia

Diagnosis is made by the history of the clinical course of the disease, as well as elevations in the following laboratory tests:

▶ C-reactive protein

▶ Rheumatoid factor

▶ Sedimentation rate

▶ Antinuclear antibody (ANA)

Treatment of Rheumatoid Arthritis

The treatment plan for RA involves the use of a combination of drugs, exercise, and pain relief measures such as heat and ice. If the interventions are not effective in providing mobility and pain relief, surgery might be required to replace the joint. The following highlights medications, comfort measures, and joint mobility interventions you need to know when testing on the topic of rheumatoid arthritis:

▶ Medications, including

  ▶ Antiarthritics (for example, etanercept [Enbrel] and infliximab [Remicade])

  ▶ Antibiotic therapy (for example, minocycline [Minocin])

  ▶ Cytotoxic agents (for example, methotrexate [Rheumatrix])

  ▶ Disease-modifying antirheumatic medications, or DMARDs (for example, hydroxycholorquine [Plaquenil])

  ▶ Gold salts

  ▶ NSAIDs

  ▶ Salycilates

  ▶ Steroids

  ▶ Sulfasalazine (Azulfidine)

  ▶ Immune modulators (for example, Arava)

▶ Application of heat and ice to the affected joints.

▶ Lightweight splints for joint rest.

▶ Plasmapheresis.

▶ Fish oil tablets to decrease inflammation.

> **CAUTION**
>
> Fish oil tablets are contraindicated in clients taking anticoagulants.

▶ A regular exercise program to maintain joint mobility. Isometric exercises of the gluteal, quadriceps, and abdominal muscles while sitting helps to maintain muscle strength and trunk stability.

Musculoskeletal Surgical Procedures

A client who has a dysfunction of the musculoskeletal system might have to undergo a surgical procedure. Surgery might be performed to relieve pain, provide stability, and improve function of the joint. The discussion that follows focuses on the care necessary for clients who have had a break in a hip, have had joint disability or damage, or who require an amputation because of disease or trauma.

Fractured Hip and Hip Replacement

Fracture of the hip is most common in white, elderly females. A fractured hip can contribute to death in the elderly due to it predisposing them to infection and respiratory complications. The most definitive symptoms associated with a fractured hip are disalignment and shortening of the affected leg. The client also cannot move the leg without pain and complains of pain in the hip and groin on the affected side. Diagnosis is made by a hip x-ray that confirms the break.

Treatment of a Fractured Hip

The treatment option for a hip fracture is to repair it by the use of internal fixation devices or prosthetic joint placement. Fractures in the trochanteric area are repaired by internal fixation devices. Femoral neck fractures with disrupted blood supply require prosthetic joints. The preoperative care of a hip fracture includes the use of Buck's traction to immobilize the hip, resulting in a reduction of muscle spasms and pain. Medications are also administered to relieve pain, relax the muscle, and prevent complications.

After the surgery, the nurse candidate needs to become familiar with assessments and specific nursing measures. The following highlights the care required after hip surgery:

▶ Assess for bleeding and shock.

▶ Monitor for deep vein thrombosis and embolisms.

▶ Encourage the use of incentive spirometry.

▶ Ambulate early, with no weight bearing on the affected leg.

▶ Joint replacement clients should sit in a recliner and not in straight chairs. The affected leg should be bent no more than 45°.

▶ When in bed, the client should be turned to the unaffected side or both sides, depending on hospital policy.

▶ For clients with prosthetic joint placement, legs must be kept abducted with no more than 90° hip flexion for four to six weeks. These clients should also be instructed to not cross their legs and not to twist or reach behind. These clients will also require elevated toilet seats.

▶ Monitor output from any existing drains. Assess the hemoglobin and hematocrit results. A blood transfusion might be necessary.

▶ Collaborate with physical therapy on mobility treatments and exercises.

Total Knee Replacement

Total knee replacements are performed for clients who have severe joint pain that makes them immobile. It is also considered when people have arthritic destruction of the articular cartilages or deformity of the knee, and in clients who are not able to walk or have limited motion due to knee instability. The goal of the surgery is twofold:

▶ Restore full flexion and extension

▶ Provide adequate strength and stability of the knee for most functional activities

Post-operative efforts for the client after total knee replacement are directed toward preventing complications and restoring mobility. The candidate should consider the nursing care requirements for this client when studying for the exam. Along with the usual medication administration (pain medication, antithrombotics, and antibiotics), these clients need specific limb care and physical therapy. The following includes the specific care of the post-operative knee replacement, use of the continuous passive motion (CPM) machine, and physical therapy regimen that are important to know for the exam:

► Keep the knee in extension to prevent contractures.

► Splint or immobilizer can be used after the pressure dressing is removed.

► Maintain the patella in alignment with the toes.

► Use two persons for transfer until the client regains muscle strength.

► Support the affected leg during a transfer.

► Follow a set protocol for movement, ambulation, and weight bearing. Dislocation of the prosthesis is not of concern as with hip replacements.

Clients are usually placed on a CPM machine in the recovery room. This device is applied early to increase circulation and range of motion of the knee joint. Flexion of the knee is an important aspect of care because, if it is not achieved, another surgery might be required. You need to know the usual guidelines for the use of the machine. The major information for use of the machine follows:

> **NOTE**
>
> CPM control machines are usually placed at the foot of the bed, beyond the reach of the client.

► On day 1, the client should be on the CPM with a setting of 0°–45°.

► The CPM machine should be on for two hours and off for one hour. Following two hours on the CPM machine, the leg should remain in extension for one hour; then resume use of the CPM machine.

Physical Therapy for Total Knee Replacement

Physical therapy is invaluable in supervising the exercises for strength and range of motion. Clients with total knee replacements are usually discharged within 3–4 days with a plan for continued exercises. An initial appointment is needed with the physical therapy department within 48–72 hours of discharge. The client usually starts with use of a walker (crutches if a younger client), and then advances to a cane. After one month, if the client can walk without a severe limp, no assistive devices are necessary.

Amputations

Amputations occur when a part of the body is removed, usually an extremity. Causes of amputations include trauma, infection and possible sepsis, peripheral vascular disease, and accidents. Amputations are done to relieve pain or improve the quality of life. They can also be required to save the patient's life.

Interventions Post Amputation Surgery

The candidate needs to be aware of the nursing care required for amputation clients. Specific problems that might occur with the client after an amputation include pain, hemorrhage, and infection. You need to be aware of the therapeutic measures to use with phantom limb pain that commonly occurs in amputation. One way to deal with phantom limb pain is to treat it as any other pain. If the pain is real, it is nontherapeutic to remind the client of the missing limb. A TENS unit might be used to relieve the pain. Other pharmacological measures for pain relief are prescribed depending on the type of pain the client describes and include: intravenous Calcimar, beta blockers, anticonvulsants, and antispasmodics.

Assessments are another important nursing measure. Monitoring for hemorrhage and infection are critical because they are major potential complications. The client will arrive after surgery with a compression bandage. Restoring mobility is very important; mobility can be fostered by collaboration with physical therapy and encouraging the use of a prosthetic limb. Additional nursing measures that focus on exercise and prevention of complications are as follows:

▶ Exercises (a trapeze bar is used to move in bed).

▶ A firm mattress is needed to make movement easier.

Prevent contractures by using the following nursing interventions:

▶ Placing the client in a prone position for 30 minutes every 3–4 hours

▶ Using a sandbag to the knee

▶ Ensuring that the residual limb stays flat on the bed

▶ Avoid sitting in a chair for over one hour

> **NOTE**
>
> The residual limb might be elevated for the first 24 hours after surgery to reduce swelling and pain.

> **NOTE**
>
> Stump wrapping: wrapping the stump can be effective in shrinking the limb, reducing the swelling, help with shaping for a prosthesis, and keeping the dressing in place. The stump is wrapped using the figure eight technique to prevent impeding blood flow.

The nurse candidate must also be aware of the psychological aspects of the loss of a limb. A disturbance in body image occurs with an amputation. The client might therefore go through the grief process.

Assistive Devices for Ambulation

Clients with musculoskeletal disorders often need devices to assist them with mobility. The following discusses how to measure and fit for three of these devices: crutches, canes, and walkers. This information will assist you in answering questions on the exam that refer to these topics.

Crutches

Crutches are prescribed for clients who need partial weight bearing or non-weight bearing assistance. A person who is to use crutches needs to have good balance, good upper body strength, and an adequate cardiovascular system. The procedure used to fit the client for crutches follows: With the crutch tip extended six inches diagonally in front of the foot, 2–3 finger widths should be allowed between the axilla and the top of the crutch to prevent nerve damage.

Five types of crutch-walking gaits exist, with the use depending on the amount of weight bearing allowed:

▶ **Two-point gait**—This permits limited weight bearing bilaterally. The right leg and left crutch move simultaneously; the left leg and right crutch move simultaneously.

▶ **Three-point gait**—Non-weight bearing or partial weight bearing is allowed on the affected leg. Both crutches and the affected leg move in unison. Body weight is supported on the unaffected leg.

▶ **Four-point gait**—This permits weight bearing on both legs. The crutches and feet move alternately. The left crutch and right foot move, and then the right crutch and left foot.

▶ **Swing through**—No weight bearing is permitted on the affected legs. Both crutches move forward and both legs swing through between the crutches. The weight is borne by the crutches.

▶ **Stairs**—This is for climbing stairs. The client leads with the unaffected leg, and the crutches and affected leg move together. For descending stairs, the client leads with the crutches and affected leg.

TIP

Go up the stairs with the good leg first, and go down the stairs with the bad leg first.

Canes

Canes are the least stable of ambulation devices and are not recommended for nonweight bearing activities. The cane does give a client greater balance and support and is recommended when this is needed. The top of the cane should be at the greater trochanter area. The cane goes on the unaffected side with no more than 30° elbow flexion. There are basically three types of canes: the four-foot adjustable (quad or hemi), the adjustable, and the offset adjustable. Here's how you adjust the cane for proper fit:

▶ To determine the proper length of the cane, the client should be standing or lying supine.

▶ The client's arm should lie straight along the side with the cane handgrip level with the greater trochanter.

▶ The cane should be placed parallel to the femur and tibia with the tip of the cane on the floor or at the bottom of the shoe heel.

Walkers

Indications for walker use include the need for balance, stability, and decreased weight bearing. This assistive device is most commonly used for older clients. Walkers provide anterior and lateral stability with a wide base of support. Proper walker adjustment allows for 20°–30° elbow flexion. The three types of walkers are the standard, the folding, and the rolling walker. The following highlights the instructions that the exam taker should be aware of for the use of a walker.

The instructions for using walkers for partial or non-weight bearing are as follows:

1. Advance the walker an arm's length.

2. Place all four legs on the floor.

3. Advance the affected leg.

4. Push the body weight through the arms.

5. Advance the unaffected leg.

The instructions for using walkers for balance and stability are as follows:

1. Advance the walker an arm's length.

2. Set all four legs on the floor.

3. Take two complete steps into the walker.

CAUTION

For safety reasons, a gait belt is necessary when initiating cane and walker use.

Diagnostic Tests for Review

The diagnostic exams that are used for the musculoskeletal system are associated with the body part involved. Fractures are easily diagnosed by an x-ray of the area. As with all diseases or disorders, the usual exams are the CBC, urinalysis, and chest x-ray. Direct visualization is obtained by the use of scopic devices—for example, arthroscopes are typically used with knees. For clients with bone weaknesses, density testing is done to measure the degree of the problem. While reviewing the diagnostic exams that follow, you should be alert for the abnormalities that correlate with specific musculoskeletal diseases, such as the elevation levels of rheumatoid factor in rheumatoid arthritis:

▶ Arthrography

▶ Arthroscopy

▶ Bone biopsy

▶ Bone density testing

▶ Bone scan

▶ CT scan

▶ Electromyography

▶ Laboratory tests, including rheumatoid factor, antinuclear antibody titer, and erythrocyte sedimentation rate (ESR)

▶ MRI

▶ Muscle biopsy

Pharmacology for Review

Medications are invaluable as a method of treatment for musculoskeletal disorders. These medications are important in preventing some of the common complications that can occur with immobility. Commonly used medications include antithrombotics and antimicrobials. The uric acid inhibitors function well in curing the disease of gouty arthritis, and the newer

DMARD classification has helped with osteoporosis. You need to focus on the drug classifications in this list and think about which drug would be used in which musculoskeletal disease:

- ▶ Analgesics
- ▶ Antiarthritics
- ▶ Anticoagulants
- ▶ Antimicrobial agents
- ▶ Antithrombotics
- ▶ Bisphosphonates
- ▶ Cytotoxics
- ▶ DMARDs
- ▶ Muscle relaxants
- ▶ NSAIDs
- ▶ Salycilates
- ▶ SERMs
- ▶ Steroids
- ▶ Uric acid inhibitors
- ▶ Vitamins

Exam Prep Questions

1. The nurse is caring for a client after a motor vehicle accident. The client has a fractured tibia, and bone is noted protruding through the skin. Which action is of priority?

   ○ **A.** Provide manual traction above and below the leg.

   ○ **B.** Cover the bone area with a sterile dressing.

   ○ **C.** Apply an Ace bandage around the entire lower limb.

   ○ **D.** Apply an immobilizer to the area.

2. The nurse has performed nutritional teaching on a client with gout who is placed on a low-purine diet. Which selection by the client would indicate a need for further teaching?

   ○ **A.** Broccoli

   ○ **B.** An orange

   ○ **C.** Chocolate cake

   ○ **D.** Fish

3. The nurse at an orthopedic joint clinic is preparing pre-operative teaching for clients scheduled for total hip replacement surgery. Which would be included in the teaching plan?

   ○ **A.** Avoid sitting in a recliner.

   ○ **B.** Make sure that commode seats are at low levels.

   ○ **C.** Avoid crossing the legs when sitting.

   ○ **D.** Physical therapy will assist with adduction leg exercises.

4. Which client would be at greatest risk for a fat emboli following a fracture?

   ○ **A.** A 50-year-old with a fractured fibula

   ○ **B.** A 20-year-old female with a wrist fracture

   ○ **C.** A 21-year-old male with a fractured femur

   ○ **D.** An 8-year-old with a fractured arm

5. An elderly female is admitted with a fractured right femoral neck. Which assessment finding is expected?

   ○ **A.** Free movement of the right leg

   ○ **B.** Abduction of the right leg

   ○ **C.** Internal rotation of the right hip

   ○ **D.** Shortening of the right leg

6. The nurse is caring for a client with osteoporosis who is being discharged on alendronate (Fosamax). Which statement would indicate effective teaching?

   ○ **A.** "I should take the medication immediately before bedtime."

   ○ **B.** "I should remain in an upright position for 30 minutes after taking the medication."

   ○ **C.** "The medication is more effective if I take it with milk or dairy products."

   ○ **D.** "If I skip a dose, I can take two tablets the next time."

7. The nurse has a client with knee surgery who is receiving patient-controlled analgesia (PCA) of meperidine (Demerol). Which assessment finding would be a priority due to the use of this device and medication?

   ○ **A.** Pulse rate 108

   ○ **B.** 100 cc of green emesis

   ○ **C.** Respiratory rate of 10

   ○ **D.** Lack of pain relief

8. A client with a below-the-knee amputation is experiencing phantom limb pain. Which action by the nurse would be most effective in relieving the pain?

   ○ **A.** Acknowledging the presence of the pain

   ○ **B.** Elevating the stump on a pillow

   ○ **C.** Applying a transcutaneous nerve stimulator unit (TENS)

   ○ **D.** Rewrapping the stump

9. A client is being evaluated for carpal tunnel syndrome. The nurse is observed asking the client to place the backs of her hands together and flex them at the same time. Which assessment is the nurse performing?

   ○ **A.** Phalen's maneuver

   ○ **B.** Tinel's sign

   ○ **C.** Kernig's

   ○ **D.** Brudzinski's

10. The nurse is caring for a client recovering from a fracture. Which diet selection would be best for this client?

    ○ **A.** Fried chicken, a loaded baked potato, and tea

    ○ **B.** Dressed cheeseburger, French fries, and soda

    ○ **C.** Tuna fish salad on sourdough bread, potato chips, and skim milk

    ○ **D.** Broiled chicken, Mandarin orange salad, and milk

Answer Rationales

1. Answer B is correct. The client has an open fracture. The priority would be to cover the wound and prevent further contamination. Manual traction should not be attempted, so answer A is incorrect. Swelling usually occurs with a fracture, making answer C an incorrect option. Preventing contamination would have priority over immobilization at this point, so answer D is incorrect.

2. Answer D is correct. Fish should be avoided on a low-purine diet. Other foods to avoid include poultry, liver, lobster, oysters, peas, spinach, and oatmeal. Answers A, B, and C are all foods included on a low-purine diet, which makes them incorrect.

3. Answer C is correct. The client with joint hip replacement should avoid adduction of the legs and flexion of the hips greater than 90° to ensure continued placement of the prosthetic joint. It is recommended for these clients to use recliners for seating instead of straight chairs, therefore A is incorrect. Commode seats will have to be raised and abduction of the legs is required, making B and D incorrect choices.

4. Answer C is correct. Fat emboli occur more frequently with long bone or pelvic fractures and usually in young adults age 20–30. Answers A, B, and D are not high-risk incidents and do not fall in the greater risk category, so they are incorrect.

5. Answer D is correct. The symptoms of this fracture include shortened, adducted, and external rotation. Answer A is incorrect because the patient usually is unable to move the leg due to pain. Answer B is incorrect because the symptom is adduction, not abduction. Answer C is wrong because it's external rotation, not internal rotation.

6. Answer B is correct. This is required to prevent esophageal problems. The medication should be taken in the morning before food or other medications with water, making answers A and C incorrect choices. It should also be taken as ordered, which makes answer D incorrect.

7. Answer C is correct. The patient is in danger of respiratory depression due to narcotic administration; therefore, this would be a priority assessment. Answer A does not relate to the PCA, so it is incorrect. Answer B is not a priority, making it wrong. Pain relief in answer D is important, but not as important as airway, so it is incorrect.

8. Answer C is correct. The TENS unit is applied for pain relief. This is the only option that actually does anything about the pain the client is experiencing. Answers A, B, and D might help the pain, but answer C would help more, so those answers are wrong.

9. Answer A is correct. This test is used to check for paresthesia in the median nerve. An abnormal result would be paresthesia within 60 seconds of performing the test. Answer B is incorrect because it is another test used in which the nurse taps over the median nerve in the wrist or uses a BP cuff inflated to the patient's systolic pressure, resulting in pain and tingling. Answers C and D are both incorrect because these are methods of assessment for menengeal irritation and have nothing to do with carpal tunnel.

10. Answer D is correct. This diet selection is the most balanced and the best to promote healing. Answers A, B, and C are not as inclusive as answer D, so they are incorrect.

Suggested Reading and Resources

▶ Brunner, L., and Suddarth, D. *Textbook of Medical-Surgical Nursing*. 12th ed. Philadelphia: Lippincott Williams & Wilkins, 2009.

▶ Hogan, M. *Child Health Nursing Reviews and Rationales*. 2nd ed. Upper Saddle River, NJ: Pearson Prentice Hall, 2007.

▶ Ignatavicius, D., Workman, S. *Medical-Surgical Nursing: Critical Thinking for Collaborative Care*. 6th ed. Philadelphia: Elsevier, 2007.

▶ Deglin, J., and Vallerand, A., *Davis Drug Guide for Nurses*. Philadelphia: F.A. Davis, 2009.

▶ Lewis, S., Heitkemper, M., Dirkson, S., O Brien, P., and Bucher, L. *Medical Surgical Nursing: Assessment and Management of Clinical Problems*. 7th ed. Philadelphia: Elsevier, 2007.

▶ Rinehart, W., Sloan, D., and Hurd, C. *NCLEX Exam Cram*. Indianapolis: Que, 2007.

▶ Lacharity, L., Kumagai, C., and Bartz, B. *Prioritization, Delegation, & Assignment*. 2nd ed. St. Louis: Mosby Elsevier, 2006, 2011.

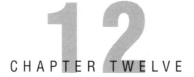

CHAPTER TWELVE

Caring for the Client with Disorders of the Endocrine System

Terms you'll need to understand

- ✓ Chvostek's sign
- ✓ Corticosteroids
- ✓ Cretinism
- ✓ Cushing's syndrome
- ✓ Dwarfism
- ✓ Endocrine
- ✓ Exophthalmoses
- ✓ Glucocorticoids
- ✓ Goiter
- ✓ Graves' disease
- ✓ Hashimoto's disease
- ✓ Hormones
- ✓ Myxedema
- ✓ Syndrome of inappropriate antidiuretic hormone (SIADH)
- ✓ Thyroid-stimulating hormone (TSH)
- ✓ Thyroid storm
- ✓ Transphenoidal hypophysectomy
- ✓ Trousseau's sign

The Endocrine System

The endocrine system is made up of a group of glands that are responsible for secretion of hormones. These hormones work in conjunction with other systems of the body to regulate various body systems. The endocrine system includes:

▶ Pituitary gland

▶ Thyroid gland

▶ Parathyroid glands

▶ Adrenal glands

▶ Pancreas

▶ Gonads

▶ Thymus

This chapter will discuss the most common disorders of the endocrine system and their treatments.

Pituitary Disorders

The pituitary gland is located adjacent to the brain in the midbrain area and works with the hypothalamus to regulate various body functions. Hormones secreted by the anterior lobe and the hypothalamus are as follows:

▶ **Growth hormone (somatrotropin) and growth hormone releasing hormone (GH-RH)**—Regulates cell division and protein synthesis

▶ **Adrenocorticotropic hormone and corticotrophin releasing hormone (PIH)**—Regulates functions of the adrenal cortex

▶ **Follicle-stimulating hormone**—Regulates ovulation

▶ **Prolactin and prolactin inhibiting hormone (PIH)**—Regulates breast milk production

▶ **Luteinizing Hormone**—Assists with ovulation

▶ **Melanocyte**—Stimulating hormone that influences melanin formation which causes color changes in the skin and hair.

▶ **Thyroid stimulating hormone and thyrotropin releasing hormone**—Regulates functional activity of the thyroid

> ▶ **Gonadotrophic hormone**—Stimulates development of ovarian follicles in females and spermatogenesis in males

The posterior pituitary regulates:

> ▶ Vasopressin— (antidiuretic hormone) (ADH)

> ▶ Oxytocin—Regulates uterine contractions and mammary function

Tumors of the Pituitary

Tumors of the pituitary tend to be benign, but due to their location they can be fatal. Depending on the area of the tumor, several problems can arise. Elevations in prolactin inhibit the secretion of gonadal steroids and gonadotropins in men and women, resulting in galactorrhea, amenorrhea, and infertility. Overproduction of growth hormone results in gigantism or acromegaly. If the disorder is noted prior to puberty, a diagnosis of *gigantism* is made. If the disorder occurs in the adult, it is known as *acromegaly*. Because growth hormone is an insulin antagonist, hyperglycemia can also occur.

Tumors of the posterior pituitary can result in syndrome of inappropriate antidiuretic hormone (SIADH) or Diabetes Insipidus (DI).

SIADH is an excessive amount of anti-diuretic hormone. This excess results in water intoxication and hyponatremia. Some causes include:

> ▶ Oat cell cancer of the lung

> ▶ Cancers of the pancreas

> ▶ Hodgkin's lymphoma

> ▶ Leukemia

> ▶ Head trauma

> ▶ Hydrocephalus

> ▶ Infections of the brain

> ▶ Brain hemorrhage

After a diagnosis is made, the client is managed with fluid restriction, especially water intake. The nurse should monitor the serum sodium and chloride levels to check for hyponatremia. Daily weights and checks for urine specific gravity should also be assessed. IV hypertonic saline solution and demeclocycline (Declomycin) is used to replace electrolytes. The nurse should monitor the client's vital signs and level of consciousness and offer nutritional support. Diuretics may be ordered to help eliminate excess water.

NOTE

Normal specific gravity is 1.010-1.030.

Diabetes insipidus is a result of a lack of antidiuretic hormone. This lack of ADH results from a lack of secretion or the kidneys' inability to regulate the amount of ADH being utilized.

Some causes include:

▶ Head trauma

▶ Pituitary tumors

▶ Craniotomy

The result of this lack of ADH is polyuria with an extremely low specific gravity. Polyuria often leads to dehydration, hypovolemia, and alterations in serum sodium levels. Serum sodium levels are often greater than 145 mg/dl. When polyuria occurs, the client experiences extreme thirst often called polydipsia.

Management includes monitoring of intake and output, daily weight, and monitoring of urine specific gravity. Medication often used to treat diabetes insipidus include Desmopressin (DDAVP), supplemental ADH, chlorpropamide (Diabenese), carbamazepine (Tegretol), and IV replacement of fluids and electrolytes.

Other pituitary tumors cause symptoms that are much like brain tumors. These symptoms include:

▶ Diminished vision due to pressure on the optic chiasm

▶ Headache and a feeling of "fullness" in the head

▶ Amenorrhea

▶ Sterility

▶ Increased growth plates

▶ Skeletal thickness

▶ Hypertrophy of the skin

▶ Enlargement of the visceral organs, such as the heart and liver

Management of the client with a pituitary tumor involves

▶ Surgery using a transphenoidal approach

▶ Radiation

▶ Chemotherapy

▶ Bromocriptine mesylate (Parlodel) and cabergoline (Dostinex), which are used to treat prolactinoma, which is a prolactin-based tumor.

NOTE

Bromocriptine mesylate (Parlodel) should not be given to a pregnant client. To decrease gastrointestinal symptoms, this drug should be given with food.

CAUTION

A client with transphenoidal surgery has no incision. An instrument is passed through the nose and the sphenoid sinuses to locate the tumor and remove it. The client often returns from surgery with nose packings in place. Assessment of the airway is the nurse's priority. The presence of a halo sign on the nasal dressing indicates the presence of cerebrospinal fluid.

Thyroid Disorders

The thyroid is located below the larynx and anterior to the trachea. The thyroid gland produces two iodine-dependent hormones (thyroxin and thyroid-stimulating hormone) that regulate the metabolic processes controlling the rate of growth, oxygen consumption, contractility of the heart, and calcium absorption.

Hypothyroidism

Hypothyroidism is caused by a deficiency of thyroid hormone. In the adult this is called _myxedema,_ and in the infant it is called _cretinism._

Signs and symptoms of hypothyroidism in the adult are as follows:

▶ Fatigue and lethargy

▶ Decreased body temperature

▶ Decreased pulse rate

▶ Decreased blood pressure

▶ Weight gain

▶ Edema of hands and feet

▶ Hair loss

▶ Thickening of the skin

Signs and Symptoms of Hypothyroidism in the Infant

As mentioned previously, hypothyroidism in an infant is called *cretinism*. The following list gives you the signs and symptoms of cretinism:

▶ Decreased respirations

▶ Changes in skin color (jaundice or cyanosis)

▶ Poor feeding

▶ Hoarse cry

▶ Mental retardation in those not detected or improperly treated

Diagnostic studies for cretinism include evaluation of T3 and T4 levels using test doses of thyroid-stimulating hormone.

Managing Hypothyroidism

Management of the client with hypothyroidism includes the replacement of thyroid hormone, usually in the form of synthetic thyroid hormone (Synthroid). The client's history should include other drugs the client is taking. Prior to administering thyroid medications, the pulse rate should be evaluated. If the pulse rate is above 100 in the adult or above 120 in the infant, the physician should be notified. Clients with hypothyroidism are more comfortable in a warm environment. Because constipation is often a problem, a high fiber diet is suggested.

Hyperthyroidism

Hyperthyroidism, or Graves' disease, results from an increased production of thyroid hormone. The most common cause of hyperthyroidism is hyperplasia of the thyroid, commonly referred to as a *goiter*. Signs and symptoms of hyperthyroidism include

▶ Increased heart rate and pulse pressure

▶ Tremors, or nervousness

▶ Moist skin and sweating

▶ Increased activity

▶ Insomnia

▶ Atrial fibrillation

▶ Increased appetite and weight loss

▶ Exopthalmos

> **CAUTION**
>
> A *thyroid storm* is an abrupt onset of the symptoms of hyperthyroidism. These symptoms result from inadequate treatment, trauma, infection, surgery, embolus, diabetic ketoacidosis, emotional upset, or toxemia of pregnancy. This collection of symptoms represents a medical emergency that requires immediate intervention.

Diagnosis of hyperthyroidism involves the evaluation of T3 and T4 levels and a thyroid scan with or without contrast media. These thyroid function studies tell the physician if the client has an adequate amount of circulating thyroid hormone. A thyroid scan can clarify the presence of or an enlargement of a tumor of the thyroid gland.

Management of the client with hyperthyroidism includes

▸ The use of antithyroid drugs (propylthiouracil or tapazole)

▸ Radioactive iodine, which can be used to test and to destroy portions of the gland

▸ Surgical removal of a portion of the gland

Prior to thyroid surgery, the client is given Lugol's solution—an iodine preparation—to decrease the vascularity of the gland. Post-operatively the client should be carefully assessed for the following:

▸ Edema and swelling of the airway (the surgical incision is located at the base of the neck anterior to the trachea)

▸ Bleeding (check for bleeding behind the neck)

▸ Tetany, nervousness, and irritability (complications resulting from damage to the parathyroid)

> **CAUTION**
>
> Because the thyroid is located anterior to the trachea, any surgery in this area may result in swelling of the trachea. For this reason it is imperative that the nurses be prepared for laryngeal swelling and occlusion of the airway. The nurse should keep a tracheostomy set at the bedside and call the doctor if the client has changes in his voice or signs of laryngeal stridor. The nurse should instruct the client to keep the head and neck as straight as possible and to support the neck when getting out of bed.

Parathyroid Disorders

The parathyroid glands are four small glands located on the thyroid gland. The primary function of the parathyroid glands is the regulation of calcium and phosphorus. Diagnosis of parathyroid disorders is based on an evaluation of serum calcium and serum phosphorus levels and 24-hour urine levels of calcium and phosphorus. Radioimmunoassay exams are used to check serum parathormone. Potential disorders of these glands include hypoparathyroidism and hyperparathyroidism.

Hypoparathyroidism

Hypoparathyroidism is an inadequate production of parathormone. This hormone is responsible for the regulation of calcium and phosphorus levels in the blood. Calcium and phosphorus levels must be maintained within normal limits to have adequate nerve function. Bone density is also maintained by the parathormone. Signs and symptoms of hypoparathyroidism include the following:

▶ Decreased blood calcium

▶ Increased blood phosphorus

▶ Neuromuscular hyperexcitability

▶ Carpopedal spasms

▶ Urinary frequency

▶ Mood changes (depression)

▶ Dry, scaly skin and thin hair

▶ Cataracts

▶ Changes in teeth (cavities)

▶ Seizures

▶ Changes in EKG (prolonged QT intervals and inverted T waves)

▶ Checking Trousseau's sign, which is carpopedal spasms (noted when the blood pressure cuff is inflated on the arm) or checking the Chvostek's sign (noted when the facial nerve [C7] and trigemmial nerve [C5] is tapped with the nurse's index finger and grimacing of the facial muscles is observed)

TIP

Here's a way to remember that the facial nerve is cranial nerve 7: Place your hand on the cheek bone and move your finger out toward the ear and down the jaw line. You will note that you have formed the number seven.

Management of the client with hypoparathyroidism involves the administration of IV calcium gluconate and long-term use of calcium salts. Vitamin D supplements can be given to increase the absorption of calcium preparations as well as calcium in the diet. Parathyroid hormone in the form of Forteo (PTH) can also be given on a long term basis. To prevent the need for life-long treatment with calcium, the client may have a parathyroid transplant (implantation of one or more parathyroid glands to another part of the body).

Hyperparathyroidism

Hyperparathyroidism is the direct opposite of hypoparathyroidism. In this disorder, you find an overproduction of parathormone. Signs and symptoms of hyperparathyroidism include

▶ Decreased blood phosphorus.

▶ Increased blood calcium.

▶ Muscle weakness.

▶ Osteoporosis.

▶ Bone pain and pathological fractures.

▶ Increased urinary output and calcium renal calculi.

▶ Nausea and vomiting.

▶ Changes in ECG (shortened QT interval and signs of heart block). Heart block involves an alteration in the conduction system of the heart. In third and fourth degree heart block there is an alteration in the heart's ability to transmit electrical impulses from the sinus node located in the right atria to the ventricle. This interference in the conduction system may cause a prolonged p-r interval and possibly deletion of atrial contractions.

Managing a client with hyperparathyroidism is accomplished by the removal of the parathyroid. Pre-operative management involves the reduction of calcium levels. Post-operative management includes

▶ Assessment of the client for respiratory distress

▶ Maintaining suction, oxygen, and a tracheostomy set at bedside

▶ Checking for bleeding (1–5 cc's is normal)

▶ Checking the serum calcium level and serum phosphorus

Adrenal Gland Disorders

Adrenal gland disorders result from insufficient production of cortisol or overproduction of cortisol. Two adrenal gland disorders include adrenocortical insufficiency (Addison's disease) and adrenocortical hypersecretion (Cushing's disease).

Adrenocortical Insufficiency (Addison's Disease)

Addison's disease can occur as a result of long-term use of steroids or the rapid cessation of corticosteroids. It may also be caused by sepsis, surgical stress, or hemorrhage of the adrenal glands (Waterhouse-Friderichsen syndrome).

Signs and symptoms associated with Addison's disease include

- Weakness

- Bronze-like pigmentation of the skin

- Decreased glucose levels

- Decreased blood pressure

- Anorexia

- Sparse axillary hair

- Urinary frequency

- Depression

- Addisonian crisis

CAUTION

The symptoms of Addisonian crisis are severe hypotension, cyanosis, and shock. This constitutes an emergency situation. The nurse should call the doctor immediately to obtain orders for medications to treat shock.

Diagnosis of Addison's disease involves an evaluation of serum sodium and chloride levels. Evaluation of ketosteroid and 17-hydroxycorticoids is also done. Adrenal function is evaluated by administering adrenocorticoid stimulating hormone (ACTH) and checking for changes in cortisol levels.

Management of the client with Addison's disease includes the use of intravenous cortisone and plasma expanders to achieve and maintain the blood pressure. Once stable, the client can be given intramuscular cortisol in the form of dexamethasone (Decadron) or orally in the form of prednisolone (Prednisone). The client with Addison's disease requires lifelong maintenance with cortisone. The client should be instructed to take the medication exactly as prescribed and to avoid sudden cessation of the drug.

Adrenocortical Hypersecretion (Cushing's Syndrome) or Cushing's Disease

The term Cushing's disease and Cushing's syndrome are often used interchangeably although they are not the same. Cushing's syndrome or Primary Cushing's Syndrome may be caused by tumors of the adrenal cortex. Secondary Cushing's Syndrome (Cushing's disease) often is caused by pituitary hypothalamus or adrenal cortex problems that result in an increased adrenocorticotropic hormone (ACTH). Long term signs and symptoms associated with Cushing's syndrome or disease include

- ▶ Pendulous abdomen
- ▶ Buffalo hump
- ▶ Moon face
- ▶ Hirsutism (facial hair)
- ▶ Ruddy complexion (dark red)
- ▶ Increased BP
- ▶ Hyperglycemia
- ▶ Osteoporosis
- ▶ Decreased serum potassium and decreased serum chloride
- ▶ Increased 17-hydroxycorticoids
- ▶ Decreased eosinophils and decreased lymphocytes

Management of the client with Cushing's syndrome is accomplished by removing part of the adrenal gland or reducing the amount of cortisone that the client is receiving. Administration of a drug such as spironolactone (Aldactone), a potassium-sparing diuretic, has also been used to reduce the amount of circulating antidiuretic hormone. The treatment for Cushing's syndrome is accomplished by decreasing the amount of cortisone that the client is receiving.

Diabetes Mellitus

Diabetes mellitus is a chronic disorder of carbohydrate metabolism, marked by hyperglycemia and glycosuria resulting in the inadequate production or use of insulin. Diabetes mellitus is believed to be multifactorial in nature (genetic, autoimmune, or insulin resistance). Signs and symptoms associated with it include

▶ **Weight loss**—Insulin is required for carbohydrates to be converted into useable glucose; a lack of insulin results in a lack of glucose with cellular starvation.

▶ **Ketonuria**—The breakdown of fats leads to the production of ketones that causes characteristic fruity breath.

▶ **Polyphagia**—Cellular starvation causes the diabetic to increase food consumption.

▶ **Polyuria**—The kidneys attempt to regulate pH by increasing urinary output of ketones and glucose.

▶ **Polydipsia**—The loss of large amounts of fluid leads to metabolic acidosis and dehydration. To compensate for the fluid loss, the client drinks large amounts of water.

▶ **Delayed wound healing**—Increased blood sugar contributes to poor wound healing.

▶ **Elevated blood glucose**—Related to decreasing function of the isles of Langerhan or insulin resistance. Normal is 70–110 mg/dl.

CAUTION

Uncorrected or improperly managed diabetes mellitus leads to coma and death.

Diagnosis of diabetes mellitus is made by checking blood glucose levels. There are several diagnostic tests that can be performed to determine the presence and extent of diabetes. The following are diagnostic tests done for determining if the client has diabetes and if the client has been compliant to treatment:

▶ **Glucose tolerance test:** The glucose tolerance test is the most reliable diagnostic test for diabetes. Prior to the glucose tolerance test, the client should be instructed to eat a diet high in carbohydrates for three days and remain NPO after midnight the day of the test. The client should come to the office for a fasting blood glucose level, drink a solution high in glucose, and have the blood tested at one and two hours after drinking the glucose solution (glucola) for a test of glucose in the serum. A diagnosis of diabetes is made when the venous blood glucose is greater than 200 mg/dl two hours after the test.

▶ **Fasting blood glucose levels:** The normal fasting blood glucose is 70–110 mg/dl. A diagnosis of diabetes can be made if the fasting blood glucose level is 140 mg/dl or above on two occasions. A blood glucose level of 800 mg/dl or more, especially if ketones are present, indicates a diagnosis of *hyperosmolar hyperglycemic nonketotic syndrome (HHNKS)*.

▶ **Two-hour post-prandial:** Blood testing for glucose two hours after a meal.

▶ **Dextrostix:** Blood testing for glucose.

▶ **Glycosylated hemoglobin assays (HbA1c):** The best indicator of the average blood glucose for approximately 90–120 days. A finding greater than 7% indicates non-compliance.

▶ **Glycosylated serum proteins and albumin levels:** Become elevated in the same way that HbA1c does. Because serum proteins and albumin turn over in 14 days, however, glycosylated serum albumin (GSA) can be used to indicate blood glucose control over a shorter time.

▶ **Urine checks for glucose:** Ketonuria occurs if blood glucose levels exceed 240 mg/dl.

▶ **Antibodies:** Checked to determine risk factors for the development of type 1 diabetes. Measurement of the cells' antibodies can also determine the rate of progression to diabetes.

Management of the client with diabetes mellitus includes the following:

▶ **Diet**—The diet should contain a proper balance of carbohydrates, fats, and proteins.

▶ **Exercise**—The client should follow a regular exercise program. He should not exercise if his blood glucose is above 240 mg/dl. He should wait until his blood glucose level returns to normal.

▶ **Medications**—Oral antidiabetic agents or insulin.

CAUTION

Because regular insulin peaks in 90–120 minutes and NPH insulin peaks in 8–12 hours, the nurse should instruct the client to draw up the regular insulin (clear) and then draw up the NPH insulin. This prevents contaminating the regular insulin with the NPH insulin.

Because Lantus and Levemir are insulins that are released slowly over an extended time, they should not be mixed in the same syringe with any other insulin. This would cause a client to experience a hypoglycemic reaction.

It is very important that the nurse be aware of the signs of hyperglycemia to teach the client and family. Signs and symptoms of hyperglycemia are

▶ Headache

▶ Nausea/vomiting

▶ Coma

- Flushed, dry skin
- Glucose and acetone in urine

> **TIP**
>
> The following statements are a couple of helpful hints for dealing with diabetes mellitus clients:
> - **Hot and dry; blood sugar high**—This means that if the diabetic's skin is hot and he is dehydrated, his blood glucose level is likely high.
> - **Cold and clammy; need some candy**—This means that if the diabetic's skin is cold and clammy, his blood glucose level is low and he needs a glucose source.

Signs and symptoms of hypoglycemia are

- Headache
- Irritability
- Disorientation
- Nausea/vomiting
- Diaphoresis
- Pallor
- Weakness
- Convulsions
- Coma
- Death

> **CAUTION**
>
> If the client fails to eat her regular bedtime snack, she might experience Somogyi's effect. This abrupt drop in the client's blood glucose level during the night is followed by a false elevation. The treatment of Somogyi's effect is to teach the client to eat a bedtime snack consisting of a protein source, such as peanut butter, and a glass of milk.

Extreme hypoglycemia can be managed with an injectable hormone called glucogon. Cake icing, orange juice, or a similar carbohydrate can be administered. The best bedtime snack is milk and a protein source, such as peanut butter, and crackers.

Diagnostic Tests for Review

The following are diagnostic tests you should review. These tests require the collection of a blood sample to determine the glucose level:

▶ **Glucose tolerance test**—The glucose tolerance test is the most diagnostic test for determining whether the client has diabetes. A high-carbohydrate diet is eaten prior to the exam. The client is told to remain NPO after midnight the day of the test and to come to the clinic for a blood sample to be collected. After a fasting blood sample is obtained, the client is told to drink a liquid containing 75 gm of glucose. A sample of blood is then collected one hour after the glucose is administered. Some physicians also obtain blood samples at two hours or more.

▶ **Fasting blood glucose**—A fasting blood glucose is an excellent method of determining an accurate estimate of the glucose level. It is obtained by asking the client to refrain from eating after midnight and coming to the clinic for a blood sample.

▶ **Dextrostix**—A glucose test that requires a sample of blood be collected, usually prior to meals.

▶ **Hgb A-1C or glycosylated hemoglobin**—A blood test done to determine the client's compliance to his diet and medication regimen. It is obtained by a collection of a blood sample.

Pharmacology Categories for Review

Several drug categories are used in the care of the client with disorders of the endocrine system. The following list highlights the drug categories you should be familiar with:

▶ Antidiabetics

▶ Calcium supplements

▶ Glucocorticoids

▶ Insulins

▶ Mineralcorticoids

▶ Plasma expanders

▶ Synthetic thyroid hormone

▶ Antithyroid medications

▶ Antidiuretic hormone

Exam Prep Questions

1. A client is admitted for removal of a goiter. Which nursing intervention should receive priority during the post-operative period?

   ○ **A.** Maintaining fluid and electrolyte balance

   ○ **B.** Assessing the client's airway

   ○ **C.** Providing needed nutrition and fluids

   ○ **D.** Providing pain relief with narcotic analgesics

2. A client is admitted for treatment of hypoparathyroidism. Based on the client's diagnosis, the nurse would anticipate an order for:

   ○ **A.** Potassium

   ○ **B.** Magnesium

   ○ **C.** Calcium

   ○ **D.** Iron

3. A client with Addison's disease will most likely exhibit which symptom?

   ○ **A.** Hypertension

   ○ **B.** Bronze pigmentation

   ○ **C.** Hirsutism

   ○ **D.** Purple striae

4. A client with Cushing's syndrome should be instructed to:

   ○ **A.** Avoid alcoholic beverages

   ○ **B.** Limit the sodium in her diet

   ○ **C.** Increase servings of dark green vegetables

   ○ **D.** Limit the amount of protein in her diet

5. The client with a suspected pituitary tumor will most likely exhibit symptoms of:

   ○ **A.** Alteration in visual acuity

   ○ **B.** Frequent diarrhea

   ○ **C.** Alterations in blood glucose

   ○ **D.** Urticaria

6. A diabetic client has been maintained on Glucophage (metformin) for regulation of his blood glucose levels. Which teaching should be included in the plan of care?

   ○ **A.** Report changes in urinary pattern.

   ○ **B.** Allow six weeks for optimal effects.

   ○ **C.** Increase the amount of carbohydrates in your diet.

   ○ **D.** Use lotions to treat itching.

7. A client with diabetes experiences Somogyi's effect. To prevent this complication, the nurse should instruct the client to:

   ○ **A.** Take his insulin each day at 1400 hours

   ○ **B.** Engage in physical activity daily

   ○ **C.** Increase the amount of regular insulin

   ○ **D.** Eat a protein and carbohydrate snack at bedtime

8. Which item should be kept at the bedside of a client who has just returned from having a thyroidectomy?

   ○ **A.** A padded tongue

   ○ **B.** An endotracheal tube

   ○ **C.** An airway

   ○ **D.** A tracheostomy set

9. Which vitamin is directly involved in the metabolism of the hormones secreted by the parathyroid?

   ○ **A.** Vitamin C

   ○ **B.** Vitamin D

   ○ **C.** Vitamin K

   ○ **D.** Vitamin B9

10. A client with acromegaly will most likely experience which symptom?

   ○ **A.** Bone pain

   ○ **B.** Frequent infections

   ○ **C.** Fatigue

   ○ **D.** Weight loss

11. A diabetic client is taking Lantus insulin for regulation of his blood glucose levels. The nurse should know that this insulin will most likely be administered:

   ○ **A.** Prior to each meal

   ○ **B.** At night

   ○ **C.** Midday

   ○ **D.** Prior to the evening meal

12. A client with polyuria, polydipsia, and polyphagia is diagnosed with diabetes mellitus. The nurse would expect that these symptoms are related to

   ○ **A.** Hypoglycemia

   ○ **B.** Hyperglycemia

   ○ **C.** Hyperparathyroidism

   ○ **D.** Hyperthyroidism

13. Which laboratory test conducted on the client with diabetes mellitus indicates compliance?

   ○ **A.** Fasting blood glucose

   ○ **B.** Two-hour post-prandial

   ○ **C.** Hgb A-1C

   ○ **D.** Dextrostix

Answer Rationales

1. Answer B is correct. A goiter is hyperplasia of the thyroid gland. Removal of a goiter can result in laryngeal spasms and airway occlusion. The other answers are lesser in priority.

2. Answer C is correct. The parathyroid is responsible for calcium and phosphorus absorption. Clients with hypoparathyroidism have hypocalcemia. Answers A, B, and D are not associated with hypoparathyroidism therefore they are incorrect.

3. Answer B is correct. Answer B is correct because a bronze pigmentation is a sign of Addison's disease. Answers A, C, and D are symptoms of Cushing's syndrome, making them incorrect.

4. Answer B is correct. A client with Cushing's syndrome has adrenocortical hypersecretion, so she retains sodium and water. The client may drink alcohol in moderation, so answer A is incorrect, and there is no need to eat more green vegetables or limit protein, so answers C and D are incorrect.

5. Answer A is correct. The pituitary is located in the middle of the skull adjacent to the optic nerve and brain. Pressure on the optic nerve can cause an increase in intracranial pressure. Clients frequently complain of headache, nausea, vomiting, and decreasing visual acuity as the intracranial pressure increases. B, C, and D are incorrect because they are not associated with a pituitary tumor.

6. Answer A is correct. Glucophage (metformin) can cause renal complications. The client should be monitored for changes in renal function. In answer B, the medication begins working immediately, so it is incorrect. In answer C, the amount of carbohydrates should be regulated with a diabetic diet, so it is incorrect. The use of lotions in answer D is unnecessary, so it is incorrect.

7. Answer D is correct. Somogyi's is characterized by a drop in glucose levels at approximately 2 a.m. or 3 a.m. followed by a false elevation. Eating a protein and carbohydrate snack before retiring prevents the hypoglycemia and rebound elevation. Answers A, B, and C are incorrect because they do not prevent Somogyi's effect.

8. Answer D is correct. Laryngeal swelling is not uncommon in clients following a thyroidectomy. A tracheostomy tray should be kept available. The ventilator is not necessary, so answer A is incorrect. The endotracheal tube is very difficult, if not impossible, to intubate if swelling has already occurred, so answer B is incorrect. The airway will do no good because the swelling is in the trachea, so answer C is incorrect.

9. Answer B is correct. Vitamin D is related to absorption of calcium and phosphorus. A, C, and D are incorrect because they are not related to the absorption of calcium and phosphorus.

10. Answer A is correct. Acromegaly is an increase in secretion of growth hormone. The growth hormones cause expansion and elongation of the bones. Answers B, C, and D are not directly associated with acromegaly, so they are incorrect.

11. Answer B is correct. This insulin, unlike others, is most frequently administered at night. Its duration is 24–36 hours. A, C, and D are incorrect they are incorrect times to administer Lantus insulin.

12. Answer B is correct. The client with hyperglycemia will exhibit polyuria, polydipsia, or increased thirst, and polyphagia, or increased hunger. A, C, and D are incorrect because they are not signs of hypoglycemia.

13. Answer C is correct. The Hgb A-1C indicates that the client has been compliant for approximately three months. Answers A, B, and D tell the nurse the client's blood glucose at the time of the test, so they are incorrect.

Suggested Reading and Resources

▶ American Diabetes Association (http://www.diabetes.org)

▶ Hogan, M. *Medical Surgical Nursing.* 2nd ed. Upper Saddle River, NJ: Pearson Prentice Hall, 2008.

CHAPTER THIRTEEN

Caring for the Client with Disorders of the Cardiovascular System

Terms you'll need to understand

- ✓ Aneurysms
- ✓ Angina pectoris
- ✓ Angioplasty
- ✓ Arterosclerosis
- ✓ Blood pressure
- ✓ Buerger's disease
- ✓ Cardiac catheterization
- ✓ Cardiac tamponade
- ✓ Cardiopulmonary resuscitation
- ✓ Cholesterol
- ✓ Conduction system of the heart
- ✓ Congestive heart failure
- ✓ Coronary artery bypass graft
- ✓ Defibrillation
- ✓ Diastole
- ✓ Electrocardiogram
- ✓ Heart block
- ✓ Hypertension
- ✓ Implantable cardioverter
- ✓ Myocardial infarction
- ✓ Pacemaker
- ✓ Raynaud's
- ✓ Systole
- ✓ Thrombophlebitis
- ✓ Varicose veins
- ✓ Ventricular fibrillation
- ✓ Ventricular tachycardia

Nursing skills you'll need to master

- ✓ Performing cardiopulmonary resuscitation (CPR)
- ✓ Monitoring central venous pressure
- ✓ Monitoring blood pressure
- ✓ Interpreting electrocardiography (ECG)

The cardiovascular system is comprised of the heart and blood vessels and is responsible for the transport of oxygen and nutrients to organ systems of the body. The heart is a cone-shaped organ made up of four chambers. The right side of the heart receives deoxygenated venous blood from the periphery by way of the superior and inferior venae cavae. The left side of the heart receives blood from the lungs and pumps the oxygenated blood to the body. The blood vessels are divided into arteries and veins. Arteries transport oxygenated blood and veins transport deoxygenated blood. In this chapter, you will discover diseases that affect the cardiovascular system, the treatment of these diseases, and the effects on the client's general health status.

Hypertension

Blood pressure is the force of blood exerted on the vessel walls. *Systolic pressure* is the pressure during the contraction phase of the heart and is evaluated as the top number of the blood pressure reading. *Diastolic pressure* is the pressure during the relaxation phase of the heart and is evaluated as the lower number of the blood pressure reading. A diagnosis of hypertension is made by a blood pressure value greater than 140/90 obtained on two separate occasions with the client sitting, standing, and lying. In clients with diabetes, a reading of 130/85 or higher is considered to be hypertension.

Accuracy of the BP reading depends on the correct selection of cuff size. The bladder of the blood pressure cuff size should be sufficient to encircle the arm or thigh. According to the American Heart Association, the bladder width should be approximately 40% of the circumference or 20% wider than the diameter of the midpoint of the extremity. A blood pressure cuff that's too small yields a false high reading, whereas a blood pressure cuff that's too large yields a false low reading.

Hypertension is classified as either primary or secondary. Primary hypertension, or essential hypertension, develops without apparent cause; secondary hypertension develops as a result of another illness or condition. Symptoms associated with secondary hypertension are improved by appropriate treatment of the contributing illness. Blood pressure fluctuates with exercise, stress, changes in position, and changes in blood volume. Medications such as oral contraceptives and bronchodilators can also cause elevations in blood pressure. Often the client with hypertension will have no symptoms at all or might complain of an early morning headache and fatigue. This silent killer, if left untreated, can lead to coronary disease, renal disease, strokes, and other life-threatening illnesses.

Management of hypertension includes a program of diet and exercise. If the client's cholesterol level is elevated, a low-fat, low-cholesterol diet is ordered. The total serum cholesterol levels should be less than 200 mg/dl and serum triglycerides should be less than 150 mg/dl. Current studies show consumption of folic acid can help to lower homocysteine levels. Lowered homocysteine levels may contribute to lowering of blood pressure. Foods such as meats, eggs, and canola oil are rich in monounsaturated fat. Safflower and sunflower oils are high in polyunsaturated oils. These oils are recommended for individuals at risk for coronary disease. The client is taught to avoid palm oil and coconut oil. If a change in diet does not lower the client's cholesterol level, the doctor might prescribe hyperlipidemic medications such as simvastatin (Zocor), gemfibrozil (Lopid), or ezetimibe (Zetia).

Medications Used to Treat Hypertension

Should diet and exercise prove unsuccessful in lowering the blood pressure, the doctor might decide to prescribe medications such as diuretics or antihypertensives. Table 13.1 includes examples of medications used to treat hypertension.

TABLE 13.1   Hypertension Drugs

Drug Category	Drug Types
Diuretics	Thiazide: Chlorothiazide (Diuril), hydrochlorothiazide (Esidrix, HydroDiuril)
	Loop diuretics: Furosemide (Lasix), ethacrynic acid (Edecrin)
	Potassium-sparing diuretics: Spironolactone (Aldactone), triamterone (Dyrenium)
Beta blockers	Propanolol (Inderal), atenolol (Tenormin), nadolol (Corgard)
Calcium channel blockers	Nifedipine (Procardia), verapamil (Calan), diltiazem hydrochloride (Cardizem)
Angiotensin converting	Captopril (Capoten), enalpril (Vasotec), lisinopril (Zestril, Prinivil) enzyme inhibitors
Angiotensin receptor blockers	Candesartan (Altacand), losartan (Cozaar), telmisartan (Micardis)

These drugs can be used alone or in conjunction with one another. Diuretics and vasodilators are often given in combination to lower blood pressure through diuresis and vasodilation. Hypertensive crisis exists when the diastolic blood pressure reaches 140. Malignant hypertension is managed with administration of IV Nitropress, nitroglycerine, Nipride, Lasix, and other potent vasodilators such as Procardia.

Heart Block

The normal conduction system of the heart is comprised of the sinoatrial (SA) node located at the junction of the right atrium and the superior vena cava. This area contains the pacing cells that initiate the contraction of the heart. The SA node is considered to be the main pacer of the heart rate. The atrioventricular (AV) node is located in the interventricular septum and receives the impulse and transmits it on to the Bundle of His, which extends down through the ventricular septum and merges with the Purkinje fibers in the lower portion of the ventricles. Figure 13.1 shows an anatomical drawing of the human heart.

Heart block is a condition in which the conduction system of the heart fails to conduct impulses normally. Heart block can occur as a result of structural changes in the conduction system, such as tumors, myocardial infarctions, coronary artery disease, infections of the heart, or toxic effects of drugs such as digoxin. First-degree AV block occurs when the SA node continues to function normally, but transmission of the impulse fails. Because of the conduction dysfunction and ventricular depolarization, the heart beats irregularly. These clients are usually asymptomatic and all impulses eventually reach the ventricles. Second-degree heart block is a block in which impulses reach the ventricles, but others do not. In third-degree heart block or complete heart block, none of the sinus impulses reach the ventricle. This results in erratic heart rates where the sinus node and the atrioventricular nodes are beating independently. The result of this type of heart block can be hypotension, seizures, cerebral ischemia, or cardiac arrest. Detection of a heart block is made by assessing the electrocardiogram. See Figure 13.2 for a graph depicting a normal electrocardiogram.

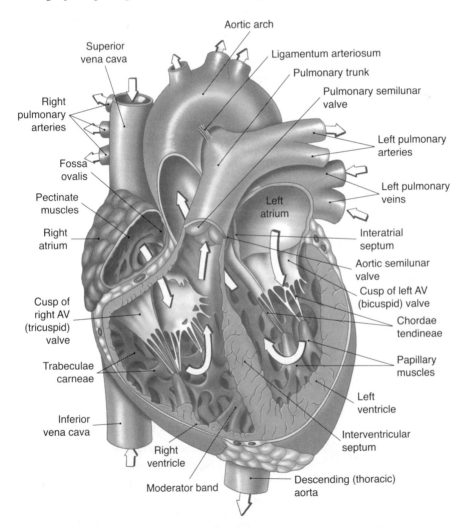

FIGURE 13.1
Anatomical drawing of the heart.

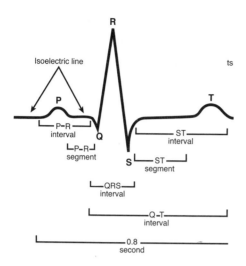

FIGURE 13.2 A normal electrocardiogram.

The P wave as shown in the graph is the SA node firing, the QRS complex is the contraction phase of the heart, and the T wave is the repolarization of the heart.

Toxicity to Medications

Toxicity to medications, such as Digoxin, can be associated with heart block. Clients taking Digitalis should be taught to check their pulse rate and to return to the physician for regular evaluation of their Digitalis level. The therapeutic level for Digoxin is 0.5–2.0 ng/ml. If the client's blood level of Digoxin exceeds 2.0 ng/ml, the client is considered to be toxic. Clients with Digoxin toxicity often complain of nausea, vomiting, and seeing halos around lights. The nurse should teach the client to check his heart rate prior to taking Digoxin. A resting pulse rate of less than 60 bpm in the adult client should alert the nurse to the possibility of toxicity. Treatment for Digoxin toxicity includes checking the potassium level because hypokalemia can contribute to Digoxin toxicity. The physician often will order potassium be given IV or orally and that the Digoxin be held until serum levels return to normal. Other medications, such as Isuprel or Atropine, and Digibind (Digoxin Immune Fab), are frequently ordered to increase the heart rate.

Malfunction of the Conduction System

Because a malfunction of the conduction system of the heart is the most common cause for heart block, a pacing mechanism is frequently implanted to facilitate conduction. Pacemakers can be permanent or temporary and categorized as demand or set. A *demand* pacemaker initiates an impulse if the client's heart rate falls below the prescribed beats per minute. A *set* pacemaker overrides the heart's own conduction system and delivers an impulse at the rate set by the physician. Frequently, pacemakers are also combined with an internal defibrillation device.

Permanent Pacemakers/Internal Defibrillators: What the Client Should Know

Clients with internal defibrillators or pacemakers should be taught to avoid direct contact with electrical equipment. Clients should be instructed to

▶ Wear a medic alert stating that a pacemaker/internal defibrillator is implanted. Identification will alert the healthcare worker so that alterations in care can be made.

▶ Take the pulse for one full minute and report the rate to the physician.

▶ Avoid applying pressure over the pacemaker/internal defibrillator. Pressure on the defibrillator or pacemaker can interfere with the electrical leads.

▶ Inform the dentist of the presence of a pacemaker/internal defibrillator or because electrical devices are often used in dentistry.

▶ Avoid having a magnetic resonance imaging (MRI). Magnetic resonance interferes with the electrical impulse of the implant.

▶ Avoid close contact with electrical appliances, electrical or gasoline engines, transmitter towers, antitheft devices, metal detectors, and welding equipment because they can interfere with the electrical conduction of the device.

▶ Be careful when using microwaves. Microwaves are generally safe for use, but the client should be taught to stand approximately five feet away from the device while cooking.

▶ Report fever, redness, swelling, or soreness at the implantation site.

▶ If a vibration or beeping tone is noted coming from the internal defibrillator, immediately move away from any electromagnetic source. Stand clear from other people because shock can affect anyone touching the client during defibrillation.

▶ Report dizziness, fainting, weakness, blackouts, or a rapid pulse rate. The client will most likely be told not to drive a car for several months after the internal defibrillator is inserted to evaluate any dysrhythmias.

▶ Report persistent hiccupping because this can indicate misfiring of the pacemaker/internal defibrillator.

Myocardial Infarction

When there is a blockage in one or more of the coronary arteries, the client is considered to have had a myocardial infarction. Factors contributing to diminished blood flow to the heart include arteriosclerosis, emboli, thrombus, shock, and hemorrhage. If circulation is not quickly restored to the heart, the muscle becomes necrotic. Hypoxia from ischemia can lead to vasodilation of blood vessels. Acidosis associated with electrolyte imbalances often occurs, and the client can slip into cardiogenic shock. The most common site for a myocardial infarction is the left ventricle. Classic signs of a myocardial infarction include substernal pain or a feeling of heaviness in the chest. However it should be noted that women, elderly clients, and clients with diabetes may fail to report classic symptoms. Women might tell the nurse that pain she is experiencing beneath the shoulder or in the back, anxiety, or a feeling of apprehension and nausea.

The most commonly reported signs and symptoms associated with myocardial infarction include

▸ Sub-sternal pain or pain over the precordium of a duration greater than 15 minutes

▸ Pain that is described as heavy, vise-like, and radiating down the left arm

▸ Pain that begins spontaneously and is not relieved by nitroglycerin or rest

▸ Pain that radiates to the jaw and neck

▸ Pain that is accompanied by shortness of breath, pallor, diaphoresis, dizziness, nausea, and vomiting

▸ Increased heart rate, decreased blood pressure, increased temperature, and increased respiratory rate

CAUTION

Angina pectoris occurs when there are vasospasms. This pain is relieved by nitroglycerine. The client should be taught to take one nitroglycerine tablet sublingually every five minutes. If the first tablet does not relieve the pain, a second can be taken, and if the pain is still not relieved, a third can be taken. If, however, the pain is not relieved after taking three tablets, one every five minutes, the client should come directly to the hospital or call an ambulance. The client should be taught to replenish his supply every six months and protect the pills from light by leaving them in the brown bottle. The cotton should be removed from the bottle because it will decrease the tablets' effectiveness. Most physicians recommend that the client take one 365 mg aspirin at the first sign of chest pain. Aspirin has an anticoagulant effect and decreases the clotting associated with heart attacks.

The nurse must always wear gloves when applying nitroglycerine cream or patches to the client. Clip hair with scissors or shave, but do not abrade area.

Diagnosis of Myocardial Infarction

The diagnosis of a myocardial infarction is made by looking at both the electrocardiogram and the cardiac enzymes. The following are the most commonly used diagnostic tools for determining the type and severity of the attack:

▸ Electrocardiogram (ECG), which frequently shows dysrhythmias

▸ Serum enzymes and isoenzymes

Other tests that are useful in providing a complete picture of the client's condition are white blood cell count (WBC), sedimentation rate, and blood urea nitrogen (BUN).

The best serum enzyme diagnostic is the creatine kinase (CK-MB) diagnostic. This enzyme is released when there is damage to the myocaridium. The Troponin T and 1 are specific to striated muscle and are often used to determine the severity of the attack. C-reactive protein (CRP) levels are used with the CK-MB to determine whether the client has had an acute MI and the severity of the attack. Lactic acid dehydrogenase (LDH) is a nonspecific enzyme that is elevated with any muscle trauma.

Management of Myocardial Infarction Clients

Management of myocardial infarction clients includes monitoring of blood pressure, oxygen levels, and pulmonary artery wedge pressures. Because the blood pressure can fall rapidly, medications such as dopamine is prescribed. Other medications are ordered to relieve pain and to vasodilate the coronary vessels—for example, morphine sulfate IV is ordered for pain. Thrombolytics, such as streptokinase, will most likely be ordered. Early diagnosis and treatment significantly improve the client's prognosis.

Clients suffering a myocardial infarction can present with dysrhythmias. Ventricular dysrhythmias such as ventricular tachycardia or fibrillation lead to standstill and death if not treated quickly.

Ventricular Tachycardia

Ventricular tachycardia is a rapid rhythm absence of a p-wave. Usually the rate exceeds 140–180 bpm. A lethal arrhythmia that leads to ventricular fibrillation and standstill, ventricular tachycardia is often associated with valvular heart disease, heart failure, hypomagnesium, hypotension, and ventricular aneurysms. Figure 13.3 shows a diagram demonstrating ventricular tachycardia.

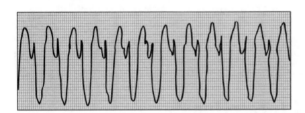

FIGURE 13.3 Evidence of ventricular tachycardia.

Ventricular tachycardia is treated with oxygen and medication. Examples of medications used to treat ventricular tachycardia are Amiodarone (Cordarone), procainamide (Pronestyl), or magnesium sulfate. These drugs are given to slow the rate and stabilize the rhythm. Lidocaine has long been established for the treatment of ventricular tachycardia; however, it should not be used in an acute MI client. Heparin is also ordered to prevent further thrombus formation but is not generally ordered with clients taking streptokinase.

Ventricular Fibrillation

Ventricular fibrillation (V-fib) is the primary mechanism associated with sudden cardiac arrest. This disorganized, chaotic rhythm results in a lack of pumping activity of the heart. Without effective pumping, no blood is sent to the brain and other vital organs. If this condition is not corrected quickly, the client's heart stops beating and asystole is seen on the ECG. The client quickly becomes faint, loses consciousness, and becomes pulseless. Hypotension or a lack of blood pressure and heart sounds are present. Figure 13.4 shows a diagram of the chaotic rhythms typical with V-fib.

Ventricular Fibrillation
(V Fib)

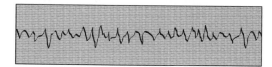

"sawtooth"

FIGURE 13.4   Ventricular fibrillation diagram.

Treatment of ventricular fibrillation is to defibrillate the client starting with 200 Joules. Three quick, successive shocks are delivered with the third at 360 Joules. If a defibrillator is not readily available, a precordial thump can be delivered. Oxygen is administered and antidysrhythmic medications such as epinephrine, amiodarone, procainamide, lidocaine, or magnesium sulfate are ordered. If cardiac arrest occurs, the nurse should initiate cardiopulmonary resuscitation and be ready to administer first-line drugs such as epinephrine.

Cardiac catheterization is used to detect blockages associated with myocardial infarctions and dysrhythmias. Cardiac catheterization, as with any other dye procedure, requires a permit. This procedure can also accompany percutaneous transluminal coronary angioplasty. Prior to and following this procedure, the nurse should

- ▶ Assess for allergy to iodine or shellfish.

- ▶ Maintain the client on bed rest with the leg straight.

- ▶ Maintain pressure on the access site for at least five minutes or until no signs of bleeding are noted. Many cardiologists use a device called Angio Seals to prevent bleeding at the insertion site. The device creates a mechanical seal anchoring a collagen sponge to the site. The sponge absorbs in 60–90 days.

- ▶ Use pressure dressing and/or ice packs to control bleeding.

▶ Check distal pulses because diminished pulses can indicate a hematoma and should be reported immediately.

▶ Force fluids to clear dye from the body.

If the client is not a candidate for angioplasty, a coronary artery bypass graft might be performed. The family should be instructed that the client will return to the intensive care unit with several tubes and monitors. The client will have chest tubes and a mediastinal tube to drain fluid and to reinflate the lungs. If the client is bleeding and blood is not drained from the mediastinal area, fluid accumulates around the heart. This is known as *cardiac tamponade*. If this occurs, the myocardium becomes compressed and the accumulated fluid prevents the filling of the ventricles and decreases cardiac output.

A Swan-Ganz catheter for monitoring central venous pressure, pulmonary artery wedge pressure monitor, and radial arterial blood pressure monitor are inserted to measure vital changes in the client's condition. An ECG monitor and oxygen saturation monitor are also used. Other tubes include a nasogastric tube to decompress the stomach, a endotracheal tube to assist in ventilation, and a Foley catheter to measure hourly output.

Following a myocardial infarction, the client should be given small, frequent meals. The diet should be low in sodium, fat, and cholesterol. Adequate amounts of fluid and fiber are encouraged to prevent constipation, and stool softeners are also ordered. Post-MI teaching should stress the importance of a regular program of exercise, stress reduction, and cessation of smoking. Because caffeine causes vasoconstriction, caffeine intake should be limited. The client can resume sexual activity in six weeks or when he is able to climb a flight of stairs without experiencing chest pain. Medications such as Viagra are discouraged and should not be taken within 24 hours of taking a nitrate because taking these medications in combination can result in hypotension. Clients should be taught not to perform the Valsalva maneuver or bend at the waist to retrieve items from the floor. The client will probably be discharged on an anticoagulant such as enoxaparin (Lovenox) or sodium warfarin (Coumadin).

CAUTION

Anticoagulants such as heparin are used. The nurse should check the partial thromboplastin time (PTT). PTT levels vary. The normal control level is approximately 30–60 seconds (this range tends to vary dependent on the laboratory methods used). The therapeutic bleeding time should be from one and a half to two times the control. The medication should be injected in the abdomen two inches from the umbilicus using a tuberculin syringe. Do not aspirate or massage. The antidote for heparin derivatives is protamine sulfate. Lovenox (enoxaparin) is a heparin derivative. There is no specific bleeding time used for Lovenox, but the platelet count should be checked prior to administration of Lovenox. The nurse should not expel the air from the syringe prior to injection of the medication.

Inflammatory Diseases of the Heart

Inflammatory and infectious diseases of the heart often are a result of systemic infections that affect the heart. Inflammation and infection might involve the endocardium, pericardium, valves, or the entire heart.

Infective Endocarditis

Infective endocarditis, also known as *bacterial endocarditis*, is usually the result of a bacterial infections, collagen diseases, or cancer metastasis. As a result, the heart is damaged and signs of cardiac decompensation results. The client commonly complains of shortness of breath, fatigue, and chest pain. On assessment, the nurse might note distended neck veins, a friction rub, or a cardiac murmur.

Treatment involves treating the underlying cause with antibiotics, anti-inflammatory drugs, and oxygen therapy. Bed rest is recommended until symptoms subside. If the valve is severely damaged by infection, a valve replacement might have to be performed. Replacement valves are xenograft (bovine [cow] or porcine [pig]), cadaver, or mechanical. If the client elects to have a mechanical valve replacement, he will have to take anticoagulants for life. Following surgery, the nurse must be alert for signs of complications. These include decreased cardiac output or heart failure, infection, and bleeding. The physician often will prescribe digoxin, anticoagulants, cortisone, and antibiotics postoperatively.

> **NOTE**
>
> A porcine valve will probably be rejected by the client who is Jewish. A bovine valve will probably be rejected by the client who is Hindu.

Pericarditis

Pericarditis is an inflammatory condition of the pericardium, which is the membrane sac around the heart. Symptoms include chest pain, difficulty breathing, fever, and orthopnea. Clients with chronic constrictive pericarditis show signs of right-sided congestive heart failure. During auscultation, the nurse will likely note a pericardial friction rub. Laboratory findings might show an elevated white cell count. ECG changes consist of an S-T segment and T wave elevation. The echocardiogram often shows pericardial effusion.

Treatment includes use of nonsteroidal anti-inflammatory drugs to relieve pain. The nurse should monitor the client for signs of pericardial effusion and cardiac tamponade that include jugular vein distention, *paradoxical pulses* (systolic blood pressure higher on expiration than on inspiration), decreased cardiac output, and muffled heart sounds. If fluid accumulates in an amount that causes cardiac constriction, the physician might decide to perform a pericardio-centesis to relieve the pressure around the heart. Using an echocardiogram or fluoroscopic monitor, the physician inserts a large-bore needle into the pericardial sac. After the procedure, the nurse should monitor the client's vital signs and heart sounds. In severe cases, the pericardium might be removed.

> **NOTE**
>
> If the client has a history of pericarditis or endocarditis and is scheduled for dental work or surgery, he/she may be placed on prophylactic antibiotics to prevent exacerbation of his/her condition.

> **CAUTION**
>
> A blood test called International normalizing ratio (INR) is often done to determine therapeutic level of oral anticoagulants. Prior to treatment the normal level is 1-2. The therapeutic range is 2–3. If the level exceeds 7, the nurse should observe the client for spontaneous bleeding.

Buerger's Disease

Buerger's disease (thromboangilitis obliterans) results when spasms of the arteries and veins occur primarily in the lower extremities. These spasms result in blood clot formation and eventually destruction of the vessels. Symptoms associated with Buerger's include pallor of the extremities progressing to cyanosis, pain, and paresthesia. As time progresses, tophic changes occur in the extremities. Management of the client with Buerger's involves the use of Buerger-Allen exercises, vasodilators, and oxygenation. The client should be encouraged to stop smoking because smoking makes the condition worse.

Thrombophlebitis

Thrombophlebitis occurs when there is an inflammation of a vein with formation of a clot. Most thrombophlebitis occurs in the lower extremities, with the saphenous vein being the most common vein affected. Homan's sign is an assessment tool used for many years by health-care workers to detect deep vein thrombi. It is considered positive if the client complains of pain on dorsiflexion of the foot. Homan's sign should not be performed routinely because it can cause a clot to be dislodged and lead to pulmonary emboli. If a diagnosis of throm-bophlebitis is made, the client should be placed on bed rest with warm, moist compresses to the leg. An anticoagulant is ordered, and the client is monitored for complications such as cellulitis. If cellulitis is present, antibiotics are ordered.

Antithrombotic stockings or sequential compression devices are ordered to prevent venous stasis. When antithrombolitic stockings are applied, the client should be in bed for a minimum of 30 minutes prior to applying the stockings. The circumference and length of the extremity should be measured to prevent rolling down of the stocking and a tourniquet effect.

Raynaud's Syndrome

Raynaud's syndrome occurs when there are vascular spasms brought on by exposure to cold. The most commonly effected areas are the hands, nose, and ears. Management includes preventing exposure, stopping smoking, and using vasodilators. The client should be encouraged to wear mittens when outside in cold weather.

Aneurysms

An *aneurysm* is a ballooning of an artery. The greatest risk for these clients is rupture and hemorrhage. Aneurysms can occur in any artery in the body and can be due to congenital malformations or arteriosclerosis or be secondary to hypertension. The following are several types of aneurysms:

▶ **Fusiform**—This aneurysm affects the entire circumference of the artery.

▶ **Saccular**—This aneurysm is an outpouching affecting only one portion of the artery.

▶ **Dissecting**—This aneurysm results in bleeding into the wall of the vessel.

Frequently, the client with an abdominal aortic aneurysm complains of feeling her heart beating in her abdomen or lower back pain. Any such complaint should be further evaluated. On auscultation of the abdomen, a bruit can be heard. Diagnosis can be made by ultrasound, arteriogram, or abdominal x-rays.

If the aneurysm is found to be approximately six centimeters or more, surgery should be scheduled. During surgery the aorta is clamped above and below and a donor vessel is anastamosed in place. When the client returns from surgery, pulses distal to the site should be assessed and urinary output should be checked. Clients who are not candidates for surgery might elect to have stent placement to reinforce the weakened artery. These stents are threaded through an incision in the femoral artery, hold the artery open, and provide support for the weakened vessel. See Figure 13.5 for a diagram of an abdominal aortic aneurysm.

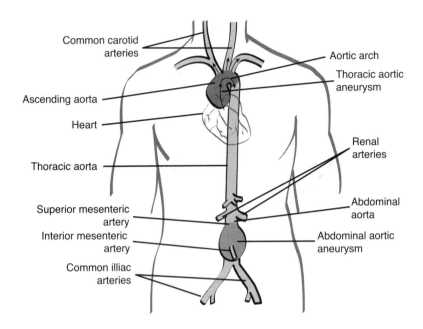

FIGURE 13.5
Abdominal aortic
aneurysm.

> **CAUTION**
>
> Avoid palpating the abdomen of the client with a suspected abdominal aortic aneurysm.

Congestive Heart Failure

When fluid accumulation occurs and the heart is no longer able to pump in an efficient manner, blood can back up. Most heart failure occurs when the left ventricle fails. When this occurs, the fluid backs up into the lungs, causing pulmonary edema. The signs of pulmonary edema are frothy, pink-tinged sputum; shortness of breath; and orthopnea. Distended jugular veins might also be present. When right-sided congestive heart failure occurs, the blood backs up into the periphery. The nurse might also note signs of pitting edema. Pitting can be evaluated by pressing on the extremities and noting the degree of pitting, how far up the extremity the pitting occurs, and how long it takes to return to the surface. Treatment for congestive heart failure includes use of diuretics, inotropic drugs such as milrinone (Primacor), and cardiotonics such as nesiritide (Natrecor). Morphine might also be ordered.

Diagnostic Tests for Review

The following diagnostic test should be reviewed prior to taking the NCLEX exam:

▶ **CBC**—A complete blood count tells the nurse the level of oxygenation of the blood, particularly the hemoglobin and hematocrit.

▶ **Chest x-ray**—Chest x-rays and other x-rays tell the nurse whether the heart is enlarged or aneurysms are present.

▶ **Arteriogram**—Arteriography reveals the presence of blockages and abnormalities in the vascular system.

▶ **Cardiac catheterization**—A cardiac catheterization reveals blockages, turbulent flow, and arteriosclerotic heart disease.

▶ **ECG interpretation**—Indicates abnormalities in the rate and rhythm of the conductions system of the heart.

▶ **Central venous pressure monitoring**—CVP indicates fluid volume status.

▶ **B-type natriuretic peptide (BNP)**—Used to diagnose heart failure in clients with acute dyspnea. It is used to differentiate dyspnea found in those with lung disorders from those with congestive heart failure.

▶ **Stress**—A stress test can be done using a treadmill. The client is asked to walk at a rapid rate to increase the work load on the heart. The client's blood pressure and heart rhythm is then observed for abnormal changes. A non-treadmill stress test is used when the client is unable to walk on the treadmill machine. This test is used to determine ischemia. A radionuclide such as Thallium or Cardiolite is injected at the peak of exercise. A creatinine should be checked to determine renal function. The client should be questioned regarding allergies to iodine or shell-fish.

Pharmacology Categories for Review

The following pharmacology categories should be reviewed prior to taking the NCLEX exam:

▶ Diuretics

▶ Cardiotonics

▶ Antihypertensives

▶ Anticoagulants

▶ Thrombolytics

▶ Inotropic

▶ Analgesics

Exam Prep Questions

1. The client presents to the clinic with a serum cholesterol of 275 mg/dl and is placed on rosuvastatin (Crestor). Which instruction should be given to the client?

   ○ **A.** Report muscle weakness to the physician.

   ○ **B.** Allow six months for the drug to take effect.

   ○ **C.** Take the medication with fruit juice.

   ○ **D.** Ask the doctor to perform a complete blood count prior to starting the medication.

2. The client is admitted to the hospital with a hypertensive crisis. Diazoxide (Hyperstat) is ordered. During administration the nurse should:

   ○ **A.** Utilize an infusion pump.

   ○ **B.** Check the blood glucose level.

   ○ **C.** Place the client in Trendelenburg position.

   ○ **D.** Cover the solution with foil.

3. A six-month-old client with a ventricular septal defect is receiving Lanoxin elixir for regulation of his heart rate. Which finding should be reported to the doctor?

   ○ **A.** A blood pressure of 126/80

   ○ **B.** A blood glucose of 110 mg/dl

   ○ **C.** A heart rate of 60 bpm

   ○ **D.** A respiratory rate of 30 per minute

4. The client admitted with angina is given a prescription for nitroglycerine. The client should be instructed to:

   ○ **A.** Replenish her supply every three months.

   ○ **B.** Take one every 15 minutes if pain occurs.

   ○ **C.** Leave the medication in the brown bottle.

   ○ **D.** Crush the medication and take it with water.

5. A 54-year-old male is admitted to the cardiac unit with chest pain radiating to the jaw and left arm. Which enzyme would be most specific in the diagnosis of a myocardial infarction?

  ○ **A.** Aspartate aminotransferase

  ○ **B.** Lactic acid dehydrogenase

  ○ **C.** Hydroxybutyric dehydrogenase

  ○ **D.** Creatine phosphokinase

6. The client is instructed regarding foods that are low in fat and cholesterol. Which diet selection is lowest in saturated fats?

  ○ **A.** Macaroni and cheese

  ○ **B.** Shrimp with rice

  ○ **C.** Turkey breast

  ○ **D.** Spaghetti and meatballs

7. The client is admitted with left-sided congestive heart failure. In assessing the client for edema, the nurse should check the:

  ○ **A.** Feet

  ○ **B.** Neck

  ○ **C.** Hands

  ○ **D.** Sacrum

8. The nurse is checking the client's central venous pressure. The nurse should place the zero of the manometer at the:

  ○ **A.** Phlebostatic axis

  ○ **B.** Point of maximum impulse (PMI)

  ○ **C.** Erb's point

  ○ **D.** Tail of Spence

9. The physician orders lisinopril (Zestril) and furosemide (Lasix) to be administered concomitantly to the client with hypertension. The nurse should:

  ○ **A.** Question the order.

  ○ **B.** Administer the medications.

  ○ **C.** Administer them separately.

  ○ **D.** Contact the pharmacy.

10. The best method of evaluating the amount of peripheral edema is:

- ○ **A.** Weighing the client daily

- ○ **B.** Measuring the extremity

- ○ **C.** Measuring the intake and output

- ○ **D.** Checking for pitting

Answer Rationales

1. Answer A is correct. The client taking antilipidemics should be encouraged to report muscle weakness because this is a sign of rhabdomyolysis. The medication takes effect within one month of beginning therapy, so answer B is incorrect. The medication should be taken with water. Fruit juice, particularly grapefruit juice, can decrease the drug's effectiveness, so answer C is incorrect. Liver function studies, not a CBC, should be checked prior to beginning the medication, so answer D is incorrect.

2. Answer B is correct. Hyperstat is given IV push for hypertensive crisis. It often causes hyperglycemia. The glucose level will drop rapidly after the medication is administered. Answer A is incorrect because this medication is given IV push. The client should be placed in dorsal recumbent position, not Trendelenburg, so answer C is incorrect. Answer D is incorrect because the medication is ordered IV push.

3. Answer C is correct. A heart rate of 60 in the six-month-old receiving Lanoxin elixir (digoxin) should be reported immediately because bradycardia is associated with digoxin toxicity. The blood glucose, blood pressure, and respirations are not associated with administration of Lanoxin, so answers A, B, and D are incorrect.

4. Answer C is correct. The client should leave the medication in the brown bottle because light deteriorates the medication. The supply should be replenished every six months, so answer A is incorrect. One tablet should be taken every five minutes times three, so answer B is incorrect. If the pain does not subside, the client should report to the emergency room. The medication should be taken sublingually and should not be crushed, so answer D is incorrect.

5. Answer D is correct. CK-MB (creatine phosphokinase muscle bond isoenzyme) is the most specific for a myocardial infarction. Troponin is also extremely reliable. Answers A, B, and C are nonspecific to myocardial infarctions, so they are incorrect.

6. Answer C is correct. Turkey contains the least amount of fat and cholesterol. Cheese, shrimp, and beef should be avoided by the client on a low cholesterol, low fat diet; therefore, answers A, B, and D are incorrect.

7. Answer B is correct. The neck veins should be assessed for distension in the client with congestive heart failure. Edema of the feet and hands do not indicate central circulatory overload, so answers A and C are incorrect. Edema of the sacrum is an indication of right-sided congestive heart failure, so answer D is incorrect.

8. Answer A is correct. The nurse should place the zero of the manometer at the phlebostatic axis (located at the fifth intercostal space mid-axillary line) when checking the central venous pressure. Answers B, C, and D are incorrect methods for determining the central venous pressure.

9. Answer B is correct. Zestril is an ACE inhibitor and is frequently given with a diuretic such as Lasix. There is no need to question the order, give the drugs separately, or contact the pharmacy, so answers A, C, and D are incorrect.

10. Answer B is correct. The best method for evaluating the amount of peripheral edema is measuring the extremity. A paper tape measure should be used rather than plastic or cloth, and the area should be marked with a pen. This provides the most objective assessment. Answers A, C, and D are not the best methods for evaluating the amount of peripheral edema, therefore they are incorrect.

Suggested Reading and Resources

▶ Ignatavicius, D., Workman, S. *Medical-Surgical Nursing: Critical Thinking for Collaborative Care*. 5th ed. Philadelphia: Elsevier, 2007.

▶ *Taber's Cyclopedic Medical Dictionary*. Philadelphia: F.A. Davis, 2005.

▶ Vanetzian, E., *Critical Thinking: An Interactive Tool for Learning Medical-Surgical Nursing*. F.A. Davis, 2005.

▶ Rinehart, W., Sloan, D., and Hurd, C. *NCLEX Exam Cram*. Indianapolis: Que, 2005.

▶ Deglin, J., and Vallerand, A., *Davis Drug Guide for Nurses*. Philadelphia: F.A. Davis, 2009.

14

Caring for the Client with Disorders of the Neurological System

---

Terms you'll need to understand

- ✓ Areflexia
- ✓ Aura
- ✓ Automatism
- ✓ Bradykinesia
- ✓ Burr holes
- ✓ Cheyne Stokes respirations
- ✓ Clonic movements
- ✓ Craniotomy
- ✓ Decerebrate posture
- ✓ Decorticate posture
- ✓ Doll's eye phenomena
- ✓ Hypocapnia
- ✓ Piloerection
- ✓ Postictal
- ✓ Pulse pressure
- ✓ Rinne test
- ✓ Sundowning
- ✓ Tonic movements
- ✓ Webber test

Nursing skills you'll need to master

- ✓ Performing neurological assessments
- ✓ Performing log roll turning technique
- ✓ Bowel and bladder training

Seizures

Seizures are episodes of abnormal motor, sensory, or autonomic activity that result from the excessive discharge of electrical impulses from cerebral neurons. All seizures affect the level of consciousness; however, the degree is dependent on the type of seizure. Most seizures occur without a cause. Any abnormality in the central nervous system (CNS) can cause seizure activity. The significant causes of a seizure you need to know for the NCLEX exam are

- ▶ Abrupt withdrawal of barbiturates
- ▶ Brain tumors
- ▶ Central nervous system infections
- ▶ Cerebrovascular disease (especially in the elderly)
- ▶ Head injuries
- ▶ High fevers
- ▶ Hypertension
- ▶ Hypoglycemia or electrolyte abnormalities

Types of Seizures

There are two main categories for classifying seizures: the *generalized* seizure and the *partial*, or *focal*, seizure. The following sections describe these two seizure categories more fully.

Generalized Seizures

With this type of seizure, the whole brain is involved in the seizure activity. Within this category, two types of seizures are identified. The first type is the *tonic-clonic*, or *grand mal*, seizure; the second is the *absence*, or *petit mal*, seizure.

Tonic-Clonic Seizures

Tonic-clonic seizures can last for up to five minutes. The following highlights the signs and symptoms of tonic-clonic seizures you need to know:

- ▶ Preictal aura (period prior to seizure activity)
- ▶ Brief episodes of apnea
- ▶ Chewing of the tongue
- ▶ Incontinence
- ▶ Loss of consciousness

▶ Loss of motor function

▶ Tonic (muscle tension) and clonic (alternating muscle contraction and relaxation) movements

NOTE

Aura can be any type of sensory sensation, such as a smell or flashing lights, that signals to the client that the seizure is about to occur. Children usually do not have an aura.

There is a risk for injury for any client involved in this type of seizure activity. You must become familiar with nursing care required for the general safety and physiological care of the client before and after the seizure. You also need to know how to accurately document the seizure because this will assist the physician with the diagnosis. You should gain knowledge of the following aspects of care and expect to see them on your exam:

▶ Assess the client's behavior and surroundings prior to the seizure.

▶ Loosen his clothing.

▶ Maintain a patent airway (oxygen, suction).

▶ Note any loss of consciousness, aura, or incontinence.

▶ Provide client safety (place padding under the client's head and move objects out of reach of the client to prevent self-injury).

▶ Time and document the seizure activity.

▶ Turn the client on his side.

▶ Oral airway may be inserted if the client has an aura and time permits.

Don't

▶ Put anything in the client's mouth after a seizure has begun.

▶ Restrain the client.

After the seizure (postictal period), the client will be lethargic, tired, and confused. Nursing care after a tonic/clonic seizure includes

▶ Allow the client to sleep.

▶ Keep the client side-lying.

▶ Orient the client to the environment.

▶ Be prepared for the client to be confused and disoriented because he's in the postictal phase after the seizure.

Absence Seizures

The second type of generalized seizure is *absence*, or *petit mal*, seizure. This type is more common in children and might improve by adolescence. There is little or no loss of consciousness, and it can be mistaken for daydreaming. Other clinical manifestations you need to know are

▶ Blank stare

▶ Twitching of the mouth

Partial Seizures

The second category of seizures is called *partial*, or *focal*, seizures. These seizure types affect one cerebral hemisphere. Mostly found in adults, these seizures respond unfavorably to medical regimens. Focal seizures are further divided into two classifications. The first type is the *simple partial* seizure, and the second is known as the *complex partial* seizure.

Simple Partial

With simple partial seizure, the client's finger or hand might shake or she might have unusual sensations, and autonomic symptoms (flushing, heart rate changes) might occur. The client often has an aura but does not lose consciousness. These seizures can be precursors to larger seizures.

Complex Partial

The second type of focal seizure is the complex partial. One of the major differentiating factors is that these clients do lose consciousness, whereas in simple partial they do not. The seizure can last for up to three minutes. Some characteristics you need to know for the exam include

▶ Automatisms (behaviors that the person is not aware of, such as hand movements and picking at clothes) might occur.

▶ These seizures are common in adults.

▶ The client has amnesia of the episode.

Treatment of Seizure Clients

The treatment of clients with seizures concentrates on stopping the seizure activity. This goal is most often accomplished by the use of anticonvulsant medications. Another method of treatment involves the insertion of a vagal nerve stimulator (VNS). In this procedure, an electrode is placed on the vagal nerve and gives intermittent stimulation to the nerve, preventing seizures. Side effects of the VNS are hoarseness and throat discomfort. Clients who continue to have seizures with treatment might require surgical removal of the section of the brain causing the seizure; however, this is a last resort.

Status Epilepticus

A person in status epilepticus has a continuation of grand mal seizures without a normal recovery period. The client does not regain consciousness between attacks, despite medical intervention. Any one seizure that lasts longer than 5 minutes or repeated seizures longer than 30 minutes are classified as status epilepticus. This disorder is life-threatening if not corrected. Possible causes of status epilepticus include sudden noncompliance of anticonvulsant medications, head trauma, and alcohol withdrawal.

Clients experiencing status epilepticus are treated as a neurological emergency. Interventions important for the nurse candidate to know are administration of oxygen, initiation of IV access, and establishment and maintenance of a patent airway (intubation by an anesthetist or a physician might be required). Medications need to be given to stop the seizure, as well as drugs to prevent another seizure. If the seizure activity continues despite efforts, general anesthesia might be required. The following highlights the drugs you need to know for this disorder: IV diazepam (Valium) or lorazepam (Ativan) to stop the seizure activity (dosage may be repeated 10 minutes after the initial administration), followed by phenobarbital and diphenyldantoin (Dilantin) or fosphenytoin (Cerebyx).

Brain Injuries

Brain injuries occur when a force is applied to the brain, causing damage. The age group at greatest risk is 15–44. An injury of this type can cause extreme emotional adjustments and disability.

Several types of brain injuries can occur. One type is a basilar skull fracture (fracture at the base of the skull). These fractures can be severe. The trademark of basilar skull fractures are the specific symptoms, which include:

▶ CSF (cerebrospinal fluid) leakage from the ear (otorrhea) or the nose (rhinorrhea)

TIP

Indicators of CSF are the halo sign (a blood stain that develops a yellowish circle around it) or drainage that tests positive for glucose.

▶ Battle's sign (ecchymosis at the mastoid area)

▶ Raccoon eyes (ecchymosis around the eyes)

> **CAUTION**
>
> There is an increased risk of infection and cerebrospinal fluid leakage with a basilar skull fracture.
>
> Patients with nondepressed or depressed skull fractures without contamination or deformities usually require only observation. Penetrating fractures usually require surgery with debridement, cleansing, and antibiotic administration.

Another type of brain injury is a hemorrhage. They are classified according to the area in the brain that's affected. The information that follows discusses the three hematomas that can develop from an injury.

Epidural Hematomas

The first type of hematoma is the *epidural*. It usually develops from an arterial bleed, which makes it more acute. An epidural hematoma occurs when there is a collection of blood between the skull and dura. The symptoms indicating an epidural hematoma involve a pattern of consciousness, a lucid interval, followed by the client being critical and then comatose.

Subdural Hematoma

The second type of hematoma is a *subdural* hematoma. It is usually venous in origin and occurs when a collection of blood is between the dura and above the arachnoid space. Subdural hematomas are subdivided into three classifications that are identified by their time of development after the injury. The following highlights these terms and how they are identified:

▶ **Acute**—Occurs within the first 2 days of injury

▶ **Subacute**—Occurs 2–14 days after the injury

▶ **Chronic**—Occurs from 14 days to several months after the injury

Treatment of Epidural and Subdural Hematomas

Clients with hematomas are treated depending on the amount of space occupied by the hematoma. If the client has increased intracranial pressure (ICP), measures included in the following section on increased ICP are used. Surgical interventions include insertion of burr holes and a craniotomy to evacuate the hematoma.

Increased Intracranial Pressure

Increased intracranial pressure can result from any alteration that increases tissue or fluid volume within the cranium. The skull is rigid with no flexibility; therefore, there is no room for any additional fluid or blood, or a space-occupying lesion. The causes of increased ICP are as follows:

▶ Accumulation of cerebrospinal fluid in the ventricles

▶ Brain tumors

▶ Central nervous system infections

▶ Cerebral edema

▶ Intracranial bleeding

The client with increased ICP exhibits specific signs and symptoms that you need to be able to recognize and report to the physician for early intervention. These clinical manifestations include

▶ Blurred vision.

▶ Changes in cognition.

▶ Changes in the level of consciousness. Early symptoms include lethargy, disorientation, confusion. Late changes include non-responsiveness, response to painful stimuli, and coma.

TIP

Changes in the level of consciousness may be the first indication of a neurological problem.

▶ Cheyne Stokes respirations.

▶ Coma.

▶ Decerebrate posture (see Figure 14.1).

NOTE

Decerebrate posture indicates brain stem dysfunction.

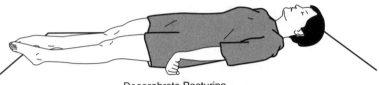

Decerebrate Posturing

FIGURE 14.1
Decerebrate posture.

▶ Decorticate posture (see Figure 14.2).

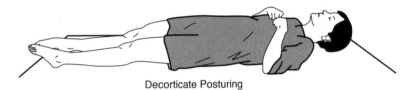

Decorticate Posturing

FIGURE 14.2
Decorticate posture.

▶ Decreased motor responsiveness.

▶ Diplopia.

▶ Doll's eye phenomena.

▶ Headache.

▶ Nausea and vomiting (usually projectile).

▶ Pupil changes.

▶ Personality and behavior changes.

▶ Seizures.

▶ Vital signs changes (also called *Cushing's triad*):

    ▶ Increased BP with a widening pulse pressure

    ▶ Decreased pulse rate

    ▶ Decreased respirations

TIP

Note that these vital sign changes are actually the opposite of shock—so if you know one, you know the other, and vice versa.

It is important for the nurse candidate to be aware of the differences of symptoms that can occur in infants. The following focuses on the clinical manifestations of increased ICP you need to know for the infant:

- Bulging fontanels

- High-pitched crying

- Irritability

- Restlessness

Treatment of ICP

Treatment of increased ICP is directed toward paths that will both prevent further increases in intracranial pressure and help in the recognition of it so that early intervention is possible. The following interventions are important for you to know for the exam:

- Keep head of bed elevated 30°.

- Keep the client well hydrated.

- Make frequent neurological assessments.

- Ensure strict intake and output to prevent overhydration.

- Prevent seizures by administering anticonvulsants when due for blood level maintenance.

- Treat nausea and vomiting.

- Maintain the client in a barbiturate coma to decrease metabolic demands as prescribed.

- Maintain hypocapnia (PCO_2 of 35-38 mm Hg) to constrict cerebral blood vessels and decrease ICP.

- Pharmacological interventions, including

  - Decadron

  - Mannitol (Osmitrol) (observe for signs of congestive heart failure due to a possible alteration of cardiac enzymes); use a filter for IV administration

  - Anticonvulsants

  - Loop diuretics

  - Avoid aspirin, narcotics, or medications that depress respirations

CAUTION

Pain medications can mask symptoms, which can make assessments inaccurate.

Neurological Assessment

The client assessment is a major component of nursing care. Early recognition of a deficit in neurological status can mean a more favorable outcome in the client's condition. The following information offers insight into three forms of assessment techniques: cranial nerve assessment, Glasgow coma scale, and intracranial pressure monitors that can be used to identify deficits in a client.

Cranial Nerve Assessment

Table 14.1 highlights the 12 cranial nerves, their names, functions, and the assessment methods.

TABLE 14.1 Assessment of Cranial Nerves

Cranial Nerve	Function	Assessment Method
1 Olfactory	Smell.	Identify common odors.
2 Optic	Visual acuity.	Snellen chart (central vision) and peripheral vision check.
3 Oculomotor; 4 Trochlear; 6 Abducens	Cranial nerves III, IV, and VI regulate eye movement, accommodation, and the elevation of the eyelids. IV is responsible for inferior and medial eye movement. VI is responsible for lateral eye movement.	Check for pupil constriction; check for accommodation and convergence as the object is brought near the eyes; check for strength of lid closure.
5 Trigeminal	Facial sensation; corneal reflex; mastication.	Identify the location of the stimulus; check jaw strength.
7 Facial	Movement of facial muscles; facial expression; tear formation; salivation; taste sensation in anterior tongue.	Check for symmetry of facial expressions; muscle strength. Identify sweet, sour, and salty taste on anterior area of the tongue.
8 Acoustic (Vestibulocochlear)	Hearing and equilibrium.	Use Weber and Rinne test for hearing loss.
9 Glossopharyngeal	Taste sensation in post third of the tongue.	Identify sweet, sour, and salty tastes on posterior area of the tongue.
10 Vagus	Pharyngeal contraction; symmetrical movement of vocal cords and soft palate; movement and secretion of thoracic and abdominal viscera.	Ask client to say "Ah"; uvula should rise midline; check ability to swallow.

TABLE 14.1 *Continued*

Cranial Nerve	Function	Assessment Method
11 Spinal Accessory	Movement of trapezius and sternocleidomastoid muscles	Have client shrug shoulders against resistance. Neck strength is checked by having the client turn the head against resistance.
12 Hypoglossal	Tongue movement	Have client stick out tongue, observe for deviations or tremors, check strength of tongue movement as it presses against tongue blade.

Glasgow Coma Scale

The Glasgow coma scale assesses neurologic status based on the client's motor, verbal, and eye-opening responses. Lower responses indicate central nervous system impairment, whereas higher responses indicate central nervous system functioning. The scale is a universal tool, which makes it a popular screening tool. The candidate should be aware of the following information for the nursing exam:

Eye Opening:

> Spontaneous opening = 4
>
> To speech = 3
>
> To pain = 2
>
> No response = 1

Best Motor Response:

> Obeys = 6
>
> Localizes pain = 5
>
> Withdraws = 4
>
> Abnormal flexion = 3
>
> Extends = 2
>
> No response = 1

Verbal Response:

> Oriented = 5
>
> Confused conversation = 4
>
> Inappropriate words = 3

Incomprehensible words = 2

No response = 1

Total Points = 3–15. A score less than or equal to 8 indicates severe coma, a score between 9 and 12 inclusive indicates a moderate coma; a score greater than or equal to 13 indicates minor coma.

Intracranial Pressure Monitors

The intracranial pressure monitor is the most invasive and accurate of the ones mentioned. It is inserted by the physician.

This is a sensing device inside the skull that is attached to a transducer. This device gives an electronic recording of intracranial pressure. The normal ICP reading is less than 20 mm Hg. The monitoring device can also be used to drain cerebrospinal fluid.

The cerebral perfusion pressure (CPP) can also be used to evaluate the client. Cerebral perfusion pressure is calculated by subtracting the ICP reading from the mean arterial pressure (MAP). A CPP above 70 is needed to have adequate brain viability. It is important for you to have the knowledge required for clients with ICP monitors in place.

Assess for complications or problems with the ICP monitor:

▶ Infection at site

▶ CSF leak

▶ Loose connection

▶ Meningitis

▶ Microhemorrhages

▶ Interpret and report results to the physician

▶ Utilize sterile technique when handling the equipment

Care of the Client with Intracranial Surgery (Craniotomy)

Neuro assessments might indicate to the physician that surgery is required. If a client has a craniotomy, post-operative care is of particular importance. The following post-operative craniotomy interventions are important for you to know:

- Monitor vital signs and neurological assessments.

- Monitor cardiac rhythm.

- Perform passive range of motion exercises on the client.

- Assist the client to turn, cough, and deep breathe every 2–3 hours.

> **CAUTION**
>
> Be careful with coughing exercises because they can increase intracranial pressure.

- Use cold application for periorbital edema and bruising.

- Prevent deep vein thrombosis by compression stocking application.

- Use the following positioning:

    - **Supratentorial surgery**—Elevate the head of the bed 30°.

    - **Infratentorial surgery**—Flat on either side. Use this position for 24–48 hours after surgery. If bone flap has been removed keep the client off of the operative side.

- Assess head dressing and drainage from wound suction devices.

- Monitor ABGs.

- Assess urinary output (note: excessive urinary output could indicate the complication of diabetes insipidus).

- Maintain the neck in a neutral position and avoid flexion of the neck and the hip.

- Assess for complications including increased intracranial pressure, hydrocephalus, pneumonia, meningitis, syndrome of inappropriate diuretic hormone, diabetes insipidus, and brain herniation.

- Use the following pharmacological interventions:

    - Anticonvulsants

    - Steroids

    - Histamine blockers

    - Prophylactic antibiotics

Cerebrovascular Accident/Stroke

Strokes or "brain attacks" are the third leading cause of death and the leading cause of disability in the United States. Risk factors for a stroke include, hypertension, long-term hypercoagability, diabetes, illicit drug use (usually cocaine), and obesity (especiallly in the abdominal area).

Ischemic and hemorrhagic strokes are the two major types of strokes.

Causes of ischemic strokes include atherosclerosis, atrial fibrillation, cocaine use, and coagulation disorders. Hemorrhagic strokes can be caused by ruptured cerebral aneurysm, uncontrolled hypertension, and a ruptured arterial venous malformation (AVM). The diagnosis of strokes are done by a CT scan or magnetic resonance imagery (MRI). It is very important to differentiate between a stroke with ischemia or hemorrhage as origin so that proper treatment can be initiated.

> **CAUTION**
>
> It is contraindicated for a client with an hemorrhagic stroke to receive anticoagulants and thrombolytics.

The clinical manifestations of a stroke are similar no matter the cause or origin and include:

- Numbness or weakness on one side of the body
- Dizziness and loss of balance or coordination
- Sudden headache (more prevalent with hemorrhagic strokes)
- Visual or perception changes
- Aphasia
- Apraxia
- Dysarthria
- Dysphagia

The treatment for strokes include patient support, non-surgical, and surgical interventions. Non-surgical treatments for ischemic strokes include thrombolytic t-PA (within three hours of occurrence of the stroke), warfarin (Coumadin), platelet inhibitors (for example, aspirin or Plavix), and heparin. Surgical interventions via a carotid endarterectomy or transluminal angioplasty may be required. For hemorrhagic strokes the focus is on prevention of complications and recovery and include: Administration of anti hypertensives, and prevention and treatment of vasospasm (calcium channel blocker administration). Surgical intervention may be a craniotomy to repair an AVM or cerebral aneurysm or removal of a clot. It is imperative for the nurse to assess for neurological status changes, maintain cerebral perfusion, administer pain medication, provide adequate oxygenation, and provide bedrest and sedation when caring for clients with a cerebrovascular accident.

Spinal Cord Injury

Spinal cord injuries (SCIs) occur most often in young men between the ages of 15 and 30. Most cord injuries occur at the 5th, 6th, or 7th cervical, or at the 12th thoracic or the 1st lumbar. These areas are weaker due to the range of mobility needed. Injuries above C4 results in loss of respiratory muscle function.

A spinal cord injury is classified as *complete* (no function below the level of injury) or *incomplete* (partial function remains). These injuries can occur from diseases—for example, tumors causing compression and damage—but the most frequent causes are trauma and falls. These clients display the following characteristics:

- Acute respiratory failure

- Compromised respiratory function

- Loss of bowel and bladder tone

- Loss of sweating and vasomotor tone

- Marked reduction in BP due to loss of peripheral vascular resistance

- Sensory and motor paralysis below the level of injury

NOTE

Acute respiratory failure is the primary cause of death in high-level cord injuries.

Treatment of Spinal Cord Injuries

Treatment of spinal cord injuries follows the paths of stabilization, monitoring and assessing, and preventing further damage. The following measures are important aspects of care:

- Stabilize respiratory and cardiovascular systems.

- Transport the client on a spinal board to prevent further damage.

- Medication administration of high-dose steroids within eight hours of injury is the front-line treatment.

▶ Perform surgical reduction and alignment. The client might be placed in traction after reduction (or initially if the client is too unstable for surgery) with the use of skeletal tongs. Three types of tongs are

  ▶ Crutchfield

  ▶ Gardner-Wells

  ▶ Vinke

> **CAUTION**
>
> Proper spinal cord alignment is essential. A physician's order is required for turning the client.

A halo vest is another type of alignment immobilization device that provides immobilization of the bone with ambulation allowed. These clients, as well as clients with tongs, require pin care per protocol with H_2O_2 or normal saline and an antibiotic cream.

Clients with thoracic and lumbar injuries might require a body cast or brace with bedrest. You must ensure that the vest is not causing pressure. Assess skin often. There should be enough space between the vest and skin for a finger to fit comfortably.

Antispastic medications can be given for spasticity. Long-term severe spasticity might require intrathecal baclofen (Lioresal) via insertion of a pump placed in the CSF.

Potential Complications with SCI Clients

Because of the damage to the spinal cord and autonomic nervous system, clients with SCIs can develop two main complications. The first complication is *spinal shock*, which occurs because of the sudden failure in the communication of the upper and lower neurons. Spinal shock can last for 3–6 weeks. Clients exhibit the following symptoms:

▶ Decreased heart rate

▶ Flaccid paralysis

▶ No reflex activity or perspiration below the level of the lesion

▶ Low blood pressure

Another complication from this syndrome is *autonomic hyperreflexia*, or *dysreflexia*. Most often seen in injuries higher than T6, this disorder usually occurs after the spinal shock has resolved. You need to be familiar with clinical manifestations, which include

▶ Bradycardia

▶ Cold, dry, pale skin below the lesion level

▶ Headache

▶ Hypertension

▶ Nasal congestion

▶ Piloerection

▶ Profuse sweating

The treatment plan for autonomic dysreflexia focuses on removing the trigger or cause and lowering the blood pressure. The immediate interventions you will need to know are

▶ Remove the triggering stimuli.

▶ Elevate the head.

▶ Check for a full bladder (the most common cause) or kinked Foley catheter tubing.

▶ Administer antihypertensive medications.

▶ Check for impaction after the episode has resolved.

Other complications associated with spinal cord injuries are mainly associated with immobility and include deep vein thrombosis and pulmonary embolus, impaired skin integrity, and contractures.

Guillain-Barré

Guillain-Barré is a rapidly ascending progressive paralysis or weakness. It can also be descending but is uncommon by this progression, and it is an acute inflammatory process. Respiratory complications are the usual cause of death, although the exact cause is unknown. It has been shown to be related to a para-infection or post-infection immune response. It frequently develops 1–3 weeks following an upper respiratory or gastrointestinal infection. It has also been linked to clients with a history of a recent immunization or allergy. A client with Guillain-Barré displays the following symptoms:

▶ Diminished or absent tendon reflexes

▶ Low-grade fever

▶ Muscle weakness that gradually moves up the arms, trunk, and face

▶ Autonomic dysfunction (hypertension, hypotension, tachycardia, bradycardia)

▶ Numbness, pain, and tingling in the extremities

Treating Clients with Guillian-Barré

The treatment phase for Guillian-Barré is directed toward performing in-depth assessments, paying particular attention to the need for assisted ventilation. Emotional support and adequate nutrition are also used. You also need to be aware of other treatment modalities, including medications such as steroids to decrease the immune response and IV immunoglobulin (must use a filter for IV delivery) and plasmapheresis. Plasmapheresis is used to remove circulating antibodies and speed the healing process.

Degenerative Neurological Disorders

Several neuro disorders have similar pathophysiological features: There is a deficit in a neurotransmitter or an impairment of nerve conduction. Table 14.2 discusses these disorders, giving you an overview of each condition. As you study this table, keep in mind that the medications for treatment in several of the disorders are used to replace the deficiencies listed in the pathophysiology section. You should study and learn this table and expect some of this information to be on the exam.

TABLE 14.2   Degenerative Neurological Disorders

Disorder	Parkinson's	Multiple Sclerosis	Myasthenia Gravis	Alzheimer's
Onset	50–60 years	20–40 years	20–50 years	30–60 years
Gender	Most prevalent in males	Most prevalent in females	Most prevalent in females	Males and females equally affected
Cause	Unknown	Unknown, but it's autoimmune or viral	Unknown, but it's autoimmune	Unknown
Area Affected	Substantia nigra in basal ganglia	White matter of brain and spinal cord	Myoneural junction of voluntary muscles	Cerebral cortex
Pathophysiology	Deficiency in dopamine, which impairs coordination and autonomic function	Impairs nerve impulse conduction, which is related to the loss of myelin sheath	Impairs transmission of impulses due to lack of acetylcholine	Loss of brain cells from the cerebral cortex and creation of neurofibrillary tangles, decreased acetylcholine
Clinical Manifestations	Muscle stiffness, non-intentional tremor, dysphagia, autonomic dysfunction, and bradykinesia	Loss of bowel and bladder control, blurry vision, paralysis	Profound muscle weakness, fatigue, respiratory failure, and lack of facial expression	Memory loss, disorientation, emotional distress, agitation, and sundowning.

TABLE 14.2 *Continued*

Disorder	Parkinson's	Multiple Sclerosis	Myasthenia Gravis	Alzheimer's
Treatment	Supportive care and medications such as levodopa Carbidopa, (Sinemet) Artane, and Cogentin	Supportive care and medications such as steroids, Immuran, interferons such as Rebif, glatiramer acetate (Copaxone), baclofen (Lioresal), and mitoxantrone (Novantrone)	Supportive care and medications such as Pyridostigmine Bromide (Mestinon), neostigmine bromide, (Prostigmin) and steroids	Supportive care and medications such as ropinirole hydrochloride (Requip), tacrine hydrochloride (Cognex), folic acid, donepezil (Aricept), and rivastigmine (Exelon)

Diagnostic Tests for Review

A part of the neurological assessment includes diagnostic exams. Routine laboratory work, such as the CBC, chest x-ray, and urinalysis will also be done. Blood cultures are also required to identify the causative agent in CNS infections. Clients with head injuries and spinal cord injuries need skull x-rays, CT scans, and MRIs to identify defects. When reviewing the diagnostic exams that follow, remember which tests are commonly done for a specific disorder. For example, the electroencephalogram is used for epilepsy and seizure activity:

▶ Angiogram

▶ Cerebral arteriogram

▶ CT scan

▶ Electroencephalogram

▶ Magnetic resonance angiography (MRA)

▶ Magnetic resonance imaging (MRI)

▶ Positron emission tomography (PET)

▶ Skull x-rays

Pharmacology for Review

Pharmacological interventions are used in most types of neurological problems. Some drug classifications are used in several disorders. For example, steroids are used in clients with multiple sclerosis, but also in head injuries and spinal cord injuries. While reviewing the drug classifications, you should recognize the most common ones, such as anticonvulsants, and realize that these drugs have a higher probability of being tested. Continue to look for the commonality in side effects of the drugs you are reviewing and focus on nursing considerations and adverse drug effects:

- ▶ Antianxiety
- ▶ Anticonvulsants
- ▶ Antimyasthenics
- ▶ Anti-Parkinson's
- ▶ Cholinesterase inhibitor
- ▶ Corticosteroids
- ▶ Diuretics
- ▶ Gamma globulins
- ▶ Immunosuppressives
- ▶ Interferons
- ▶ Muscle relaxers
- ▶ Osmotic diuretics

Exam Prep Questions

1. A client is admitted with a head injury. Which vital sign assessment is most indicative of increased intracranial pressure?

   ○ **A.** BP 120/80, pulse 120, respirations 20

   ○ **B.** BP 180/98, pulse 50, temperature 102° F

   ○ **C.** BP 98/60, pulse 132, temperature 97.6° F

   ○ **D.** BP 170/90, pulse 80, respirations 24

2. The nurse is caring for a client with a head injury who has an intracranial pressure monitor in place. Assessment reveals an ICP reading of 66. What is the nurse's best action?

   ○ **A.** Notify the physician.

   ○ **B.** Record the reading as the only action.

   ○ **C.** Turn the client and recheck the reading.

   ○ **D.** Place the client supine.

3. A client has developed diabetes insipidus after removal of a pituitary tumor. Which finding would the nurse expect?

   ○ **A.** Polyuria

   ○ **B.** Hypertension

   ○ **C.** Polyphagia

   ○ **D.** Hyperkalemia

4. The nurse is caring for a client with a head injury who has increased ICP. The physician plans to reduce the cerebral edema by reversing dilation of cerebral blood vessels. Which physician prescription would the nurse expect to accomplish this?

   ○ **A.** Hyperventilation per mechanical ventilation

   ○ **B.** Insertion of a ventricular shunt

   ○ **C.** Furosemide (Lasix)

   ○ **D.** Solu medrol

5. A client is admitted with Parkinson's disease. The client has been taking Carbidopa/levodopa (Sinemet) for one year. Which clinical manifestation would be the most important to report?

    ○ **A.** Dry mouth

    ○ **B.** Spasmodic eye winking

    ○ **C.** Dark urine

    ○ **D.** Dizziness

6. The nurse caring for a client with myasthenia gravis recognizes which of the following as the priority?

    ○ **A.** Fall risks

    ○ **B.** Acute pain

    ○ **C.** Airway clearance

    ○ **D.** Mobility impairments

7. A client with a T6 injury six months ago develops facial flushing and a BP of 210/106. After elevating the head of the bed, which is the most appropriate nursing action?

    ○ **A.** Notify the physician.

    ○ **B.** Assess the client for a distended bladder.

    ○ **C.** Apply oxygen at 3 L/min.

    ○ **D.** Increase the IV fluids.

8. The nurse is performing an admission history for a client recovering from a stroke. Medication history reveals the drug clopidogrel (Plavix). Which clinical manifestation alerts the nurse to an adverse effect of this drug?

    ○ **A.** Epistaxis

    ○ **B.** Abdominal distention

    ○ **C.** Nausea

    ○ **D.** Hyperactivity

9. Which assessment finding is most indicative of increased ICP in a client admitted with a basilar skull fracture?

    ○ **A.** Nausea and vomiting

    ○ **B.** Headache

    ○ **C.** Dizziness

    ○ **D.** Papilledema

10. A client with angina is experiencing migraine headaches. The physician has prescribed sumatriptan succinate (Imitrex). Which nursing action is most appropriate?

   ○ **A.** Call the physician to question the prescription order.

   ○ **B.** Try to obtain samples for the client to take home.

   ○ **C.** Perform discharge teaching regarding this drug.

   ○ **D.** Consult social services for financial assistance with obtaining the drug.

Answer Rationales

1. Answer B is correct. Vital signs correlating with increased intracranial pressure are an elevated BP with a widening pulse pressure, a slow pulse rate, and an elevated temperature with involvement of the hypothalamus. Answer C relates to hypovolemia, so it is incorrect. Answers A and D do not relate to increased intracranial pressure and are therefore incorrect.

2. Answer A is correct. Normal ICP is less than 15. 66 is a high reading, and the physician should be notified. Answer B would be the action if the reading was normal, so it is incorrect. Answers C and D would not be appropriate actions, so they are wrong.

3. Answer A is correct. Clients with diabetes insipidus have excessive urinary output due to a lack of antidiuretic hormone. Answers B, C, and D are not exhibited with diabetes insipidus, so they are incorrect.

4. Answer A is correct. Hyperventilation is utilized to decrease the PCO_2 to 27–30, producing cerebral blood vessel constriction. Answers B, C, and D can decrease cerebral edema, but not by constriction of cerebral blood vessels; therefore, they are wrong.

5. Answer B is correct. Spasmodic eye winking could indicate a toxicity or overdose and should be reported to the physician. Other signs of toxicity include involuntary twitching of muscles, facial grimaces, and severe tongue protrusion. Answers A, C, and D are incorrect because they are side effects of the drug.

6. Answer C is correct. Clients with myasthenia gravis have problems with the muscular activity of breathing. Answers A, B, and D are not the priority, so they are wrong.

7. Answer B is correct. The client is experiencing autonomic hyperreflexia, which can be caused by a full bowel or bladder. Answer A is not the appropriate action before the assessment of the bladder, so it is incorrect. There is no evidence in the stem to support the need for oxygen, so answer C is incorrect. Answer D is not appropriate at this time and might serve to further increase the BP, making it wrong.

8. Answer A is correct. Plavix is an antiplatelet. Bleeding could indicate a severe effect. Answers B, C, and D are not associated with Plavix's undesired effects, so they are incorrect.

9. Answer D is correct. Papilledema is a hallmark symptom of increased intracranial pressure. Answers A, B, and C are not as conclusive as papilledema, so they are wrong.

10. Answer A is correct. Imitrex results in cranial vasoconstriction to reduce pain, but it can also cause vasoconstrictive effects systemically. This drug is contraindicated in clients with angina, and the physician should be notified. Answers B and D are incorrect because they are inappropriate actions from the information given. Answer C is appropriate, but answer A is most appropriate.

Suggested Reading and Resources

▶ Broyles, B., Reiss, B., Evans, M., *Pharmacological Aspects of Nursing Care*. 7th ed. New York: Thomson Delmal Learning, 2007.

▶ Kee, J. *Laboratory and Diagnostic Tests with Nursing Implications*. New York: Prentice Hall, 2010.

▶ Lacharity, L., Kumagai, C., and Bartz, B. *Prioritization, Delegation, & Assignment*. 2nd ed. St. Louis: Mosby Elsevier, 2006, 2011.

▶ Brunner, L., and Suddarth, D. *Textbook of Medical-Surgical Nursing*. 12th ed. Philadelphia: Lippincott Williams & Wilkins, 2009.

▶ Hogan, M. *Child Health Nursing Reviews and Rationales*. 2nd ed. Upper Saddle River, NJ: Pearson Prentice Hall, 2007.

▶ Deglin, J., and Vallerand, A., *Davis Drug Guide for Nurses*. Philadelphia: F.A. Davis, 2009.

▶ Lewis, S., Heitkemper, M., Dirkson, S., O Brien, P., and Bucher, L. *Medical Surgical Nursing: Assessment and Management of Clinical Problems*. 7th ed. Philadelphia: Elsevier, 2007.

▶ Rinehart, W., Sloan, D., and Hurd, C. *NCLEX Exam Cram*. Indianapolis: Que, 2007.

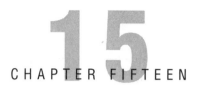

Caring for the Client with Psychiatric Disorders

Terms you'll need to understand

- ✓ Anorexia nervosa
- ✓ Attention deficit hyperactive disorder
- ✓ Bipolar disorder
- ✓ Bulimia nervosa
- ✓ Conduct disorder
- ✓ Conversion
- ✓ Delusion
- ✓ DSM-IV-TR
- ✓ Dysthymic disorder
- ✓ Electroconvulsive therapy
- ✓ Extrapyramidal side effect

- ✓ Hallucination
- ✓ Hypertensive crisis
- ✓ Hypochondriasis
- ✓ Neuroleptic malignant syndrome
- ✓ Neurosis
- ✓ Neurotransmitter
- ✓ Pain disorder
- ✓ Personality disorder
- ✓ Psychosis
- ✓ Schizophrenia
- ✓ Somatization disorder

Nursing skills you'll need to master

- ✓ Administering medication
- ✓ Performing mental status assessment
- ✓ Maintaining a therapeutic milieu
- ✓ Obtaining vital signs

- ✓ Assessing for side effects of psychotropic drugs
- ✓ Assisting with alternative therapies

The past decade has been an exciting time for psychiatric nursing. Technological advances have given us the ability to study not only the physical structure of the brain, but also how chemical messengers (known as *neurotransmitters*) affect our mood and behavior. The depiction of the hopelessness of mental illness has been partly done away with by the release of movies like *A Beautiful Mind* (2001). Finally, the discovery of newer and more effective drugs has made it possible for many of those with mental illness to lead more normal lives.

Although it is not possible to cover all the psychiatric disorders described in the *Diagnostic and Statistical Manual of Mental Disorders (DSM-IV-TR)*, we will review the most commonly diagnosed disorders: anxiety-related disorders, personality disorders, psychotic disorders of schizophrenia and bipolar disorder, substance abuse, and disorders of childhood and adolescence.

Alzheimer's disease and other degenerative neurological disorders are discussed in Chapter 14, "Caring for the Client with Disorders of the Neurological System."

Anxiety-Related Disorders

These types of disorders were formerly referred to as *neurotic disorders* and include the following categories:

- Dissociative identity disorder
- Generalized anxiety disorder
- Obsessive-compulsive disorder
- Panic disorder
- Phobic disorder
- Post-traumatic disorder
- Somatoform disorder

Anxiety disorders are characterized by feelings of fear and apprehension accompanied by a sense of powerlessness. Anxiety-related disorders are listed on Axis I of the *DSM-IV-TR*.

Generalized Anxiety Disorder

Generalized anxiety disorder (GAD) is the most common form of anxiety disorder and frequently is accompanied by depression and somatization or the development of phobias.

The client with GAD worries excessively over everything, and the stress this creates eventually affects every aspect of life. The client with GAD might try to gain a sense of control by retreating from anxiety-producing situations or by self-medication with drugs or alcohol.

Genetics and alterations in neurotransmitters seem to be the primary causes for GAD. Studies show a higher occurrence in those with an affected twin. Neurophysiology research suggests that alterations in serotonin, norepinephrine, and gamma-aminobutyric acid can account for some cases of generalized anxiety disorder.

Post-traumatic Stress Disorder

Post-traumatic stress disorder (PTSD) develops after exposure to a clearly identifiable threat. The nature of the threat is so extreme that it overwhelms the individual's usual means of coping.

PTSD is characterized according to the onset as either *acute* or *delayed*. Acute PTSD occurs within six months of the event, whereas delayed PTSD occurs six months or more after the event. Symptoms of PTSD include

- ▶ Blunted emotions
- ▶ Feelings of detachment
- ▶ Flashbacks
- ▶ Moral guilt
- ▶ Numbing of responsiveness
- ▶ Survivor guilt

Additional symptoms include increased arousal, anxiety, restlessness, irritability, sleep disturbances, and problems with memory and concentration. Individuals with PTSD frequently have problems with depression and impulsive self-destructive behaviors, including suicide attempts and substance abuse.

Post-traumatic stress disorder is common in survivors of combat, natural disasters, sexual assault, or catastrophic events.

CAUTION

Clients with PTSD who use cocaine or amphetamines are more vulnerable to paranoia and psychosis than those who do not use stimulants.

Dissociative Identity Disorder

Dissociative identity disorder (DID), formerly referred to as *multiple personality disorder*, is characterized by the existence of two or more identities or alter personalities that control the individual's behavior.

The traditional view of DID is that dissociation acts as a defense against an overwhelming sense of anxiety that is both painful and emotionally traumatic. The alter personality contains feelings associated with the trauma, which is often related to physical, emotional, or sexual abuse.

Each alter personality is different from the other, having its own name, ways of behaving, memories, emotional characteristics, and social relationships. Overwhelming psychological stress can cause the onset of a dissociative fugue. The major feature of a dissociative fugue is unexpected travel from home with the appearance of one of the alter personalities. The travel and behavior might seem normal to the casual observer who is unfamiliar with the client's history.

> **NOTE**
>
> The following films offer good depictions of dissociative identity disorder: *The Three Faces of Eve* (1957), *Sybil* (1976), and *Identity* (2003). These films are older, so you might have to check with a movie store that specializes in older films.

Somatoform Disorder

Somatoform disorder is characterized by the appearance of physical symptoms for which there is no apparent organic or physiological cause. The client with a somatoform disorder continuously seeks medical treatment for a physical complaint even though he has been told there is no evidence of physical illness. Somatoform disorders include

- ▶ Conversion disorder
- ▶ Hypochondriasis
- ▶ Pain disorder
- ▶ Somatization disorder

Panic Disorder

Panic disorder is characterized by sudden attacks of intense fear or discomfort that peaks within 10–15 minutes. Clients with panic disorder might complain of not being able to breathe, of feeling they are having a heart attack, or that they are "going crazy." Panic attacks can occur during sleep or in anticipation of some event. In some instances, clients with panic disorder develop agoraphobia, or fear of having a panic attack in a place where they cannot escape. As a result, they restrict activities outside the safety of their home.

Genetic and environmental factors appear to be involved in the development of panic disorder. Other findings suggest that there are alterations in the benzodiazepine receptor sites.

Phobic Disorders

Phobic disorders are expressed as intense, irrational fears of some object, situation, or activity. A person with a phobic disorder experiences anxiety when he comes in contact with the situation or feared object. Although the client recognizes that the fear is irrational, the phobia persists. According to the *DSM-IV-TR* the three major categories of phobic disorders are

▶ Agoraphobia

▶ Social phobia

▶ Specific phobia

There are no clearly identifiable factors in the development of phobic disorders.

Obsessive-Compulsive Disorder

Obsessive-compulsive disorder (OCD) is characterized by the presence of recurrent persistent thoughts, ideas, or impulses and the repetitive rituals that are carried out in response to the obsession. Persons with OCD know that their actions are irrational; still they must carry them out to avoid overwhelming anxiety. Unfortunately, this continual preoccupation interferes with normal relationships. The client with OCD is often viewed by others as rigid, controlling, and lacking spontaneity.

> **NOTE**
>
> The main character in the movie *As Good As It Gets* (1997) is an excellent example of the client with OCD. Remember what happened when his schedule was upset?

There is some evidence that OCD, like other anxiety disorders, is related to genetic transmissions or alterations in serotonin regulation.

Treatment of anxiety disorders depends on the diagnosis and severity of symptoms. Some disorders, such as panic disorder and obsessive-compulsive disorder, respond to treatment with antidepressant medication. Others, such as post-traumatic stress disorder and phobic disorder, benefit from cognitive behavioral therapy and desensitization.

Nursing interventions in caring for the client with an anxiety disorder include administering antidepressant medication, helping the client become aware of situations that increase anxiety, helping the client recognize the overuse of certain defense mechanisms, and teaching cognitive behavioral methods for reducing anxiety.

> **CAUTION**
>
> You should review your psychiatric nursing textbook for a discussion of the most commonly used defense mechanisms as well as cognitive behavioral methods used to reduce anxiety.

Personality Disorders

The second major category of reality-based disorders focuses on the client with faulty personality development.

Unlike clients with an anxiety disorder, who believe that everything is wrong with them, clients with personality disorders seldom seek treatment. They see nothing wrong with their behavior and therefore see no need to change. Personality disorders are listed on Axis II of the *DSM-IV-TR*.

Personality disorders refer to pervasive maladaptive patterns of behavior that are evident in the perceptions, communication, and thinking of an individual. The *DSM-IV-TR* divides personality disorders into three clusters according to the predominant behaviors:

▶ **Cluster A**—Includes odd, eccentric behavior

▶ **Cluster B**—Includes dramatic, erratic, emotional behavior

▶ **Cluster C**—Includes anxious, fearful behavior

Of these three clusters, those with dramatic, erratic behavior pose the greatest threat to others.

Each cluster contains from three to four identifiable personality disorders. The clusters and identified personality disorders of each are outlined in the following sections.

Cluster A

Cluster A disorders include paranoid, schizoid, and schizotypal personality disorders. Although these represent different personalities, they all involve behavior that is odd or eccentric in nature.

Paranoid Personality Disorder

Paranoid personality disorder is characterized by rigid, suspicious, and hypersensitive behavior. Persons with paranoid personality disorder spend a great deal of time and energy validating their suspicions. Unlike those with paranoid schizophrenia, the client with paranoid personality does not have fixed delusions or hallucinations. However, transient psychotic features can appear when the client experiences extreme stress, and the client might be hospitalized because of uncontrollable anger toward others.

Schizoid Personality Disorder

This disorder is characterized by shy, aloof, and withdrawn behavior. The client with schizoid personality disorder prefers solitary activities and is often described by others as a hermit. This client might be quite successful in situations where little interaction with others is required. Although the client with schizoid personality disorder is reality oriented, she often fantasizes or daydreams.

Schizotypal Personality Disorder

Like schizoid personality disorder, this disorder is found more often in relatives of those with schizophrenia. Their behaviors are similar to those of the client with schizoid personality—that is, they are shy, aloof, and withdrawn. However, clients with schizotypal personality disorder display a more bizarre way of thinking. They often appear similar to clients with schizophrenia but with less frequent and less severe psychotic symptoms. Because they are sensitive to the reactions of and possible rejection by others, clients with schizotypal and schizoid behavior avoid social situations.

Cluster B

This disorder set includes the histrionic, narcissistic, antisocial, and borderline personality disorders. Persons with these identified disorders tend to be overly dramatic, attention seeking, and manipulative with little regard for others.

Histrionic Personality Disorder

This disorder is diagnosed most often in females. Sometimes referred to as *southern belle syndrome*, the picture of the histrionic female is one who is overly seductive, excitable, immature, and theatrical in her emotions. These behaviors are not genuine but are used to manipulate others. The client with histrionic personality disorder tends to form many shallow relationships that are always short lived.

Narcissistic Personality Disorder

This disorder is summarized by the expression "It's all about me." Characterized by self-absorption, persons with narcissistic personality have grandiose ideas about their wealth, power, and intelligence. They believe that they are superior to others and that, because they are superior, they are entitled to certain privileges and special treatment. Although they appear nonchalant or indifferent to the criticism of others, it is only a cover-up for deep feelings of resentment and rage. Clients with narcissistic personality tend to rationalize or blame others for their self-centered behavior.

Antisocial Personality Disorder

This is characterized by a pattern of disregard for the rights of others and a failure to learn from past mistakes. These clients frequently have a history of law violations, which usually begin before age 15. Common behaviors in early childhood include cruelty to animals and people, starting fires, running away from home, truancy, breaking and entering, and early substance abuse. Persons with antisocial personality disorder are often described as charming, smooth talking, and extremely intelligent—characteristics that allow them to take advantage of others and escape prosecution when caught.

Persons with antisocial personality disorder do not feel remorse for wrongs committed and respond to confrontation by using the defense mechanisms of denial and rationalization.

NOTE

You might want to check out a number of older movies that depict the features of those with antisocial personality disorder. *Primal Fear* (1996) and *Monster* (2003) are good examples.

Borderline Personality Disorder

Borderline personality disorder, the most commonly treated personality disorder, is seen most often in females who have been victims of sexual abuse. These clients have many of the same traits as those with histrionic, narcissistic, and antisocial personality disorder; thus, they have a difficult time identifying their feelings. Like many victims of sexual abuse, this client relies on dissociation as a means of coping with stress. This dissociation results in *splitting*. Splitting is a very primitive defense mechanism that creates an inability to see self and others as having both good and bad qualities. Clients with borderline personality disorder tend to see themselves and others as all good or all bad. Feelings of abandonment and depression can escalate to the point of self-mutilation and suicidal behavior. These clients usually require hospitalization and treatment with antidepressant medication as well as counseling for post-traumatic stress disorder.

NOTE

Fatal Attraction (1987) is an excellent movie for reviewing the characteristics of borderline personality disorder.

Cluster C

Cluster C disorders include the avoidant, dependent, and obsessive-compulsive personality disorders, which are characterized by anxious, fearful behavior.

Avoidant Personality Disorder

Avoidant personality disorder is used to describe clients who are timid, withdrawn, and hypersensitive to criticism. Although they desire relationships and challenges, clients with this disorder feel socially inadequate, so they avoid situations in which they might be rejected. They tend to lack the self-confidence needed to speak up for what they want and so are seen as helpless.

Dependent Personality Disorder

Dependent personality disorder is characterized by an extreme need to be taken care of by someone else. This dependency on others leads to clinging behavior and fear of separation from the perceived caretaker. Clients with dependent personality disorder see themselves as inferior and incompetent, and they frequently become involved in abusive relationships. These abusive relationships are usually maintained because of a fear of being left alone.

Obsessive-Compulsive Personality Disorder

This disorder describes the individual who is a perfectionist, overly inhibited, and inflexible. Clients with obsessive-compulsive personality disorder are preoccupied with rules, trivial details, and procedures. They are cold and rigid with no expression of tenderness or warmth. They often set standards too high for themselves or others to make and, because they are fearful of making mistakes, tend to procrastinate. Clients with obsessive-compulsive personality disorder put off making decisions until all the facts are in; thus, they might do good work but not be very productive.

> **NOTE**
>
> Although they share some common traits, obsessive-compulsive anxiety disorder and obsessive-compulsive personality disorder are two different diagnoses.

Managing Clients with Personality Disorders

The management of the client with a personality disorder depends on the diagnosis. Pharmacological interventions are generally not appropriate for these clients. However, if there is a coexisting diagnosis such as depression or anxiety, medication will be ordered. The nurse caring for the client with a personality disorder should set limits on the client's behavior while at the same time conveying a sense of acceptance of the individual. Many clients with personality disorders have disturbed personal boundaries; therefore, it is important to maintain a professional rather than friendly relationship.

Psychotic Disorders

Psychotic disorders involve alterations in perceptions in reality. Common symptoms include hallucinations, delusions, and difficulty organizing thoughts. Psychotic symptoms are present in clients with schizophrenia, bipolar disorder, dementia, and drug intoxication or withdrawal. This section reviews two of the most common psychotic disorders: schizophrenia and bipolar disorder. Psychosis associated with drug use and withdrawal is covered later in the chapter.

Schizophrenia

This disorder is most often diagnosed in late adolescence or early adulthood, although symptoms might have been present at a much earlier age. The disorder equally affects both males and females; however, males seem to have an earlier onset of symptoms. Theories offered regarding the cause of schizophrenia include genetics, environmental factors, and biological alterations in the neurotransmitters serotonin and dopamine.

Clients with schizophrenia are best known for their odd appearance and behavior, which are sometimes summarized by the 4 *A's*. The 4 A's include

▶ **Affect**—Described as flat, blunted, or inappropriate

▶ **Autism**—Preoccupation with self and a retreat into fantasy

▶ **Association**—Loosely joined unrelated topics

▶ **Ambivalence**—Having simultaneous opposing feelings

The *DSM-IV-TR* classifies schizophrenia into subtypes based on the client's history and presenting symptoms:

▶ Catatonic

▶ Disorganized

▶ Paranoid

▶ Residual

▶ Undifferentiated

In addition to the subtypes, schizophrenia is classified as having either positive or negative symptoms. *Positive* symptoms of schizophrenia are those such as delusions and hallucinations; *negative* symptoms are those such as social withdrawal and failure to communicate with others. One of the main differences in the newer antipsychotic medications is that they work on both the negative as well as the positive symptoms of schizophrenia. The older medications worked primarily on clearing the hallucinations and delusions.

> **NOTE**
>
> You might want to refer to your nursing textbook for a more complete description of the subtypes and symptoms associated with positive and negative schizophrenia. Although there are overlapping symptoms, some have unique features. For instance, the client with catatonic schizophrenia exhibits waxy flexibility or stupor.

Nursing interventions in the care of the client with schizophrenia include

▶ Providing a quiet, supportive environment

▶ Establishing a trusting relationship

▶ Administering antipsychotic medication

▶ Observing for side effects of antipsychotic medication

▶ Assisting with the activities of daily living

▶ Attending to the client's physical needs, including nutrition and hydration

Instead of allowing the client to retreat to his room, the nurse should provide simple recreational activities such as painting.

> **NOTE**
>
> It is best to avoid challenging activities that can confuse and overwhelm the client.

The nurse shouldn't argue or try to change the client's delusional thinking; instead, redirecting the client to a reality-based subject will be more effective and less upsetting. In instances where the client is having hallucinations, the nurse should respond to the client's feelings and at the same time reinforce what is real. For example, the nurse should acknowledge the client's fear at hearing voices when no one is there but then point out that the voices are not real and that the medication will soon help eliminate the voices.

The discovery of newer, more effective medications in the past decade has enabled many persons with schizophrenia to remain in their homes and communities for longer periods of time than the older medications. These medications are often referred to as atypical or novel. Atypical antipsychotics, such as risperidone, can be given in smaller doses, produce fewer side effects, and help manage the negative symptoms of schizophrenia more effectively than the older antipsychotics (such as chlorpromazine).

> **NOTE**
>
> The mainstay in the management of the client with schizophrenia is medication. Refer to the chapter on psychopharmacology in your psychiatric nursing textbook for more information on the typical and atypical antipsychotics.

> **CAUTION**
>
> Antipsychotic medication carries the risk of neuroleptic malignant syndrome, a potentially fatal adverse reaction. Symptoms of neuroleptic malignant syndrome include malignant hyperthermia or extreme temperature elevation, in some instance as high as 107° F. The medication should be immediately discontinued and an antiparkinsonian medication given.
>
> Older antipsychotic medications have many side effects and adverse reactions associated with their use, including extrapyramidal effects. Some of these are severe enough to warrant discontinuing the drug and administering medication to reverse their effects.

Schizophrenia is a chronic illness and, although the medications improve the client's quality of life, they do not cure the disease. The prognosis for the client with schizophrenia is based on the subtype, severity of symptoms, and compliance with treatment.

Bipolar Disorders

This refers to a group of psychotic disorders that are evident in extreme changes in mood or affect. These disorders, like schizophrenia, are believed to be caused by alterations in serotonin, dopamine, and norepinephrine. Most clients with bipolar disorder have the type known as *bipolar I*, in which the client experiences periods of acute mania and major depression.

Acute Mania

Manic episodes are essential to a diagnosis of bipolar I disorder. During a manic episode, the client experiences profound changes in mood. These mood changes are described as elevated, expansive, or irritable. Additional symptoms associated with acute mania include

- ▶ Delusions of grandeur
- ▶ Flight of ideas
- ▶ Increased motor activity
- ▶ Increased risk taking and promiscuity
- ▶ Use of profanity
- ▶ Uncontrolled spending
- ▶ Failing to sleep or eat for long periods of time

When lim[...] [...]t's behavior, he typically reacts with sarcasm and belligerenc[...]

Nu[...] [...]nia include providing a quiet, nonstimulating [...]

[...] [...]haustion. Most will have weight loss due to [...] best be met by providing high-calorie, [...]hile moving about. Nursing inter-[...]stabilize the mood. Medications

con[...] [...]roic acid, and carbamezepine.
Olanz[...] [...]n to be effective in treating clients
with acut[...]

> **CAUTION**
>
> Lithium is not a drug, [...] [...]e mood of the client with acute mania. During the initiation of lithium therapy, l[...] [...]drawn twice weekly and then every 2–3 months during long-term therapy.
>
> The therapeutic range for lithium [...].5 mEq/Liter.* Lithium levels greater than 1.5 mEq/iter can produce signs of toxicity that can be fa[...] Symptoms of lithium toxicity include muscle weakness, confusion, ataxia, seizures, cardio-respiratory changes, and multiple organ failure. A standard treatment for lithium toxicity is the administration of intravenous normal saline.
>
> *The therapeutic range for lithium may vary slightly according to laboratory methods used.

Major Depression

Major depression, the other side of bipolar I disorder, is characterized by a depressed mood lasting at least two weeks. Symptoms of major depression include feelings of worthlessness, diminished ability to concentrate, anorexia, sleep disturbances, and recurrent thoughts of death or suicide. A diagnosis of mental disorder or substance abuse is among the most significant risk factors for suicide.

> **CAUTION**
>
> The depressed client should be assessed for the presence of suicidal ideation and suicidal plan. Harmful objects should be removed from the client's environment, and the client should be placed on basic suicide precautions with constant observation by the nursing staff. The nurse must remember that the greatest risk for suicide exists when the client seems to be improving.

Nursing interventions for the client with major depression include providing a safe environment, meeting the client's physiological needs, reinforcing the client's sense of worth, assisting with electroconvulsive therapy, and administering antidepressant medications. Currently, the most frequently prescribed antidepressants are selective serotonin reuptake inhibitors (SSRIs). Less frequently prescribed medications include monoamine oxidase inhibitors (MAOIs).

> **CAUTION**
>
> The use of SSRIs with MAOIs, selective MAOIs, tryptophan, and St. John's wort is contraindicated. Serotonin syndrome, a potentially fatal condition, can occur as a result of drug interaction. Symptoms of serotonin reaction include confusion, hypomania, agitation, hyperthermia, hyperreflexia, tremors, rigidity, and gastrointestinal upset. The medication should be discontinued immediately. The physician will order medication to block the serotonin receptors, and artificial ventilation might be required. Most clients show improvement within 24 hours of discontinuing the SSRI.

Substance Abuse

Substance abuse is defined as the excessive use of a drug that is different from societal norms. These drugs can be illegal, as in the case of heroin, or legal, as in the case of alcohol or prescription drugs. Symptoms of substance abuse include

- Absenteeism
- Decline in school or work performance
- Frequent accidents
- Increased isolation
- Slurred speech
- Tremors

The primary substance abuse problem in the United States is alcohol addiction.

Alcoholism

Alcoholism is responsible for more than 100,000 deaths each year in the United States. Many of these deaths are the result of accidents. Premature death from cirrhosis, cardiovascular disease, esophageal varices, and cancer has also been linked to heavy alcohol consumption. It is important for the nurse to recognize the stages of alcohol withdrawal to keep the client safe. Symptoms of withdrawal usually begin about 6–8 hours after the client's last drink, or when the amount consumed is less than usual. Four stages of alcohol withdrawal are generally recognized. The stages of withdrawal and the symptoms associated with each stage are as follows:

▶ **Stage 1 (6–8 hours after last use)**—Symptoms include anxiety, anorexia, tremors, nausea and vomiting, depression, headache, increased blood pressure, tachycardia, and profuse sweating.

▶ **Stage 2 (8–12 hours after last use)**—Symptoms include confusion, disorientation, hallucinations, hyperactivity, and gross tremors.

▶ **Stage 3 (12–48 hours after last use)**—Symptoms include severe anxiety, increased blood pressure, profuse sweating, severe hallucinations, and grand mal seizures.

▶ **Stage 4 (3–5 days after last use)**—Symptoms of delirium tremens include confusion, insomnia, agitation, hallucinations, and uncontrolled tachycardia. In spite of treatment, the client might die from cardiac complications.

NOTE

Although each stage has an expected timeframe and behaviors during the withdrawal, you should keep in mind that withdrawal is highly individual.

TIP

The Addiction Research Foundation Chemical Institute Withdrawal Assessment-Alcohol (CIWA-Ar) is a useful instrument for quickly assessing the client's withdrawal status (see Figure 15.1).

Nursing interventions for the client with alcohol withdrawal include maintaining a safe environment, providing nutritional supplements, providing additional fluids to prevent dehydration, and administering pharmacological agents to prevent delirium tremens.

CAUTION

The nurse should teach the client taking Antabuse (disulfiram) to avoid alcohol or substances containing alcohol. Contact with alcohol while taking Antabuse (disulfiram) can produce headache, nausea and vomiting, tachycardia, chest pain, convulsions, cardio-respiratory collapse, and death.

Assessment of Alcohol Withdrawal

Patient:_____Date:_____Time:_____:_____

Pulse or heart rate,taken for one minute:_____ Blood pressure:_____/_____

Nausea and vomiting. Ask "Do you feel sick to your stomach? Have you vomited?"
Observation:
  0–No nausea and no vomiting
  1–Mild nausea with no vomiting
  2–
  3–
  4–Intermittent nausea with dry heaves
  5–
  6–
  7–Constant nausea, frequent dry heaves, and vomiting
Tremor. Ask patient to extend arms and spread fingers apart.
Observation:
  0–No tremor
  1–Tremor not visible but can be felt, fingertip to fingertip
  2–
  3–
  4–Moderate tremor with arms extended
  5–
  6–
  7–Severe tremor, even with arms not extended
Paroxysmal sweats.
Observation:
  0–No sweat visible
  1–Barely perceptible sweating; palms moist
  2–
  3–
  4–Beads of sweat obvious on forehead
  5–
  6–
  7–Drenching sweats
Anxiety. Ask "Do you feel nervous?"
Observation:
  0–No anxiety (at ease)
  1–Mildly anxious
  2–
  3–
  4–Moderately anxious or guarded, so anxiety is inferred
  5–
  6–
  7–Equivalent to acute panic states as occur in severe delirium or acute schizophrenic reactions
Agitation.
Observation:
  0–Normal activity
  1–Somewhat more than normal activity
  2–
  3–
  4–Moderately fidgety and restless
  5–
  6–
  7–Paces back and forth during most of the interview or constantly thrashes about

Tactile disturbances. Ask "Do you have any itching, pins-and-needles sensations, burning, or numbness, or do you feel like bugs are crawling on or under skin?"
Observation:
  0–None
  1–Very mild itching, pins-and-needles, sensation, burning, or numbness
  2–Mild itching, pins-and-needles sensation, burning, or numbness
  3–Moderate itching, pins-and-needles sensation, burning or numbness
  4–Moderately severe hallucinations
  5–Severe hallucinations
  6–Extremely severe hallucinations
  7–Continuous hallucinations
Auditory disturbances. Ask "Are you more aware of sounds around you? Are they harsh? Do they frighten you? Are you hearing anything that is disturbing to you? Are you hearing things you know are not there?"
Observation:
  0–Not present
  1–Very mild harshness or ability to frighten
  2–Mild harshness or ability to frighten
  3–Moderate harshness or ability to frighten
  4–Moderately severe hallucinations
  5–Severe hallucinations
  6–Extremely severe hallucinations
  7–Continuous hallucinations
Visual disturbances. Ask "Does the light appear to be too bright? Is its color different? Does it hurt your eyes? Are you seeing anything that is disturbing to you? Are you seeing things you know are not there?"
Observation:
  0–Not present
  1–Very mild sensitivity
  2–Mild sensitivity
  3–Moderate sensitivity
  4–Moderately severe hallucinations
  5–Severe hallucinations
  6–Extremely severe hallucinations
  7–Continuous hallucinations
Headache, fullness in head. Ask "Does your head feel different? Does it feel like there is a band around your head?"
Do not rate for dizziness or lightheadedness; otherwise, rate severity.
  0–Not present
  1–Very mild
  2–Mild
  3–Moderate
  4–Moderately severe
  5–Severe
  6–Very severe
  7–Extremely severe
Orientation and clouding of sensorium. Ask "What day is this? Where are you? Who am I?"
Observation:
  0–Orientated and can do serial additions
  1–Cannot do serial additions or is uncertain about date
  2–Date disorientation by no more than two calendar dates
  3–Date disorientation by more than two calendar days
  4–Disoriented for place and/or person

Total score:_____(maximum = 67):_____Rater's initials_____

FIGURE 15.1 Clinical Institute Withdrawal Assessment for Alcohol (CIWA-Ar) scale.

Other Commonly Abused Substances

Other commonly abused substances include sedative-hypnotics, opiates, stimulants, hallucinogens, and cannabis. Tables 15.1–15.5 list the signs of use, signs of withdrawal, signs of overdose, and treatments for several of these substances.

Sedative-Hypnotics

Sedative-hypnotics are potent central nervous system depressants. This group, which includes barbiturates and benzodiazepines, is capable of producing both physiological and psychological dependence. Drugs in this category are regulated by the Controlled Substances Act. Table

15.1 highlights important signs and treatments related to clients abusing sedative-hypnotic drugs.

TABLE 15.1   Signs and Treatments Related to Sedative-Hypnotic Abuse

Signs of use	Slurred speech, unsteady gait, drowsiness, decreased blood pressure, irritability, inability to concentrate
Signs of withdrawal	Nausea and vomiting, tachycardia, diaphoresis, tremors, and seizures
Signs of overdose	Cardiovascular and respiratory depression, seizures, shock, coma, death
Treatment of overdose	Activated charcoal and gastric lavage, mechanical ventilation and dialysis as needed

CAUTION

Withdrawal from barbiturates should be done by slow taper to avoid fatal seizures.

Opiates

This refers to a group of drugs used for their analgesic effects. These drugs include the natural opiates morphine and codeine as well as synthetic opiates such as meperidine and methadone. Opiates produce both physiological and psychological addiction. One of the most abused opiates, heroin, has no legal medical use. Others are regulated by the Controlled Substances Act. Table 15.2 highlights signs and treatments related to clients abusing opiates.

TABLE 15.2   Signs and Treatments Related to Opiate Abuse

Signs of use	Constricted pupils, decreased respirations, decreased blood pressure, euphoria, impaired attention span, impaired judgment
Signs of withdrawal	Anorexia, irritability, runny nose, nausea, bone pain, chills
Signs of overdose	Dilated pupils, respiratory depression, seizures, coma, death
Treatment of overdose	Narcan (a narcotic antagonist that reverses the central nervous system depression)

Stimulants

Stimulants excite various areas of the central nervous system. Some stimulants, such as the amphetamine and nonamphetamine groups, are used to treat attention deficit hyperactivity disorder and weight loss. Cocaine is used to control local bleeding and is an ingredient in some eye medications. Others, such as caffeine and alcohol, are widely accepted for social use. Stimulants are physiologically addicting; therefore, the more potent ones are regulated by the Controlled Substances Act. Table 15.3 highlights signs and treatments related to clients abusing stimulants.

TABLE 15.3   Signs and Treatments Related to Stimulant Abuse

Signs of use	Euphoria, grandiosity, dilated pupils, tachycardia, elevated blood pressure, nausea and vomiting, paranoia, hallucinations, violent outbursts
Signs of withdrawal	Agitation, disorientation, insomnia, depression, suicidal ideation
Signs of overdose	Ataxia, hyperpyrexia, respiratory distress, seizures, cardiovascular collapse, coma, death
Treatment of overdose	Provide respiratory and cardiac support, treatment of hyperpyrexia and seizures

Hallucinogens

Hallucinogens are capable of distorting perceptions of reality. Hallucinogens include those that occur naturally, such as mescaline and psilocybin, as well as those that are synthetically produced, such as LSD. There is no evidence of physiological dependence with hallucinogens; however, they can produce tolerance and psychological dependence. Table 15.4 highlights signs and treatments related to clients abusing hallucinogens.

TABLE 15.4   Signs and Treatments Related to Hallucinogens Abuse

Signs of use	Dilated pupils, tachycardia, diaphoresis, irregular eye movement, grandiosity, hallucinations
Signs of withdrawal	None known
Signs of overdose	Psychosis, possible hypertensive crisis, hyperthermia, seizures
Treatment of overdose	Provide a quiet environment and sedation for anxiety

Cannabis

Cannabis ranks second among the drugs abused in the United States. Marijuana, which is composed of the dried leaves, stems, and flowers of the hemp plant (Cannabis sativa), is the most prevalent cannabis preparation. Hashish is derived from the flowering tops of the plant. Medical uses for marijuana include the management of glaucoma, treatment of the nausea that accompanies cancer therapy, and an appetite stimulant for clients with AIDS-related anorexia. Physical dependence and tolerance have been found in chronic users. Table 15.5 highlights signs and treatments related to clients abusing cannabis.

TABLE 15.5   Signs and Treatments Related to Cannabis Abuse

Signs of use	Tachycardia, increased appetite, euphoria, slowed perception of time
Signs of withdrawal	Irritability, restlessness, insomnia, tremors, sweating, gastrointestinal upset
Signs of overdose	Fatigue, paranoia, psychosis
Treatment of overdose	Treatment of presenting symptoms

Disorders of Childhood and Adolescence

These disorders refer to the emotional and behavioral alterations that become evident in the early years of life. In this section, we review five of these disorders:

- ▶ Conduct disorder

- ▶ Oppositional defiant disorder

- ▶ Attention deficit hyperactive disorder

- ▶ Autistic disorder

- ▶ Eating disorders

Other emotional disorders, such as major depression and schizophrenia, were covered in previous sections of this chapter.

Conduct Disorder

Conduct disorder is characterized by persistent patterns of behavior in which the rights of others are violated. Early in life, some say by the age of three, the child with conduct disorder is observed to be cruel and physically aggressive with people and animals. The child later develops antisocial behavior that includes destruction of property, truancy, and substance abuse. When confronted with their behavior, children with conduct disorder show a lack of guilt or remorse and frequently blame others for their acts. Conduct disorder gives way to an adult diagnosis of antisocial personality disorder.

Oppositional Defiant Disorder

Oppositional defiant disorder is characterized by persistent patterns of negativistic, hostile, and defiant behavior. Unlike the child with conduct disorder, the child with oppositional defiant disorder does not violate the rights of others. The behaviors of the child diagnosed with oppositional defiance are more likely to be argumentative, uncooperative, annoying, and spiteful.

Attention Deficit Hyperactive Disorder

Attention deficit hyperactive disorder (ADHD) is characterized by persistent patterns of hyperactivity, impulsivity, and inattention. The disorder, which is more common in boys, often goes unrecognized until the child enters school. The child with ADHD typically has problems following directions and lacks the attention necessary to complete assigned tasks. Theories as to the cause of ADHD include genetics, exposure to environmental lead, dietary influences, and alterations in dopamine and norepinephrine levels. Impairments in social, academic, and occupational functioning are common in those with ADHD.

The approach to the treatment of ADHD is threefold. Children with ADHD need counseling to help them develop positive self-esteem and gain the social skills necessary for making and keeping friends. These children also need educational interventions to help them succeed in school. Finally, children with ADHD can benefit from medication that helps control the symptoms of the disorder.

Autistic Disorder

Autistic disorder, Asperger's syndrome, Rett's disorder, and childhood disintegrative disorder make up a set of disorders referred to as pervasive developmental delay. The majority of cases of pervasive developmental delay are children with autistic disorder or simple autism. Although symptoms often begin between 18–24 months, most children are diagnosed between the ages of 6 and 11 years. The cause of autism is not known though there have been several theories including genetic transmission, immune responses, neuroanatomical changes, and alterations in the neurotransmitters dopamine and serotonin. There is a higher incidence in male children as well as children with Down syndrome and phenylketonuria.

Clinical manifestations commonly observed in the child with autism include:

▶ Impaired social interaction

▶ Impaired communication

▶ Problems adapting to new situations

▶ Impaired attention span

▶ Speech difficulties or delays in speech

▶ Absence of babbling by one year of age and absence of speech by two years of age

▶ Inability to respond to social or emotional cues in a normal manner

▶ Presence of rigid, obsessive behaviors

▶ Head banging, twirling in circles, self-biting

▶ Abnormal and exaggerated responses to sensory stimuli

Interventions for the child with autism include teaching and rewarding appropriate behaviors, encouraging positive, adaptive coping skills, and facilitating effective communication. Medications are not a part of the treatment of autism, but they can be used to treat associated behavioral disorders.

Eating Disorders

Eating disorders refer to the separate disorders of anorexia nervosa and bulimia nervosa. Both disorders, which are more common in females, have increased in incidence in the past three decades.

Anorexia Nervosa

Anorexia nervosa is defined as a morbid fear of obesity characterized by a preoccupation with food while refusing to eat. The client with anorexia nervosa sustains significant weight loss through strict dieting, excessive exercising, self-induced vomiting, and the abuse of laxatives and diuretics.

Bulimia Nervosa

Bulimia nervosa is characterized by the uncontrolled compulsive ingestion of enormous amounts of food in a short period of time. High-calorie, high-carbohydrate snacks that can be ingested quickly are preferred. The binging episode, which occurs in secret, is followed by feelings of guilt that are relieved only by a period of purging.

Nursing interventions for the client with an eating disorder include stabilizing the client's physical condition. Complications from fluid and electrolyte imbalance and muscle wasting are often life-threatening. When the client's physical condition is stable, treatment modalities using behavior modification, individual therapy, and family therapy are begun. Although there are no specific medications to treat eating disorders, selective serotonin reuptake inhibitors have been effective in treating bulimia nervosa.

Diagnostic Tests for Review

The diagnostic tests for a client admitted with a psychiatric diagnosis include many of the tests used for clients with any hospital admission. Other tests are necessary for monitoring the client's response to certain medications. For example, the client with lithium will continue to show signs of mania until a therapeutic level is reached. Some of the diagnostics requested for the client on a behavioral health unit include

- CBC
- Complete metabolic panel
- Lithium level
- Urinalysis

Pharmacology Categories for Review

The client with a psychiatric diagnosis usually receives one or more of the psychotropic medications. Some conditions, such as ADHD, are treated with central nervous system stimulants or antidepressants. The categories of psychotropic medications commonly prescribed are

▶ Anticonvulsants

▶ Antidepressants

▶ Antipsychotics

▶ Mood stabilizers

▶ Selective norepinephrine reuptake inhibitors (ADHD)

▶ Stimulants (ADHD)

Exam Prep Questions

1. A client with paranoid personality disorder monopolizes group activities with complaints that the staff is out to get him. The nurse should:

   ○ **A.** Point out that his suspicions are unfounded.

   ○ **B.** Ask the client to return to his room for awhile.

   ○ **C.** Tell the client that he is upsetting others.

   ○ **D.** Talk with the client in a nonchallenging manner.

2. The nurse is caring for a preschool-aged child admitted with a diagnosis of suspected child abuse. During painful procedures, the child remains quiet and watchful. When planning the care of a victim of child abuse, the nurse should give priority to:

   ○ **A.** Arranging playtime with same-age children

   ○ **B.** Scheduling the same caregiver each day

   ○ **C.** Asking how the injury occurred

   ○ **D.** Praising the child for grown-up behavior

3. An adolescent hospitalized with conduct disorder has been seen taking items from the nurse's station. The most therapeutic response by the nurse would be to:

   ○ **A.** Confront the client with his behavior and maintain limit setting.

   ○ **B.** Request stimulant medication to control his behavior.

   ○ **C.** Recognize that the client is not responsible for his actions.

   ○ **D.** Tell the client he will be punished for stealing.

4. The nurse is preparing to discharge a client who is receiving Nardil. The nurse should tell the client to:

   ○ **A.** Wear protective clothing and sunglasses outside.

   ○ **B.** Avoid medications containing pseudoephedrine.

   ○ **C.** Drink six to eight glasses of water a day.

   ○ **D.** Avoid foods that are high in purine.

5. The nurse caring for a client with mania understands that the client's behavior is a way of avoiding feelings of despair. The expression of behaviors opposite to those being experienced is an example of which defense mechanism?

   ○ **A.** Conversion

   ○ **B.** Splitting

   ○ **C.** Sublimation

   ○ **D.** Reaction formation

6. The morning staff of an inpatient psychiatric unit has just completed the change of shift report. The nurse should give priority to assessing the client:

   ○ **A.** With schizophrenia having auditory hallucinations

   ○ **B.** Scheduled for electroconvulsive therapy

   ○ **C.** With a lithium level of 1.8 meq/L

   ○ **D.** Receiving chlorpromazine with a WBC of 7,500

7. A client taking Zoloft tells the nurse that she has also been taking St. John's wort. The nurse should report this information to the doctor because:

   ○ **A.** The two substances have opposing effects.

   ○ **B.** The amount of medication may be reduced.

   ○ **C.** Herbals only provide a placebo effect.

   ○ **D.** It will be necessary to increase the dosage.

8. The nurse is observing the movements of a client receiving Thorazine. The client continually paces and rocks back and forth when sitting. The nurse recognizes that the client is experiencing:

   ○ **A.** Oculogyric crisis

   ○ **B.** Akathesia

   ○ **C.** Dystonia

   ○ **D.** Bradykinesia

9. Which nursing diagnosis is least likely to apply to the client admitted with a diagnosis of borderline personality disorder?

   ○ **A.** Risk for self-injury

   ○ **B.** Identity disturbance

   ○ **C.** Self-esteem disturbance

   ○ **D.** Sensory-perceptual alteration

10. A client addicted to morphine is being treated for withdrawal symptoms. The drug commonly administered for opiate withdrawal is:

   ○ **A.** Tranxene

   ○ **B.** Methadone

   ○ **C.** Narcan

   ○ **D.** Antabuse

Answer Rationales

1. Answer D is correct. One of the most therapeutic actions the nurse can take with the paranoid client is to spend time with him but not challenge his delusions. Answer A would challenge his delusions and make him more convinced that he is right, so it is incorrect. Answers B and C would isolate the client and increase his paranoid thinking, so they're incorrect.

2. Answer B is correct. Assigning a consistent caregiver will best meet the child's need for safety and security. Playtime will be therapeutic for the child, but it does not have to be with same-age children, so answer A is incorrect. Answer C is too threatening to the child who has been abused, so it is incorrect. Answer D does not allow the child the chance to respond in an expected way, so it is incorrect.

3. Answer A is correct. Management of the client with conduct disorder includes explaining the rules of the unit and maintaining limits on behavior. There is a loss of privileges if the client continues to violate unit rules. Answer B is incorrect because stimulants do not control antisocial behavior. The client with conduct disorder is responsible for his actions; therefore, answer C is incorrect. Answer D is threatening, so it is incorrect.

4. Answer B is correct. Drug interactions between an MAOI and pseudoephedrine can result in hypertensive crisis. Answer A refers to the client receiving antipsychotic medications such as Thorazine, so it is incorrect. Answers C and D do not apply to MAOIs, so they are incorrect.

5. Answer D is correct. Reaction formation is the outward expression of feelings that are opposite to those experienced. Answer A refers to the development of physical symptoms in response to inner conflict, so it is incorrect. Answer B refers to the defense mechanism used by those with borderline personality disorder, so it is incorrect. Answer C is incorrect because it's the channeling of unacceptable thoughts and behaviors into socially acceptable behaviors.

6. Answer C is correct. The client's lithium level is in the toxic range. Answers A and B should be seen next therefore they are incorrect. Answer D has a normal WBC and can be seen last, so it is incorrect.

7. Answer B is correct. St. John's wort has an antidepressant effect so it might be necessary to reduce the current medication dosage. Answers A, C, and D are incorrect statements, so they're incorrect.

8. Answer B is correct. The client's movements are an example of akathesia. Answers A, C, and D are also extrapyramidal side effects of Thorazine, but they involve different movements, so they're incorrect.

9. Answer D is correct. The client with borderline personality is least likely to have sensory-perceptual alteration. Answers A, B, and C do apply to the client with borderline personality disorder, so they're incorrect.

10. Answer B is correct. Methadone is given for the treatment of opiate withdrawal. Answer A is given for the treatment of alcohol withdrawal, so it's incorrect. Answer C is given for opiate and narcotic overdose, so it is incorrect. Answer D is aversive therapy for the treatment of alcoholism, so it's incorrect.

Suggested Reading and Resources

▶ Kneisl, C., and Trigoboff, E. *Contemporary Psychiatric Mental Health Nursing.* 2nd ed. Upper Saddle River, NJ: Pearson Prentice Hall, 2009.

▶ Townsend, M. *Essentials of Psychiatric Mental Health Nursing.* 4th ed. Philadelphia: F.A. Davis, 2008.

▶ Lehne, R. *Pharmacology for Nursing Care.* 7th ed. Philadelphia: Elsevier, 2009.

▶ Ball, J., and Bindler, R. *Pediatric Nursing: Caring for Children.* 4th ed. Upper Saddle River, NJ: Pearson Prentice Hall, 2008.

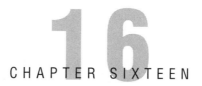

CHAPTER SIXTEEN

Caring for the Maternal/Infant Client

Terms you'll need to understand

- ✓ Abortion
- ✓ Alpha-fetoprotein
- ✓ Amenorrhea
- ✓ Braxton Hicks contractions
- ✓ Caput succedaneum
- ✓ Cervix
- ✓ Cesarean section
- ✓ Chadwick's sign
- ✓ Colostrum
- ✓ Condylomata acuminata
- ✓ Contraception
- ✓ Decelerations
- ✓ Disseminated intravascular coagulation
- ✓ Dystocia
- ✓ Ectopic pregnancy
- ✓ Epidural anesthesia
- ✓ Estriol
- ✓ Fetal monitoring
- ✓ Fundus
- ✓ Goodell's sign
- ✓ Hegar's sign
- ✓ HELLP
- ✓ Herpes
- ✓ Human papillomavirus (HPV)
- ✓ Hydatidiform mole
- ✓ Hyperbilirubinemia
- ✓ Hyperemesis gravidarum
- ✓ Isoimmunization
- ✓ Leopold's maneuvers
- ✓ Linea nigra
- ✓ McDonald's sign
- ✓ Multigravida
- ✓ Nagel's rule
- ✓ Nullipara
- ✓ Oligohydramnios
- ✓ Oxytocin
- ✓ Papanicolaou smear
- ✓ Para
- ✓ Pica
- ✓ Polyhydramnios
- ✓ Preeclampsia
- ✓ Premature rupture of membranes
- ✓ Preterm labor
- ✓ Prostaglandin
- ✓ Pulmonary surfactant
- ✓ Rubella
- ✓ Sexually transmitted infections
- ✓ TORCH
- ✓ Toxic Shock Syndrome
- ✓ Toxoplasmosis
- ✓ Ultrasonography
- ✓ Wharton's jelly

Nursing skills you'll need to master

- ✓ Performing pediatric heelstick
- ✓ Checking for cervical dilation
- ✓ Performing fetal monitoring

This chapter focuses on the health needs of the obstetric client and newborn. Methods of birth control, prenatal care, and diseases affecting women are also discussed. After reviewing this chapter, the nurse should be able to answer commonly asked questions and provide teaching for the client and family.

Signs of Pregnancy

Signs of pregnancy include presumptive signs, probable signs, and positive signs. *Presumptive* signs are subjective and can be associated with some other gynecological alteration. *Probable* signs can be documented and are more conclusive; however, these signs can also be associated with conditions other than pregnancy. *Positive* signs establish the diagnosis of pregnancy.

Presumptive Signs

Presumptive signs of pregnancy are those signs and symptoms that lead the client to believe she is pregnant but that are not conclusive. Symptoms that make the client suspect pregnancy include

- Amenorrhea
- Breast sensitivity
- Chadwick's sign
- Fatigue
- Fingernail changes
- Urinary frequency
- Weight gain

Probable Signs

Probable signs of pregnancy are more conclusive than presumptive signs, but are still not definitive. Even though the client believes she is pregnant, more tests should be done to determine if pregnancy exists. The probable signs of pregnancy are:

- Ballottement—Ballottement is easy flexion of the uterus when the examiner's finger pushes against the uterus and detects the presence of the fetus by return impact.
- Chadwick's sign—Chadwick's sign is the bluish discoloration of the vagina and cervix.
- Goodell's sign—Goodell's sign is softening of the cervix.

- ▶ Hegar's sign—Hegar's sign is softening of the portion of the cervix between the uterus and vaginal portion of the cervix.

- ▶ Positive pregnancy test—Rising Hcg levels prompts a positive pregnancy test.

- ▶ Uterine enlargement—Occurs as the fetus grows.

Positive Signs

There are only three definite signs of pregnancy. These signs are

- ▶ Fetal heart tones

- ▶ Leopold's maneuver, which is manual external palpation of the fetal outline

- ▶ Ultrasound of the fetal outline

Prenatal Care

Early prenatal care provides the nurse the opportunity to teach the client and family members. Systematic physical exam and health history provide information needed to treat and prevent fetal anomalies. Screening tests are performed during the prenatal visit to detect diseases that affect the mother and fetus. It has been found that the earlier the pregnant client begins to visit the doctor, the better the outcome for the mother and newborn. In this section, you will discover prenatal topics and information that might be tested on the NCLEX exam.

Prenatal Diet and Weight Maintenance

During the prenatal period, the nurse should encourage the client to eat foods high in vitamins and minerals. A weight gain of approximately 36 pounds is allowable, and weight reduction during pregnancy is generally discouraged. Prior to pregnancy, the client should be encouraged to increase the intake of foods high in vitamins such as B9 (folic acid). The ingestion of folic acid has been credited to a reduction of neural tube defects. Prenatal diagnostic studies can be performed to detect neural tube defects and other conditions.

Alpha-Fetoprotein Screening

Alpha-fetoprotein levels can be done on mother's blood between 16 and 20 weeks gestation. Alpha-fetoprotein levels are considered a screening tool and are not diagnostic. This level can be tested by obtaining a blood sample from the mother. Alpha-fetoprotein is a glucoprotein produced by the fetal yolk sac, gastrointestinal tract, and liver. This protein passes through the placenta to the maternal circulation and is excreted through fetal circulation. Normal ranges for each week of pregnancy are measured.

If abnormal levels are detected, the physician will probably perform an amniocentesis. An amniocentesis can be performed as early as 16 weeks gestation. An ultrasound exam of the uterus is performed prior to the amniocentesis to locate the placenta and the pockets of amniotic fluid. The client having an abdominal ultrasound is instructed to drink large amounts of fluids to fill the bladder and not to void until after the ultrasound exam. When the fetus is visualized and pockets of amniotic fluid are found, the client is instructed to void. When an amniocentesis is performed a sample of amniotic fluid is then removed using a large bore needle. The client is instructed to remain in the clinic for approximately two hours and to report any bleeding or cramping.

NOTE

The client having an amniocentesis prior to 20 weeks gestation should be instructed not to void until after the amniocentesis. A full bladder helps to push the uterus up in the abdominal cavity, thereby providing access to pockets of amniotic fluid. After 20 weeks, the client should be asked to void prior to the amniocentesis because there is an increased risk of damaging the bladder with the amniocentesis needle.

Note that clients having a vaginal ultrasound should be instructed to void prior to the exam. Please note that this is different than the preparation for a client having an abdominal ultrasound.

Other Prenatal Diagnostic Tests

Diagnostic studies can also be done from examination of amniotic fluid. Although amniocentesis is an invasive procedure with risk, the benefits of early diagnosis are many. Following the amniocentesis, the client should be told to report any cramping or bleeding and avoid lifting objects heavier than five pounds for several days. Some of the tests that can be performed on the amniotic fluid are lecithin/sphingomyelin (L/S) ratios, which detect lung maturity; estriol levels, which indicate fetal distress; and creatinine levels, which indicate renal function. Teratogenic effects of drugs and disease can also be detected by checking the amniotic fluid. Some examples of teratogenic agents are

- Accutane
- Alcohol
- Cytomegalovirus
- Herpes
- LSD
- Rubella virus
- Syphilis

▶ Tetracycline

▶ Toxoplasmosis

NOTE

TORCHS is a syndrome that includes toxoplasmosis, rubella, cytomegalovirus, herpes, and syphilis.

Assessing Fetal Heart Tones

The fetal heart tone should be checked frequently to measure the viability and status of circulating blood to the fetus. This noninvasive technique can be obtained by use of a fetoscope or tocomonitor.

Fetal heart tones can be heard with a fetoscope at approximately 18–20 weeks and with a Doppler ultrasound at approximately 12 weeks.

Ultrasonography

Ultrasonography is done to determine fetal age and can be a useful tool in determining fetal abnormalities. If a vaginal ultrasound is performed, the client is instructed to void prior to the test. If an abdominal ultrasound is performed, the client is instructed not to void until after the test.

Signs of Complications of Pregnancy

There are many complications of pregnancy. The nurse should instruct the client to report to a doctor if she has any of the following symptoms:

▶ **Persistent vomiting**—Hyperemesis gravidarum (nausea and vomiting after the first trimester) can lead to fluid and electrolyte imbalances.

▶ **Vaginal bleeding**—Can be an indication of placenta previa (placenta over cervix, which produces painless bleeding), abruptio placenta (separation of the placenta before the third stage of labor, which produces painful bleeding), or a threatened abortion.

▶ **Abdominal pain**—Can indicate a threatened abortion, an ectopic pregnancy (pregnancy outside the body of the uterus; if it ruptures, peritonitis results), or abruptio placenta.

▶ **Incompetent cervix**—Causes a spontaneous abortion. This problem is corrected by performing a McDonalds' cerclage or Shirodkar procedure to close the cervix.

▶ **Vertigo, headache, or edema of the hands and face**—Can indicate preeclampsia.

▶ **Premature rupture of membranes**—Can indicate premature labor and lead to infections.

▶ **Chills and fever**—Can be an indication of a urinary tract infection or sepsis.

▶ **Excessively rapid uterine enlargement**—Can indicate a hydatidiform mole.

NOTE

A **hydatidiform mole** is a rapid proliferation of cells within the uterus due to trophoblastic disease. A complete molar pregnancy results from fertilization of an egg whose nucleus has been lost. The rapid cell growth can be associated with chorionic carcinoma. The client with a hydatidiform mole is treated by performing a dilation and curettage. The client should be instructed not to become pregnant for at least a year following a hydatidiform mole because a rising human chorionic gonadotropin (HCG) level will stimulate cancer cell growth.

Types of Abortions

An abortion is the loss of the fetus prior to the time when it can live outside the uterus. Several types of abortions can be experienced by the client:

▶ **Elective abortion**—Evacuation of the fetus. There are several types of elective abortions, but all of them require early diagnosis of the pregnancy.

▶ **Threatened**—Produces spotting. The treatment is bed rest. If bleeding or cramping continues, the client should contact the physician immediately because the doctor might order tocolytic medications such as magnesium sulfate, bethrine, or yutopar.

▶ **Inevitable**—If there are no fetal heart tones and parts of the fetus are passed, the client is said to be experiencing an inevitable abortion. This type of abortion produces bleeding and passage of fetal parts. The treatment is a dilation and curettage (D&C).

▶ **Incomplete**—In an incomplete abortion, fetal demise exists but part of the conception is not passed. The treatment is a dilation and evacuation (D&E).

▶ **Complete**—In a complete abortion, all parts of the conception are passed. There is no treatment.

▶ **Septic**—A septic abortion includes the presence of infection. The treatment is administering antibiotics.

▶ **Missed**—In a missed abortion, there is fetal demise but there is no expulsion of the fetus. The treatment is an induction of labor or a surgical removal of the fetus.

Complications of all types of abortion include bleeding and infection. The client should be taught to report to the doctor any bleeding, lethargy, or elevated temperature.

Complications Affecting Pregnancy

Several conditions can affect the outcome of pregnancy. This section covers diabetes in pregnancy, problems with elevated blood pressure, bleeding disorders, cord prolapse, abruptio placenta, sexually transmitted infections, and preterm labor.

Diabetes in Pregnancy

Screening tests are done on all clients when they are seen in the prenatal clinic. The best diagnostic test for diabetes is the glucose tolerance test. See Chapter 12, "Caring for the Client with Disorders of the Endocrine System," for a description of the glucose tolerance test. Clients with diabetes, and their newborns, are at risk for complications during pregnancy. Newborns of diabetic mothers tend to be large for gestational age. Because glucose crosses the placenta, whereas insulin does not, these newborns tend to gain weight. At birth they appear pudgy, ruddy, and lethargic. The high glucose environment impedes lung development and, although they are large for gestational age, they are often premature. Complications of maternal diabetes on the newborn include

▶ Congenital heart defects such as patent ductus arteriosus

▶ Polyhydramnios

▶ Premature delivery

▶ Respiratory distress syndrome

▶ Hypoglycemia

Fluctuations in maternal blood sugar can result in fetal brain damage or sudden fetal death due to ketosis. The pregnant client with diabetes should be taught to check her blood glucose levels frequently during the day. Levels over 120 mg/dl should be reported to the doctor.

Newborns of diabetic mothers might be delivered by Cesarean section due to their large sizes. They should be assessed immediately after delivery for hypoglycemia by performing a dextrostix. The blood is usually obtained by performing a heel stick. The newborn should be stuck on the lateral aspect of the heel. Blood tests should be performed to detect hypocalcemia, hypokalemia, and acidosis.

Preeclampsia

Preeclampsia is an abnormality found only in pregnancy. The diagnostic criteria are an elevated blood pressure, facial edema, and proteinuria. Clients with preeclamsia tend to have infants that are low birth weight for gestational age. These newborns can also suffer from respiratory distress syndrome and congenital heart defects such as patent ductus arteriosus. Clients with mild preeclampsia are treated with bed rest and a low sodium diet. A diagnosis of severe preeclampsia is made if

- The blood pressure is equal to or greater than 160/110 on two occasions at least six hours apart with the woman at bed rest.

- Proteinuria is found to be greater than or equal to five grams in a 24-hour urine specimen.

- Oliguria equal to or less than 400ml in a 24-hour period is present.

- Cerebral or visual disturbances are reported.

- Epigastric pain is present.

- Pulmonary edema or cyanosis is reported.

- HELLP syndrome is diagnosed.

NOTE

HELLP syndrome means hemolysis, elevated liver enzymes, and low platelets. This syndrome results in an enlarged liver and associated bleeding. If it's not treated, the client can die as a result of bleeding. The treatment for this problem is early delivery of the fetus.

Management of severe preeclampsia include

- Complete bed rest

- Moderation in sodium

- Magnesium sulfate

Magnesium sulfate, or magnesium gluconate, is the treatment of choice. A therapeutic level of 4.8–9.6 mg/dl is achieved by controlled infusion of intravenous magnesium sulfate. Magnesium sulfate is a vasodilator that rapidly lowers the blood pressure.

Complications associated with the use of $MgSO_4$ include maternal hypotension, oliguria, and apnea. Hourly intake and output should be done to access for oliguria.

Common side effects of $MgSO_4$ infusion are drowsiness and hot flashes. Every effort should be made to prevent seizures. A quiet, dark environment must be maintained and visitors should be restricted. The client should be assessed for signs of toxicity, which include hyporeflexia, oliguria, and decreased respirations. Magnesium levels should be checked approximately every six hours and the results reported to the doctor.

The treatment for magnesium sulfate toxicity is the administration of calcium gluconate. Calcium gluconate should be kept at the bedside along with an airway and tracheotomy set.

Disseminated Intravascular Coagulation

Disseminated intravascular coagulation (DIC) can occur in many disorders; however, pregnancy is a high risk time for the development of DIC. This bleeding disorder is caused when clotting factor is consumed, causing widespread external and internal bleeding. Bleeding can be evident from the gastrointestinal tract, kidneys, and vagina. The diagnostic tool for DIC is the presence of fibrin split compound. Treatment includes heparin administration to treat clotting, Amicar to stabilize bleeding, electrolyte replacement, blood transfusions , and administration of oxygen. Hourly intake and output should also be monitored carefully. Early diagnosis is imperative if the prognosis is to be improved.

Cord Prolapse

Umbilical cord prolapse occurs when the umbilical cord is expelled with rupture of the membranes. If pressure is exerted on the cord by the presenting fetal part, fetal hypoxia results. Treatments include placing the client in Trendelenburg position or knee-chest position, rapid IV infusion of normal saline or lactated Ringer's solution, and oxygen administration. Vital signs and fetal heart tones are evaluated, and the client is readied for a Cesarean section. If the cord remains outside the uterus, drying will occur, causing loss of oxygen-carrying capacity. Treatment with sterile saline soaks is recommended until a Cesarean section can be performed.

Abruptio Placenta

Abruptio placenta is the separation of the placenta from the uterine wall prior to the third stage of labor. This premature separation results in bleeding. A board-like abdomen and abdominal pain are often noted. Vital signs often reveal hypotension. The treatment for abruption is delivery of the fetus.

Placenta Previa

Placenta previa is the result of implantation of the placenta over the cervix. When cervical dilation occurs, the placenta is delivered first. The symptom of placenta previa is painless bleed. The treatment of placenta previa is delivery of the fetus by Cesarean section.

Maternal Infections

Infections during pregnancy are responsible for significant mortality and morbidity. Vaginal cultures to check for *beta streptococcus* infection are done to prevent contact of the newborn with the infection during birth. If the bacteria is found to be present, the mother is given antibiotics during labor. Sexually transmitted infections are detrimental to the mother and fetus and should be treated promptly. Table 16.1 highlights some infections you should be aware of.

TABLE 16.1   Sexually Transmitted Infections

Disease	Symptoms	Diagnosis	Treatment
Syphilis (caused by the spirochete Treponema pallidum)	Primary stage: Chancre, regional lymph node enlargement that disappears within six weeks. Secondary stage: Malaise, low-grade fever, sore throat, headache, muscle aches, generalized rash, and pustules that disappear in 4–12 weeks. Tertiary stage: Benign lesions of skin and mucosa and heart and central nervous system involvement.	VDRL, RPR, FTA-ABS (fluorescent treponemal antibody absorption test; it's most sensitive to all stages).	Penicillin or other antibiotics.
Gonorrhea (caused by gram-negative bacteria Neisseria gonorrhea; onset occurs 3–10 days after exposure)	Males: Dysuria and yellowish-green discharge. Females: Dysuria, vaginal discharge, no symptoms in many; late in course of the illness, pelvic inflammatory disease can occur.	Culture of discharge.	Penicillin, tetracycline, Rocephin 125 mg IM in a single dose with Vibramycin 100 mg twice daily for one week.
Chlamydia trachomatis (caused by a bacteria; onset occurs in 1–3 weeks)	Males: Urethritis, dysuria, frequent urination, discharge. Females: Frequent urination and mucopurulent cervicitis.	Gram stain of the discharge.	Vibramycin 100 mg twice daily. Azithromycin one gram and treat the client and partner.

TABLE 16.1 *Continued*

Disease	Symptoms	Diagnosis	Treatment
Genital herpes (HSV2) (caused by a virus; incubation period is 2–4 weeks)	Local symptoms are caused by blisters, which erupt and leave shallow ulcers that disappear after 2–6 weeks. Systemic symptoms include fever, malaise, anorexia, painful inguinal lymph nodes, and dysuria. HSV harbors in one or more of the nerve ganglia. Physical and emotional stress trigger recurrent episodes. (If there is an active lesion during labor, a Cesarean section is performed because direct contact can lead to transmission of the virus to the infant.)	Direct visualization of lesions and a viral culture.	Antiviral medications such as acyclovir. Acyclovir can be used during pregnancy.
Condylomata acuminate (caused by human papilloma virus [HPV] that is transmitted by skin-to-skin contact; the presence of HPV has been linked to vaginal and cervical cancers)	A dry wart located on vulva, cervix, rectum, or vagina.	Visualization, biopsy, and Pap smear.	Antiviral medications, Podophyllin 20% in tincture of benzoin (Podophyllin is not recommended for pregnant clients because this drug can cause birth defects). Antineoplastics such as 5-FU have been used successfully. Imiquimod cream (Aldara0), Trichloroacetic acid (TCA) can be used during pregnancy. Recently, the FDA has approved Gardasil (Human papilloma virus vaccine), a vaccine for the prevention of types 6, 11, and 18 HPV. This vaccine is recommended for girls ages 9-26. The medication is given by injection in three doses, The first at a time suggested by the client's physician, the second two months later, and the third six months after the first dose.

(continues)

TABLE 16.1 *Continued*

Disease	Symptoms	Diagnosis	Treatment
Human immuno-deficiency virus/acquired immuno-deficiency syndrome (acquired primarily through blood and other body fluids)	Seroconversion to HIV occurs in approximately 10 weeks. Many opportunistic illness can affect the client, including parasitic infections (enterocolitis), bacterial (tuberculosis), viral infections (cytomegalovirus), fungal infections (candidiasis), and malignancies (Kaposi's sarcoma).	ELISA; western blot; viral T-cell count. A T-cell count of less than 200 indicates that the client is at risk for opportunistic diseases. Load/burden; a viral load of less than 400 copies/mL indicates the client is relatively free of circulating virus. A white blood cell count less than 3200 requires evaluation. Presence of opportunistic infections.	Antiviral medications: Nucleoside analog transcriptase inhibitors (AZT, primarily Zidovudine, is given to the pregnant client and the infant after delivery). Non-nucleoside reverse transcriptase inhibitors. Protease inhibitors. Highly active antiretroviral therapy (HAART), previously known as an AIDS cocktail, is a combination of these medications given in conjunction with other medications used to treat anemia and infections. Bactrim (sulfamethoxazole) is used to treat Pneumocystis carinii pneumonia (PCP). Blood and body fluids should be cleaned up with a hypochlorite solution (1 part bleach and 10 parts water).

Preterm Labor

Premature labor can be managed with hypnotics or sedatives. Several medications stop contractions, including

▶ **Brethine (terbutaline sulfate)**—A commonly used bronchodilator that is contraindicated in clients with cardiovascular disease because it causes tachycardia and in clients with diabetes because it elevates the blood glucose levels.

▶ **Magnesium sulfate**—A drug used to treat preeclampsia. It can also help to decrease uterine contractions. If this drug is given to treat premature contractions, the client should be monitored for magnesium toxicity.

> **NOTE**
>
> Clients receiving magnesium sulfate should have a Foley catheter inserted to monitor the output hourly. The client should be assessed for hypotension and respiratory distress.

Preterm is defined as a delivery that occurs prior to 37 weeks gestation. These infants exhibit several characteristics, including low birth weight (less than 1500 gms), lack of lanugo, absence of sucking pads, and in males undescended testes. Premature infants are prone to rapid heat loss through conduction, convection, radiation, and evaporation. Additional complications include respiratory distress syndrome, pneumothorax, necrotizing enterocolitis, bronchopulmonary dysplasia, and bleeding disorders. Careful management of the infant during bathing and drying should be taken because intracranial bleeding is a potential danger. Premature infants are best managed in neonatal intensive care units where respiratory status is supported through mechanical ventilation and treatment with applied surfactant.

Intrapartal Care

Labor is defined as the process by which the fetus is expelled from the uterus and the time period immediately after. Five factors influence the labor process:

▶ **Passageway**—The birth canal, which consists of the uterus, bony pelvis, and vagina.

▶ **Passenger**—The baby. This consideration during the intrapartal period involves evaluation and management of distress.

▶ **Powers**—The mother's body's power to expel the fetus; it consists of the uterine contractions.

▶ **Position**—The position the mother assumes during labor; it can make a difference in the decent of the fetus and the mother's comfort.

▶ **Psychological response**—The psychological response of the mother makes a difference in the labor experience. If the mother is prepared and in control, it is much more likely that the labor process will proceed smoothly.

The intrapartal period is divided into stages and phases of labor, as covered in the following sections.

Stages of Labor

The stages of labor describe the process of dilation and decent of the baby. The four stages of labor are

▶ **Stage 1**—Closed cervix to 10 centimeters dilation of the cervix

▶ **Stage 2**—From complete cervical dilation to delivery of the baby

▶ **Stage 3**—From delivery of the baby to delivery of the placenta

▶ **Stage 4**—From delivery of the placenta until completion of the recovery period

Phases of Labor

The first stage of labor is divided into three phases of labor:

▶ **Phase 1**—Early labor or prodromal (0–3 cm dilation)

▶ **Phase 2**—Active labor (4–7 cm dilation)

▶ **Phase 3**—Transition (8–10 cm dilation)

Important Terms You Should Know

Several terms associated with labor and delivery are listed here. You should know these for the exam:

▶ **Presentation**—The part of the fetus that engages and presents first at delivery (cephalic presentation, or head presentation, is the most common type of presentation).

▶ **Position**—The relationship of the presenting part to the mother's pelvis. For example, left occiput anterior (LOA) means that the back of the baby's head is anterior to the pelvis and tilted to the left side. Right occiput anterior (ROA) means that the back of the baby's head is anterior and tilted to the right side; occiput anterior (OA) means that the back of the baby's head is directly to the front of the mother's pelvis. See Figure 16.1 for a diagram of the fetal positions.

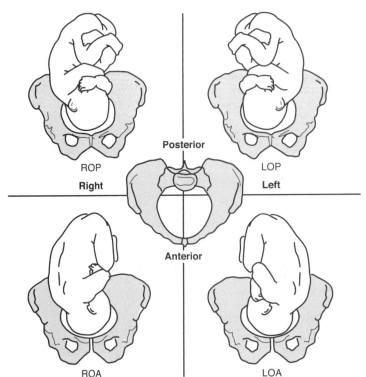

FIGURE 16.1 Fetal positions.

▶ **Fetal lie**—The relationship of the fetus to the long axis of the mother. This can be determined by performing Leopold's maneuvers. Leopold's maneuver is a technique performed by the healthcare provider by palpating the maternal abdomen to determine where the fetal back, legs, head, and so on are located. This technique is a noninvasive way of estimating the fetal lie and whether the baby is engaged or in the true pelvis.

▶ **Dystocia**—This term is associated with a difficult or extremely painful labor and delivery.

▶ **Effacement**—This is the thinning of the cervix.

▶ **Dilation**—This is the opening of the cervix.

▶ **Precipitate delivery**—This term is associated with a rapid labor and delivery. The client with precipitate delivery is at risk for uterine rupture, vaginal lacerations, amniotic emboli, and postpartal hemorrhage. Fetal complications include hypoxia and intracranial hemorrhage.

▶ **Station**—This refers to the relationship of the presenting part to the maternal ischial spines (0 station is at the ischial spines).

Prelabor Testing

Several tests can be performed to predict possible complications to the fetus and mother:

▶ **Non-stress test**—This test is used to determine fetal response to cyclical periods of rest and activity. A fetal monitor is applied for approximately 90 minutes. During this time, the client is instructed to press the response button each time the baby moves. Normal fetal response is an increase in fetal heart rate of 15 beats per minute. A reassuring or positive reading indicates a positive fetal outcome.

▶ **Oxytocin challenge test (contraction stress test)**—This test is used to determine fetal response to contractions. The length of time for an OCT is generally 90–120 minutes. Contractions are stimulated by beginning an infusion of Pitocin. Ten units of pitocin are diluted in 1000 ml of IV fluid, begun at three milliunits per minute, and increased every 15 minutes until three contractions in 10 minutes are observed. If fetal bradycardia (FHT is less than 110 bpm) or tachycardia (FHT is greater than 160 bpm) is observed or if the blood pressure of the mother rises above normal, the test is considered positive or abnormal. A positive reading can indicate that labor might not be advisable. After the exam, the pitocin is discontinued.

NOTE

If the physician decides to induce labor, the pitocin can be continued and prostaglandin gel can be used to ripen or soften the cervix.

CAUTION

Pitocin should always be infused using a pump or controller.

Fetal Monitoring

Fetal monitoring can be done continuously by using an external tocodynamometer monitor. External monitoring is a noninvasive procedure that allows the nurse to observe the fetal heart tones and uterine contractions. Internal fetal monitoring is recommended if fetal heart tones and contractions cannot be evaluated externally. The duration of a contraction is evaluated by measuring from the beginning of a contraction to the end of the same contraction. The frequency of a contraction is evaluated by measuring from the beginning of one contraction to the beginning of the next contraction or from the peak of one contraction to the peak of the next contraction.

Bradycardia is a deceleration of fetal heart tones. Decelerations are associated with fetal hypoxia. The three types of decelerations are

> ▶ **Early decelerations**—Transitory drops in the fetal heart rate caused by head compression. If the client is complete and pushing and the baby is in a cephalic presentation, this finding is relatively benign. An early deceleration mirrors in depth and length the contraction. If there is a rapid return to the baseline fetal heart rate and the fetal heart rate is within normal range, no treatment is necessary. Figure 16.2 shows graphs of early decelerations.

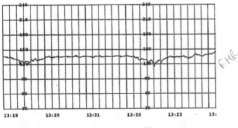

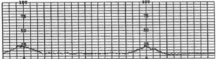

FIGURE 16.2 Early decelerations.

Note there is a drop in the fetal heart rate prior to the peak of the contraction. If there is average variability and rapid return to the baseline fetal heart rate, no treatment is necessary.

▶ **Variable deceleration**—V-shaped transitory decreases in the fetal heart rate that occur anytime during the contraction. Variable decelerations can also occur when no contractions are present. Variable decelerations are caused by cord compression. Two possible causes of variable decelerations are a prolapsed cord and a cord that is entangled or wrapped around the fetal neck (nuchal cord). Because hypoxia can result from the cord being compressed, intervention is required. Treatment of variable decelerations includes placing the mother in Trendelenburg position, oxygen administration, IV fluids, and notification of the physician. If fetal distress continues, the client should be prepared for a C-section. Figure 16.3 shows graphs of variable decelerations.

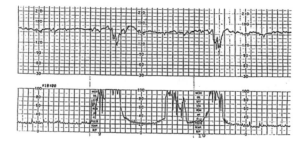

FIGURE 16.3   Variable decelerations.

Note the drop in the fetal heart tones that are V-shaped and do not correlate to the contractions. These decelerations are caused by cord compression. The treatment is to turn the client to the side, turn off pitocin, and apply oxygen. Contact the doctor if these continue after treatment.

▶ **Late decelerations**—Drops in the fetal heart rate late in the contraction are caused by utero-placental insufficiency. These decelerations are U-shaped and mirror the contractions. Late decelerations are ominous because they result in fetal hypoxia. Treatment of late decelerations includes discontinuation of pitocin, applying oxygen, and changing the mother's position. The recommended position is left side-lying. If late decelerations continue despite interventions, the physician should be notified to expedite delivery. Figure 16.4 shows graphs of late decelerations.

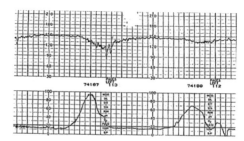

FIGURE 16.4   Late decelerations.

Note the drop in the fetal heart rate after the peak of the contraction caused by utero-placental insufficiency. The treatment is to turn off pitocin if infusing, administer oxygen, and turn the client on her side or change position. Left side-lying is best. If this pattern continues, contact the doctor.

Pharmacologic Management of Labor

Several methods are used to relieve the pain of labor, including

▶ **Sedatives**—Examples: Stadol (butorphanol) and Nubain (nalbuphine) are two agonist medications commonly used in labor. These drugs provide pain relief with little suppression of fetal heart tones. To decrease the amount of medication crossing the placental barrier, the medication should slowly be administered via IV push during a contraction. Phenergan (promethezine) can also be used to treat nausea associated with labor.

▶ **Nerve blocks**—Several types of nerve blocks are useful in labor. The following six items are examples of nerve blocks:

  ▶ **Local infiltration**—This uses xylocaine for an episiotomy.

  ▶ **Pudendal block**—Useful for the second stage of labor, episiotomy, and birth, this blocks nerve impulses to the perineum, cervix, and vagina.

  ▶ **Subarachnoid (spinal) anesthesia**—This is injected through the third, fourth, or fifth lumbar interspace into the subarachnoid space. It is useful in relieving uterine pain. Because complete anesthesia is achieved, the client should be observed for hypotension and bradycardia. She will probably be unable to assist with pushing during the third stage of labor.

NOTE

Leakage of spinal fluid can result in a headache. The client should be maintained supine following delivery for eight hours, and fluids should be encouraged. If a spinal headache occurs following spinal anesthesia, the doctor might perform a blood patch. A blood patch is done by injecting maternal blood into the space where spinal fluid is being lost. This allows for quicker replenishing of spinal fluid and restoration of equilibrium.

  ▶ **Epidural block**—This is useful for uterine labor pain. This type of anesthesia is commonly used in laboring clients because it does not suppress the fetal heart rate and does not result in complete anesthesia. The client is able to assist with pushing but is relatively free of pain. Maternal hypotension is a complication. Two thousand milliliters of IV fluid should be given immediately prior to an epidural or spinal anesthesia to prevent hypotension. This increase in the amount of circulating volume helps prevent the associated hypotension. If hypotension occurs, the nurse should increase the IV infusion, apply oxygen, and reposition the client on her left side. Platelet counts should be monitored. Obstetric clients having epidural anesthesia often complain of shivering; explain to the client that this is expected and provide extra blankets.

▶ **Spinal/epidural narcotics**—Narcotics can be administered into the spinal or epidural space. Fentanyl or morphine is commonly used. Side effects include nausea, itching, urinary retention, and respiratory distress.

▶ **General anesthesia**—This is rarely used for the laboring client and if used is reserved for Cesarean section deliveries.

Postpartum Care

To reduce bleeding and improve uterine tone, the nurse should massage the fundus often. *Lochia rubra*, or bright red bleeding, occurs after delivery and lasts approximately three days. *Lochia serosa*, or blood and serous fluid, is usually noted on the third or fourth postpartum day. *Lochia alba*, or the white or clear discharge, can last several weeks following delivery. Allowing breast feeding immediately after delivery is encouraged because it stimulates oxytocin release and uterine contractions. Another advantage of early breast feeding is the production of colostrum. Colostrum, the first liquid secreted from the breast, contains antibodies and nutrients that are needed by the infant.

Urinary retention often increases postpartal bleeding and is a problem during the early postpartal period, especially in clients who have epidural or spinal anesthesia for relief of labor pain. If the nurse notes that the fundus is deviated to the side, the bladder is probably distended. Encourage the client to void, or insert a French or Foley catheter to empty the bladder and enhance uterine contractions.

Terms Associated with the Normal Newborn

The following terms are associated with normal newborns. You should be familiar with these terms for the exam:

▶ **Acrocyanosis**—This is a bluish discoloration of the hands and feet of the newborn.

▶ **APGAR scoring**—This permits a rapid assessment of the need for resuscitation based on five signs. This survey is done at one and five minutes. Table 16.2 demonstrates the measures for APGAR scoring.

▶ **Caput succedaneum**—This is an edema that crosses the suture line on the baby's scalp.

▶ **Cephalohematoma**—This is blood that does not cross the suture line on the baby's scalp.

▶ **Hyperbilirubinemia**—An elevation in the infant's bilirubin level caused by an immature liver. The bilirubin level is checked by obtaining a blood sample via heel stick or by use of a bilirubinometer. This device uses a handheld battery-powered instrument to detect jaundice. Levels of 12mg/dl may require phototherapy. Preparation of the infant for phototherapy include covering the eyes and genitals. Increasing fluids and feedings is encouraged to facilitate the excretion of bilirubin through the gastrointestinal tract and urinary system.

▶ **Milia**—These are tiny, white bumps that occur across the newborn's nose.

▶ **Mongolian spots**—These are darkened discolorations that occur on the sacral area of dark-skinned infants.

TABLE 16.2 APGAR Scoring

Heart Rate	Respiration	Reflexes	Cry Reflex Irritability	Color
0 = Absent	0 = Absent	0 = Absent, flaccid	0 = Absent	0 = Blue
1 = Slow <100	1 = Slow, weak cry	1 = Some flexion of extremities	1 = Grimace	1 = Pink body, blue extremities
2 = Over 100	2 = Good cry	2 = Good reflexes, active movement	2 = Cry	2 = Pink

Rh Incompatibility

Problems with hemolysis occur if the mother is Rh negative and the fetus is Rh positive. Maternal and fetal blood do not mix in utero until the third stage of labor when the placenta separates from the wall of the uterus. At that time, a fetal-maternal transfusion can occur. This mixing of incompatible blood types causes isoimmunization and a transfusion reaction.

Usually no problems are seen in the first pregnancy. If, however, the mother becomes pregnant with another Rh positive fetus, her body will react as if the fetus were a foreign object and destroy the baby's red blood cells. This destruction is known as erythroblastosis fetalis.

To prevent isoimmunization, the mother should be given Rhogam during pregnancy as early as 20 weeks or postpartally within the first 48–72 hours. *Kernicterus* is the condition that results when unconjugated bilirubin crosses the blood-brain barrier. This often results in conditions such as cerebral palsy. Infants with pathologic jaundice should be assessed for alertness, presence of a high-pitched cry, a decreased sucking reflex, hydrops fetalis, and seizure activity. Treatment for pathological jaundice involves exchange transfusion either in utero or immediately after delivery.

Physiologic jaundice is a benign condition resulting from an immature liver. As the amount of conjugated bilirubin builds in the baby's blood, the infant becomes jaundice. This jaundice does not become evident until 48–72 hours and, although it does cause the infant to be irritable, it does not cause brain damage. Treatment of physiological jaundice includes placing the baby under a bili-light. Clothing should be removed and the eyes and genitals covered to prevent damage to fragile tissue. Feedings and fluids should be increased to promote defecation and urination. The infant should be turned often and vital signs should be monitored frequently.

Contraception

Contraception is the voluntary prevention of pregnancy. This can be accomplished using several methods (see Table 16.3).

TABLE 16.3   Contraception Methods

Method Name	Description	Effectiveness
Coitus interruptus	Withdrawal of the penis from the vagina before ejaculation.	Not very effective and should be discouraged. It does not prevent STDs.
Abstinence	Voluntarily refraining from sexual intercourse.	Very reliable if the client abstains from sexual intercourse and there is no presence of ejaculatory fluid.
Rhythm method	The client is instructed to refrain from intercourse during ovulation.	Very reliable if the client has adequate knowledge of ovulation. Ovulation usually occurs 12–18 days after the first day of the menstrual cycle. The client's temperature decreases and then sharply rises at the time of ovulation.
Cervical mucus method	The cervical mucus method is also called the Billings Method and the Creighton Model. This method helps the client determine whether ovulation has occurred. If the mucus is slippery, the client should abstain from sexual intercourse until ovulation is past.	Adequate amounts of thin cervical mucus is required for the sperm to have motility. This method of birth control is less effective than many others because it requires the client to make a judgment of the consistency of the mucus.

(continues)

TABLE 16.3 *Continued*

Method Name	Description	Effectiveness
Barrier methods	Condom/Diaphragm: One concern with the use of a diaphragm is the occurrence of Toxic Shock Syndrome, a potentially life-threatening problem caused by bacterial invasion of the uterus. To prevent the occurrence of this problem, the woman should be taught to clean the diaphragm after each use and remove it after eight hours. She should not use the diaphragm during menses. Signs of TSS include hypotension, fever, dizziness, and a rash. Treatment includes antibiotics. Condoms are the only method of birth control that is also helpful in preventing sexually transmitted infections. Latex condoms are recommended.	Very reliable. Latex condoms also help decrease the incidence of STDs. The condom should be removed from the vagina while the penis is still erect. Diaphragms should be resized if the client gains or loses 10 pounds, has abdominal surgery, or has a baby. The diaphragm is used in conjunction with spermicidal gel or cream and should be left in for six–eight hours after intercourse. The client should not douche after intercourse.
Hormonal methods	Birth control pills, such as Depo-Provera and Norplant.	Very reliable if taken consistently. If the client misses a pill, she should be instructed to take it as soon as she remembers. If she misses more than two, another method of contraception such as a condom should be used until the end of the cycle. If antibiotics are taken, oral contraceptives might be ineffective.
Intrauterine device (IUD)	Several types exist. These prevent implantation, not fertilization.	Very reliable. They should not be used in clients with a history of pelvic inflammatory disease (PID), diabetes, or bleeding disorders.
Sterilization (tubal ligation and vasectomy)	Tubal fulguration in females is the destruction of a portion of the fallopian tube by an electric current. A vasectomy is cutting the vasa deferentia to prevent the passage of sperm.	Very reliable.

Diagnostic Tests for Review

The following are diagnostic tests you should review before taking the NCLEX exam. These tests are performed to determine potential problems in the obstetric client and the fetus:

▶ 24-hour urine to determine renal disease

▶ Alpha feto-protein to determine neural tube defects

▶ CBC to indicate anemia or infections

- Estriol levels to determine fetal well-being

- Ferning test/nitrazine testing to confirm amniotic fluid

- Glucose tolerance test to determine whether an elevated blood glucose exists, and possibly diabetes

- L/S ratio to determine lung maturity

- Pap smear to detect cervical cancer

- Ultrasound/amniocentesis to determine fetal anomalies

- Urinalysis to detect kidney infections

Pharmacology Categories for Review

Several pharmacological agents are used to treat the pregnant client. You will need to review these prior to taking the NCLEX exam:

- Analgesics

- Anesthetics

- Antibiotics

- Antihypertensives

- Antivirals

- Hormonal preparations

- Insulin

- Narcotics

- Surfactants

- Tocolytics

- Vasodilators

Exam Prep Questions

1. A client is admitted to the labor and delivery unit in active labor. During examination, the nurse notes a papular lesion on the perineum. Which initial action is most appropriate?

   ○ **A.** Document the finding.

   ○ **B.** Report the finding to the doctor.

   ○ **C.** Prepare the client for a C-section.

   ○ **D.** Continue primary care as prescribed.

2. A client with a diagnosis of HPV is at risk for which of the following?

   ○ **A.** Hodgkin's lymphoma

   ○ **B.** Cervical cancer

   ○ **C.** Multiple myeloma

   ○ **D.** Ovarian cancer

3. During the initial interview, the client reports that she has a lesion on the perineum. Further investigation reveals a small blister on the vulva that is painful to touch. The nurse is aware that the most likely source of the lesion is:

   ○ **A.** Syphilis

   ○ **B.** Herpes

   ○ **C.** Gonorrhea

   ○ **D.** Condylomata

4. A client visiting a family planning clinic is suspected of having an STD. The most diagnostic test for all stages of treponema pallidum (syphilis) is the:

   ○ **A.** Venereal Disease Research Lab (VDRL)

   ○ **B.** Rapid plasma reagin (RPR)

   ○ **C.** Florescent treponemal antibody (FTA-Abs)

   ○ **D.** Thayer-Martin culture (TMC)

5. A 15-year-old primigravida is admitted with a tentative diagnosis of HELLP syndrome. Which laboratory finding is associated with HELLP syndrome?

   ○ **A.** Elevated blood glucose

   ○ **B.** Elevated platelet count

   ○ **C.** Elevated creatinine clearance

   ○ **D.** Elevated hepatic enzymes

6. The nurse is assessing the deep tendon reflexes of a client with preeclampsia. Which method is used to elicit the biceps reflex?

   ○ **A.** The nurse places her thumb on the muscle inset in the antecubital space and taps the thumb briskly with the reflex hammer.

   ○ **B.** The nurse loosely suspends the client's arm in an open hand while tapping the back of the client's elbow.

   ○ **C.** The nurse instructs the client to dangle her legs as the nurse strikes the area below the patella with the blunt side of the reflex hammer.

   ○ **D.** The nurse instructs the client to place her arms loosely at her side as the nurse strikes the muscle insert just above the wrist.

7. A primigravida with diabetes is admitted to the labor and delivery unit at 34 weeks gestation. Which doctor's order should the nurse question?

   ○ **A.** Magnesium sulfate 4 gm (25%) IV

   ○ **B.** Brethine 10 mcg IV

   ○ **C.** Stadol 1 mg IV push every 4 hours PRN for pain

   ○ **D.** Ancef 2 gm IVPB every 6 hours

8. A diabetic multigravida is scheduled for an amniocentesis at 32 weeks gestation to determine the L/S ratio and phosphatidyl glycerol level. The L/S ratio is 1:1 and the presence of phosphatidylglycerol is noted. The nurse's assessment of this data is:

   ○ **A.** The infant is at low risk for congenital anomalies.

   ○ **B.** The infant is at high risk for intrauterine growth retardation.

   ○ **C.** The infant is at high risk for respiratory distress syndrome.

   ○ **D.** The infant is at high risk for birth trauma.

9. Which observation in the newborn of a diabetic mother would require immediate nursing intervention?

   ○ **A.** Crying

   ○ **B.** Wakefulness

   ○ **C.** Jitteriness

   ○ **D.** Yawning

10. The nurse caring for a client receiving intravenous magnesium sulfate must closely observe for side effects associated with drug therapy. An expected side effect of magnesium sulfate is:

    ○ **A.** Decreased urinary output

    ○ **B.** Hypersomnolence

    ○ **C.** Absence of knee jerk reflex

    ○ **D.** Decreased respiratory rate

11. The client has elected to have epidural anesthesia to relieve labor pain. If the client experiences hypotension, the nurse's first action should be:

    ○ **A.** Place her in Trendelenburg position.

    ○ **B.** Slow the IV infusion.

    ○ **C.** Administer oxygen per nasal cannula.

    ○ **D.** Speed the IV infusion of normal saline.

Answer Rationales

1. Answer B is correct. Any lesion should be reported to the doctor. This can indicate a herpes lesion. Clients with open lesions related to herpes are delivered by Cesarean section because there is a possibility of transmission of the infection to the fetus with direct contact to lesions. It is not enough to document the finding, so answer A is incorrect. The physician must make the decision to perform a C-section, making answer C incorrect. It is not enough to continue primary care, so answer D is incorrect.

2. Answer B is correct. The client with HPV is at higher risk for cervical and vaginal cancer related to this STI. She is not at higher risk for the cancers mentioned in answers A, C, and D, so those are incorrect.

3. Answer B is correct. A lesion that is painful is most likely a herpetic lesion. A chancre lesion associated with syphilis is not painful, so answer A is incorrect. Gonorrhea does not present as a lesion but is exhibited by a yellow discharge, so answer C is incorrect. Condylomata lesions are painless warts, so answer D is incorrect.

4. Answer C is correct. The FTA-Abs is the most sensitive to all stages of syphilis. VDRL and RPR are screening tests done for syphilis, so answers A and B are incorrect. The Thayer-Martin culture is done for gonorrhea, so answer D is incorrect.

5. Answer D is correct. The criteria for HELLP is hemolysis, elevated liver enzymes, and low platelet count. An elevated blood glucose level is not associated with HELLP, so answer A is incorrect. Platelets are decreased in HELLP syndrome, not elevated, so answer B is incorrect. The creatinine levels are elevated in renal disease and are not associated with HELLP syndrome, so answer C is incorrect.

6. Answer A is correct. Answer B elicits the tricep reflex, so it's incorrect. Answer C elicits the patella reflex, making it incorrect. Answer D elicits the radial nerve reflex, so it's incorrect.

7. Answer B is correct. Brethine is used cautiously because it raises the blood glucose levels. Answers A, C, and D are all medications that are commonly used in the diabetic client, so they are incorrect.

8. Answer C is correct. When the L/S ratio reaches 2:1, the lungs are considered to be mature. The L/S ratio does not indicate congenital anomalies, so answer A is incorrect. The infant is not at risk for intrauterine growth retardation, so answer B is incorrect. The infant will most likely be small for gestational age and will not be at risk for birth trauma, so answer D is incorrect.

9. Answer C is correct. Jitteriness is a sign of seizure in the neonate. Crying, wakefulness, and yawning are expected in the newborn, so answers A, B, and D are incorrect.

10. Answer B is correct. The client is expected to become sleepy, have hot flashes, and lethargy. A decreasing urinary output, absence of the knee jerk reflex, and decreased respirations indicate toxicity, so answers A, C, and D are incorrect.

11. Answer D is correct. If the client experiences hypotension after an injection of epidural anesthetic, the nurse should turn her to the left side, apply oxygen by mask, and speed the IV infusion. If the blood pressure does not return to normal, the physician should be contacted. Epinephrine should be kept for emergency administration. Placing the client in Trendelenburg position allows the anesthesia to move up above the respiratory center, thereby decreasing the diaphragm's ability to move up and down and ventilate the client, so answer A is incorrect. The IV rate should be increased, not decreased, making answer B incorrect. The oxygen should be applied by mask, not cannula, so answer C is incorrect.

Suggested Reading and Resources

- Rinehart, W., Sloan, D., and Hurd, C. *NCLEX Exam Cram*. Indianapolis: Que, 2005.

- McKinney, E., Stone, James, S., Murray, S., and Ashwill, J. *Maternal-Child Nursing*. 2nd ed. Philadelphia: Saunders, 2005.

17

Caring for the Pediatric Client

Terms you'll need to understand

✓ Aganglionic

✓ Atresia

✓ Autosomal recessive disorder

✓ Congenital anomaly

✓ Craniofacial

✓ Dysplasia

✓ Enteropathy

✓ Extravasation

✓ Fistula

✓ Hyperpnea

✓ Hyperpyrexia

✓ Lordosis

✓ Meconium ileus

✓ Neural tube defect

✓ Palliative

✓ Polycythemia

✓ Respiratory synctial virus

✓ Sex-linked disorder

✓ Steatorrhea

✓ Stenosis

✓ Stridor

Nursing skills you'll need to master

✓ Performing sterile dressing changes

✓ Calculating pediatric medication dosage

✓ Administering medications to infants and children

✓ Using intravenous pumps and burettes

✓ Applying pediatric urine collector

✓ Instilling eye drops and ear drops

✓ Determining intake and output

✓ Applying mummy and clove hitch restraints

✓ Providing care for the client with traction and casts

There are few areas in nursing more challenging or more rewarding than working with children and their families. Most nurses who work with pediatric clients will jokingly tell you that one of the first things that attracted them to the specialty was the brightly painted walls with the likes of Charlie Brown, Linus, and Snoopy or the fact that they get to wear cartoon-imprinted uniforms. But taking care of a sick child involves more than reading a bedtime story or making a balloon from a surgical glove. The pediatric nurse combines the knowledge of disease process with an understanding of how illness and injury affect normal growth and development and uses the best of her communication skills to help parents cope. This chapter reviews normal growth and development and the most common alterations in child health. As you review normal growth and development, you should consider ways in which nurses help children stay healthy through accident prevention and immunizations. Your pediatric textbook lists guidelines for accident prevention as well as the recommended schedule for childhood immunizations. The recommended schedule for childhood immunizations is also included in Appendix A, "Things You Forgot," which you can find on the CD.

Growth and Development

Growth and development refers to the numerous changes that take place over a lifetime. For the nurse, growth and development represents a guide for assessing and providing care to children from birth through adolescence. Key elements include physical growth, development of gross motor and fine motor skills, and socialization through play. Although there are individual differences in growth and development, Tables 17.1–17.4 provide useful information regarding overall developmental changes.

Infant (28 Days to 1 Year)

The infancy stage is marked by rapid changes in growth and development. In fact, there is no other time in life when changes occur so quickly and dramatically. Body weight triples and length increases by 50% in the first year of life (aren't we glad that doesn't continue!). Infant reflexes are replaced with fine motor and gross motor skills. These skills occur in an orderly fashion in a head-to-toe and center-to-peripheral sequence, which is referred to as *cephalocaudal—proximodistal development*. Table 17.1 summarizes infant development elements that are important for you to know for the exam.

TABLE 17.1 Key Elements in the Development of Infants

Type of Development	Characteristics
Physical growth and development	Weight: The birth weight (average is 7–9 pounds) doubles by approximately six months of age and triples by one year of age. Length: The length at birth (average is 19–21 inches) increases by one inch per month during the first six months of life. By one year of age, the birth length has increased by 50%. Head circumference: The head circumference at birth (13–14 inches) increases to an average of 17 inches by six months and 18 inches at one year of age. The posterior fontanel closes by approximately two months of age; the anterior fontanel closes by approximately 18 months of age. As the brain matures, the infant's reflexes (Moro, tonic neck, Babinski, stepping, and rooting) are replaced by purposeful movements that influence motor development. Chest circumference: The lateral diameter becomes greater than the anteroposterior diameter. By one year of age, the circumferences of the head and the chest are approximately the same.
Development of gross motor and fine motor skills	1–3 months: The infant can lift the head, grasp and hold objects for a brief period of time, and roll from side to back. The eyes become more coordinated, and the infant can focus on objects. 3–6 months: The infant gains head control, rolls from abdomen to back, sits with support, and can move her hand to her mouth. The lower central incisors erupt and, by six months of age, new foods are added to the infant's diet, including crackers, melba toast, rice cereal, vegetables, fruits, meat, and egg yolk. 9 months: The infant can sit without support, transfer objects from hand to hand, bang cubes together, play patty-cake, creep on hands and knees, and pull herself to a standing position. Upper lateral incisors begin to appear. 12 months: The infant cruises well, can walk with one hand being held, begins to take her first steps alone, can sit down from a standing position unassisted, can turn pages in a book, and recognizes familiar pictures like animals (likes to make animal sounds). The use of a pincer grasp allows placement and retrieval of small objects. The one-year-old has from six to eight deciduous teeth.
Socialization	1–3 months: The infant smiles, recognizes the primary caregiver, and vocalizes by cooing. 3–6 months: The infant now socializes by imitating sounds and laughing aloud. 9 months: The infant now reaches for familiar people, can say "mama" and "dada," and responds to simple verbal requests. 12 months: The infant shows affection (blows kisses on request), explores away from parents, and seeks a security blanket or favorite toy when upset. The infant plays alone (solitary play) and enjoys mobiles, busy boxes, soft cuddle toys, and soft picture books.

Toddler (1–3 Years)

By the end of the first year of life, the infant has acquired the skills necessary for mobility. Sitting up and pulling to a standing position give rise to the more advanced gross motor skills of walking, running, and climbing. These skills, along with advancing fine motor development, allow the child to explore his environment as he tries to find out how things work. In the midst of toddlerdom is the stage known as the *terrible twos*, in which the most often-heard word from both parent and child is *no*. Everyday is a new adventure for the toddler and getting into things is a way of life. Parenting the toddler involves allowing exploration while setting limits, overcoming the struggles of toilet training, and (in some cases) managing sibling rivalry. Table 17.2 highlights important developmental elements for toddlers.

TABLE 17.2 Key Elements in the Development of Toddlers

Type of Development	Characteristics
Physical growth and development	Weight: On average, the birth weight quadruples by the time the toddler is age 2 1/2 years. Weight gain slows to an average of 4–6 pounds per year. Height: The toddler is approximately one-half his adult height by the age of 2 1/2 years. Head circumference: The anterior fontanel closes. The head circumference is about 19 inches by 15 months of age and about 20 inches by 2 years of age. Brain growth increases to 90% of the adult size. Chest circumference: The chest circumference is greater than the head circumference, giving the toddler a more adult appearance.
Development of gross motor and fine motor skills	12–18 months: The toddler can kick a ball forward, walk up steps, build a tower of two or four cubes, use a spoon, drink from a cup, push and pull toys, remove clothes, and scribble with crayons or pencils. 19–24 months: The toddler can run, jump in place, throw a ball overhand, kick a ball forward without falling, walk up and down steps with two feet on each step, build a tower of four or six cubes, copy a vertical line, wash and dry his hands, gains bowel control, and helps dress himself. 2–3 years: The toddler can balance on one foot, jump with both feet, take a few steps on tiptoe, ride a tricycle, build a tower of eight cubes, and copy vertical and horizontal lines. Day time bladder control has been achieved. The toddler at this age can give his first and last name and name a friend and one color.
Socialization	12–18 months: At this age, the toddler imitates housework, points to at least one named body part (nose, eyes, and so on), and has a vocabulary of 10 words. 19–24 months: At this age, the toddler has understandable speech, can combine three or four words, has a vocabulary of 300 words, and can name pictures. 2–3 years: At this age the toddler has a vocabulary of 900 words. The toddler plays beside another child with little or no interaction in a fashion known as parallel play. Toddlers enjoy nesting toys, picture books, push-pull toys, riding toys, pounding boards, sand, soap bubbles, talking toys, balls, dolls, and dress-up clothes.

Preschooler (3–5 Years)

If toddlers are best known for the terrible twos, the preschooler should be known as a delightful paradox. He loves secrets and yet he will share all the family secrets with a total stranger. He can recite the sweetest of prayers and yet swear like a sailor. He can be brutally honest and yet invent the tallest of tales. He explores his world; imitates the adults in it; and yet lives in the fantasy world of adventure figures, becoming them from time to time. No one has more fun than the preschooler, who will run with total abandonment through the largest, muddiest puddle of water. Many of his baby features have given way to those of the older child. The potbelly of the toddler disappears and is replaced by a thinner, more athletic preschooler's body. Unfortunately, the potbelly will reappear when you least want it—and you can count on the preschooler to point it out to you in case you didn't notice. Although physical growth slows a bit, cognitive and language development continue at a rapid rate, preparing the child for a major life event: entering school. Table 17.3 summarizes important elements that are key to the development of preschoolers.

TABLE 17.3 Key Elements in the Development of Preschoolers

Type of Development	Characteristics
Physical growth and development	Weight: The average weight gain is about five pounds per year so that the three-year-old weighs about 37 pounds, the four-year-old about 42 pounds, and the five-year-old about 47 pounds.
	Height: The average increase in height is about 2–3 inches per year, which is mostly due to an elongation of the legs rather than the trunk. The average three-year-old is 37 inches tall, the average four-year-old is 40 inches tall, and the average five-year-old is 43 inches tall.
	Head and chest circumference: Unlike the squatty, potbellied appearance of the toddler, the physical proportions of the preschooler are more like that of the adult. The preschooler is usually slender and agile and takes great pride in showing off for others.
Development of gross motor and fine motor skills	3 years: The three-year-old can pedal a tricycle, jump in place, broad jump, balance on one foot, walk up and down steps using alternating feet, build a tower of 9 or 10 cubes, copy a circle, put facial features on a circle, and feed and dress himself.
	4 years: The four-year-old can balance on one foot for five seconds, walk heel to toe, catch a ball, throw a ball overhand, skip and hop on one foot, use scissors, lace shoes, copy a square, and add three parts to a stick figure.
	5 years: The five-year-old can skip and hop on alternate feet, throw and catch a ball, jump rope, jump from a height of 12 inches, balance on alternate feet with eyes closed, tie shoelaces, use scissors, begin to print a few letters or numbers, copy a diamond and triangle, and draw a stick figure with seven to nine parts.

(continues)

TABLE 17.3   *Continued*

Type of Development	Characteristics
Socialization	3 years: The three-year-old has a vocabulary of about 900 words and can use complete sentences of 3–4 words, asks many questions, and begins to sing songs. 4 years: The four-year-old understands time in relation to daily events, prizes independence, takes pride in her accomplishments, enjoys entertaining others, shares family secrets with outsiders, and commonly has an imaginary friend. Four year olds use sentences and have a vocabulary of 1,500 words. Egocentrism, or the inability to envision situations from perspectives other than their own, is a key feature of this age group. 5 years: The five-year-old has a vocabulary of approximately 2,100 words and can use sentences with 6–8 words. He asks the meaning of words and has many questions. At this age, the child can name the days of the week and the months of the year. The preschooler enjoys associative play, group play with similar or identical activities but without organization or rules. Preschoolers enjoy wading pools, tricycles, wagons, dolls, books with pictures, musical toys, finger paints, and toys that imitate objects used by adults.

School Age (6–12 Years)

School age begins with the child's entrance into the school environment, which has a profound effect on the child's development and relationship to the outside world. The freedom of expression enjoyed by the preschooler is less tolerated in the classroom, and the child learns to conform to social expectations. Associative play gives way to cooperative play in which following the rules is a must with little or no tolerance for those who do not. It is a time of leaders and followers as well as the emergence of in crowds and out crowds. Children with special learning needs, the overweight, those with physical limitations, and the poor often find themselves in the out crowd, making the school years a time of loneliness and frustration. In a few instances, this has later given way to school violence with tragic results. Parents and teachers can help by making children more sensitive to the needs of others and by providing opportunities for all children to achieve their potential. Table 17.4 highlights development milestones for the school-aged child.

TABLE 17.4   **Key Elements in the Development of School-Age Children**

Type of Development	Characteristics
Physical growth and development	Weight: During the period known as school age, the child gains an average of 6–8 pounds a year, reaching an average of 85–90 pounds by age 12 years. Height: Between the ages of 6 and 12, children grow an average of two inches per year. By age 12, the child should be approximately five feet tall. Head and waist circumference: Head and waist circumference decrease in relation to standing height. Leg length increases, and the child takes on a more mature appearance. Permanent tooth eruption is complete by 12 years of age.

TABLE 17.4 *Continued*

Type of Development	Characteristics
Development of gross motor and fine motor skills	6–8 years: The child has boundless energy, which is motor channeled into activities such as swimming, skating, biking, dancing, and sports. Fine motor skills become more developed as dexterity becomes more refined. Among the skills acquired during the early school years are the ability to read, tell time, and use simple math. 9–12 years: The child uses tools and equipment well, follows direction, is enthusiastic at work and at play, and looks for ways to earn money.
Socialization	6–8 years: During these years interest in group activities heighten and the child wants to be with peers. Participation in group activities such as scouting begin. 9–12 years: The older school-age child loves secrets and might help organize secret clubs. The school-age child participates in cooperative play or activities that are organized with rules. Play activity is mostly with same-sex groups, but with some mix in the later years. The school-age child enjoys board games, video games, music, and sporting activities that are shared with others.

Adolescence (12–18 Years)

Adolescence is a time of rapid growth with the peak growth spurt spanning 24–36 months. Secondary sex characteristics appear, with physical and sexual maturity occurring in late adolescence.

Growth in height generally ceases by age 17 in girls and age 18–20 in boys. Boys generally gain more in height and weight than girls. In early adolescence (12–15 years), the teen is usually uncoordinated with awkward movements due to the increasing length of the legs and the size of the feet. In later adolescence (16–18 years), the teen has increased coordination with more graceful movement. This no doubt accounts for the perfecting of athletic ability in high school and college.

The teen years represent a time of developmental crisis for the adolescent as well as the parents. The adolescent is usually on an emotional roller coaster, with highs and lows and periods of sociability and isolation. The desire for increased independence and changing roles within the family often leads to parent-child conflicts. Peer relationships are all-important and friendships can replace the influence parents have had during the childhood years. Adolescents enjoy music, sports, video games, and activities where there are others of the same age.

TIP

You should review nursing textbooks for Erikson's Theory of Psychosocial Development, Kohlberg's Theory of Moral Development, and Piaget's Theory of Cognitive Development as they relate to normal growth and development.

Congenital Anomalies

Congenital anomalies are also known as *birth defects*, and they refer to deviations in normal development that are evident at the time of birth or shortly thereafter. Congenital anomalies can be caused by genetic or environmental factors and include gastrointestinal, musculoskeletal, neurological, and cardiovascular defects. Some congenital defects are not physical malformations but are evident as inborn errors in metabolism and mental retardation. This section includes a review of the most common congenital anomalies, their management, and the reaction of parents to the birth of an infant with defects in physical development.

Anomalies of the Gastrointestinal System

These disorders can involve any portion of the gastrointestinal tract from the mouth to the anus. Incomplete development during embryonic development can result in atresia, malrotation, malposition, or failure of embryonic structures to close. The most common disorders of the gastrointestinal tract are

▶ Cleft lip and cleft palate

▶ Esophageal atresia/tracheoesophageal atresia

▶ Imperforate anus

▶ Hirschsprung disease

▶ Biliary atresia

Cleft Lip and Cleft Palate

Cleft lip and cleft palate are craniofacial deformities that involve the lip, hard palate, or soft palate. These can occur as separate malformations or occur together. Surgical repair of a cleft lip is generally performed between one and three months of age, whereas cleft palate repairs are performed between six months and two years of age depending on whether the defect involves the hard palate or soft palate.

> **CAUTION**
>
> Lip repair is performed earlier than palate repair to facilitate feeding and promote parental-infant bonding. The nurse should assess the amount and quality of parental interaction with the infant because the bonding process can be negatively affected by the infant's appearance.

Preoperatively the nurse should teach the parents to feed the infant using a Breck feeder or flanged nipple. The infant should be fed slowly to prevent aspiration and should be burped more frequently to prevent gastric distention. The infant's weight should be closely monitored.

CAUTION

Postoperatively the nurse should give priority to assessing the respiratory status of the infant. Surgical correction of the soft tissue of the mouth and palate can result in airway obstruction.

Additional postoperative care includes feeding the infant using a Breck feeder to prevent stress on the suture line caused by sucking. The mouth and suture line are cleansed of formula residue using sterile water. The suture line of the lip is cleaned using half-strength hydrogen peroxide. The suture line is reinforced with a Logan bar, which lessens stress on the suture line caused by crying. Elbow restraints prevent the infant placing his hands near his face or mouth.

NOTE

A multidisciplinary team is involved in the care of the infant with cleft lip/cleft palate. This team can include the physician, nurse, orthodontist, speech therapist, otolaryngologist, and social worker.

Esophageal Atresia or Tracheoesophageal Fistula

Esophageal atresia (EA) is a failure of the esophagus to develop a continuous passage, and tracheoesophageal fistula (TEF) is an abnormal opening between the trachea and esophagus. These can occur alone or in combination. Symptoms of EA and TEF include

▶ The presence of maternal polyhydramnios (excessive amniotic fluid)

▶ Excessive mucus and drooling in the newborn

▶ Coughing, choking, and cyanosis with the first feeding

▶ An x-ray of the esophagus that confirms the presence of a blind pouch at each end, widely separated with no connection (EA) or the presence of an abnormal connection between the trachea and esophagus (TEF)

Prior to surgical correction, intravenous fluids are started and the infant is positioned to facilitate drainage of secretions. Frequent suctioning of secretions from the mouth and pharynx decreases the likelihood of aspiration. A double lumen catheter placed in the esophageal pouch is attached to intermittent low suction. Keeping the infant's head in an upright position makes it easier to remove collected secretions.

NOTE

Aspiration pneumonia is so common that prophylactic antibiotics are usually started.

The surgical correction of esophageal atresia can be performed in one operation or staged in one or two operations. Surgical correction of TEF involves a thoracotomy, a division and ligation of the TEF, and an end-to end anastomosis. If the repair is to be done in stages, a gastrostomy tube is inserted to permit tube feedings. Prior to feeding, the gastrostomy tube is elevated and secured above the level of the infant's stomach. This allows gastric contents to pass into the duodenum and lessens the likelihood of aspiration. Gastrostomy feedings are continued until the esophageal anastomosis is healed. Oral feedings are begun about one week postoperatively and are started with sterile water followed by small, frequent feedings of formula.

Esophageal atresia and tracheoesophageal fistula are associated with several other anomalies, including congenital heart disease, anorectal malformations, and genitourinary anomalies. The prognosis depends on the preoperative weight, associated congenital anomalies, and prompt diagnosis. Premature and low birth weight infants as well as those with severe respiratory complications have poorer prognoses.

Imperforate Anus

This deformity includes a number of malformations in which there is no obvious anal opening or where an abnormal opening exists between the anus and the perineum or genitourinary system. A routine part of neonatal assessment includes checking for patency of the anus and rectum and noting the passage of meconium.

> **CAUTION**
>
> Passage of meconium does not always indicate anal patency—particularly in females—because a fistula might be present, allowing evacuation of the meconium. In males meconium might pass through a fistula in the midline. This can appear as ribbonlike meconium at the base of the scrotum or near the base of the penis.

Surgical repair depends on the extent of the malformation. The imperforate anal membrane is removed, followed by dilation. More extensive surgery is required for the infant with perineal defects. Postoperatively, the infant should be positioned to prevent pressure on the perineal sutures.

Hirschsprung Disease (Congenital Aganglionic Megacolon)

This anomaly refers to the absence of nerve stimulation to the bowel, which produces normal peristalsis. Although it accounts for about 25% of all cases of neonatal bowel obstruction, it might not be diagnosed until later in infancy or childhood. Hirschsprung disease is more common in males and is frequently associated with other congenital anomalies such as Down syndrome. The symptoms of Hirschsprung disease depend on the amount of bowel involved, the occurrence of complications, and the age at time of diagnosis.

Symptoms in the newborn include failure to pass meconium within the first 24–48 hours, refusal to feed, abdominal distention, and intestinal obstruction. During infancy, symptoms include the failure to gain weight, constipation, abdominal distention, and episodes of vomiting. In childhood the symptoms become chronic and include poor appetite; poor growth; abdominal distention; infrequent passage of foul-smelling, ribbonlike stools; and palpable fecal masses.

CAUTION

The presence of fever, bloody diarrhea, and severe lethargy should alert the nurse to the possibility of enterocolitis, a potentially fatal condition.

The diagnosis of Hirschsprung disease is made using a barium enema, rectal biopsy, and anorectal manometry (a procedure that records the pressure response of the internal anal sphincter). In the case of Hirschsprung disease, the internal sphincter fails to relax.

In some cases the child with Hirschsprung disease can be managed with dietary modifications such as increasing fluid and fiber intake. Management also includes the administration of occasional enemas using isotonic or normal saline solutions. These solutions can be purchased without a prescription or can be prepared by adding one level measuring teaspoon of noniodized salt to one pint of tap water.

CAUTION

The use of tap water, concentrated salt solutions, soap solutions, or phosphate preparations is discouraged because frequent use of nonisotonic solution can lead to water intoxication and the dilution of serum electrolytes.

Most children with Hirschsprung disease require surgical correction. The child's fluid and electrolyte is stabilized, and a temporary colostomy is performed to relieve the obstruction and allow the bowel to return to normal. Following the initial surgery, a complete corrective surgery is performed. Several surgeries are used; however, one of the most common includes a pull-through procedure in which the end of the normal bowel is pulled through the muscular sleeve of the rectum. The temporary colostomy is closed at the same time. Postoperative nursing care includes assessing the client for abdominal distention and for the return of bowel sounds and the passage of stool. The abdominal wound is assessed and cared for the same as any abdominal wound.

Biliary Atresia

This problem causes fibrosis of the intrahepatic and extrahepatic bile ducts and gradually results in liver failure. Most affected infants are full term and appear healthy at birth. Jaundice, dark urine, clay-colored stools, and hepatomegaly occur early in the disease. Later symptoms are associated with the development of cirrhosis and splenomegaly.

Treatment of biliary atresia includes surgical procedures that allow drainage of the bile (hepatic portoenterostomy or Kasai procedure) and orthotopic liver transplantation, now considered to be the definitive therapy for biliary atresia.

CAUTION

Jaundice that exists longer than two weeks of age accompanied by elevations in direct (conjugated) bilirubin points to the possibility of biliary atresia.

Anomalies of the Musculoskeletal System

These disorders affect the development and ossification of bones and joints. The most common skeletal disorders are developmental hip dysplasia (DHD) and congenital clubfoot.

Developmental hip dysplasia most commonly involves subluxation or incomplete dislocation of the hip. The disorder can affect one or both hips; if only one hip is involved, it is most often the left hip. Although the cause is unknown, certain factors such as gender, family history, intrauterine position, method of delivery, and postnatal positioning affect the risk of DHD. Females are affected more often than males, and there is an increased incidence if one of the parents or a sibling had the disorder. DHD is more common in the infant with frank breech presentation and delivery by Cesarean section.

NOTE

DHD is found more often in groups that use cradle boards or papoose boards for carrying the infant (such as Native Americans) than those groups that carry the infant on the back or on the hips (such as Asians).

Symptoms of DHD in the infant 2–3 months of age include laxity in the hip joint and the presence of the Ortolani click—the audible sound that is made when the affected hip is abducted. Other signs include shortening of the affected limb (Allis sign) and asymmetrical thigh and gluteal folds. Symptoms of DHD in the older child include delays in walking, the presence of extra gluteal folds, and a positive Trendelenburg sign when weight bearing. If both hips are affected, the child develops a waddling gait and lordosis.

Early diagnosis and correction of DHD are important because correction becomes more difficult as the child ages. Correction in the infant less than six months of age involves the use of a Pavlik harness. This device prevents hip extension or adduction and is worn continuously for about 3–6 months. Failure to diagnose the condition before the child begins to stand results in apparent contractures of the hip adductor and flexor muscles. Correction at this point involves traction, open or closed reduction, and the application of a hip spica cast.

> **CAUTION**
>
> The infant is growing rapidly, so the straps of the Pavlik harness should be checked every 1–2 weeks for needed adjustments because vascular or nerve damage can occur with improper positioning.

Congenital Clubfoot

Also known as *talipes equinovarus*, this problem is a structural deformity in which the foot is turned inward, causing the child to walk on the outer border of the foot. Congenital clubfoot can be classified as *positional* (due to intrauterine crowding), *teratologic* (associated with other congenital anomalies), or *true* clubfoot (due to a bony abnormality). The affected foot is usually smaller and shorter than the unaffected foot. If the defect is unilateral, the affected limb is smaller with atrophy of the calf muscle.

Treatment begins in the nursery or shortly after birth with the application of casts. The cast is changed and the affected limb is manipulated weekly for the first 6–12 weeks. Surgical correction involves pin fixation and the release of tight joints and tendons followed by casting for 2–3 months. After the cast is removed, a varus-prevention brace is worn.

Anomalies of the Central Nervous System

Central nervous system (CNS), or neural tube defects, make up the largest group of congenital anomalies. The incidence of neural tube defects has been drastically reduced by supplementing the mother's diet with folic acid prior to conception. Avoiding extremes of temperature during early fetal development has likewise reduced the risk of neural tube defects.

> **CAUTION**
>
> The pregnant client should avoid external heat exposure, such as hot tubs and saunas, because these have been identified as factors that increase the risk of neural tube defects.

Spina Bifida

This disordered is marked by a failure of the bony spine to close. It is the most common defect of the central nervous system. There are two types of spina bifida: spina bifida occulta and spina bifida cystica. Of these two types, spina bifida cystica, an external sac-like protrusion, causes the greatest CNS damage.

The major forms of spina bifida cystica are *meningocele* (the defect contains the meninges and spinal fluid) and *myelomeningocele* (the defect contains the meninges, nerve tissue, and spinal fluid). Unlike the child with a meningocele, who usually has no neurological deficit, the child with a myelomeningocele often has serious neurological deficit.

In most instances, myelomeningocele occurs in the lumbar or lumbosacral area. Regardless of where the defect is located, higher and larger defects result in more neurological damage.

The defect, which is usually enclosed in a thin membrane, should be protected from trauma as well as contamination with urine and stool, which can cause infection. Any stool or urine near the sac is gently removed using sterile saline, and the sac is examined for signs of leakage.

> **CAUTION**
>
> During the preoperative period, the nurse should give priority to preventing injury to or drying of the sac. The sac should be covered with a sterile, nonadherent dressing moistened with sterile normal saline. Dressings are changed every 2–4 hours. The newborn should be placed prone with the hips slightly flexed and elevated (low Trendelenburg) to prevent stretching of involved nerves.

Surgical correction usually takes place within the first 24–72 hours of life to prevent local infection and trauma to the exposed tissues. Several neurosurgical and reconstructive procedures are used for skin closure. Complications of myelomeningocele include the development of hydrocephalus, urinary tract infection, meningitis, pressure sores, and contractures.

> **CAUTION**
>
> Symptoms of meningitis in the infant include temperature instability, poor feeding, high-pitched cry, and bulging fontanels. Symptoms of meningitis in the child include fever, projectile vomiting, headache, and visual disturbances.

Anomalies of the Cardiovascular System

Cardiovascular disorders are classified as congenital heart defects and acquired heart disorders. *Congenital* heart defects involve structural defects in the anatomy of the heart and blood vessels that are apparent at birth or shortly thereafter. These affect the function of the heart and are evident in the development of congestive heart failure and hypoxemia. *Acquired* heart disorders refers to disease processes that affect the structure and function of the heart. Acquired heart disease can be the result of bacterial infection, autoimmune response, environmental factors, or heredity. This section focuses on two congenital heart defects: coarctation of the aorta and Tetralogy of Fallot. A review of two acquired heart diseases—rheumatic fever and Kawasaki disease—follows later in the chapter.

Congenital Heart Defects

Heart defects are the major cause of death during the first year of life, with the exception of those infants who die from prematurity. In most cases, the cause of congenital heart defects (CHD) remains unknown. However, certain maternal risk factors have been identified:

▶ Alcoholism

▶ Maternal age over 40

▶ Rubella during pregnancy

▶ Type 1 diabetes

CHD is more likely to be diagnosed when the infant is several weeks old than at the time of birth.

> **NOTE**
>
> The rapid heart rate of the infant, the instability of the circulatory system, and the fact that many newborns have a benign murmur present for the first few days of life often delay diagnosis. It is more likely that a congenital heart defect will be diagnosed when the infant is several weeks old.

Symptoms of CHD in the infant and child depend on the type and severity of the defect but include

▶ Cyanosis with feeding

▶ Clubbing of the fingers and toes

▶ Dyspnea

▶ Failure to gain weight

▶ Fatigue

▶ Respiratory congestion

Complications of CHD include delayed growth and development, polycythemia, clot formation, and congestive heart failure.

> **CAUTION**
>
> Early signs of congestive heart failure include tachycardia while sleeping, profuse sweating (especially on the scalp), fatigue, irritability, respiratory distress, and weight gain.

Congenital heart disease is classified according to whether the defect is acyanotic (without cyanosis) or cyanotic (with cyanosis). Acyanotic defects include patent ductus arteriosus, atrial septal defect, ventricular septal defect, and coarctation of the aorta. Cyanotic defects include transposition of the major vessels, truncus arteriosus, and Tetralogy of Fallot.

> **CAUTION**
>
> At this point, you might want to review heart structure and normal circulation in a nursing textbook as well in an anatomy and physiology textbook. It is difficult to understand the abnormal if you don't know the normal.

As you probably realize, the content area of congenital heart disease is quite large, so we'll focus on two defects (one acyanotic and one cyanotic) because of the uniqueness of the symptoms associated with these two conditions.

Coarctation of the Aorta

This refers to a narrowing within the aorta that alters blood flow to the extremities. Symptoms of coarctation of the aorta (COA) include elevated blood pressure and bounding pulses in the upper extremities and diminished blood pressure and weak or absent pulses in the lower extremities. Infants who develop congestive heart failure require hospitalization for stabilization of the blood pressure and treatment of acidosis. Older children with COA might complain of dizziness; headache; fainting; and nosebleed, which can indicate that the blood pressure is higher than usual.

Correction of COA involves resection of the coarcted portion with an end-to-end anastomosis of the aorta or by enlargement of the narrowed portion using either a prosthetic graft or a graft taken from the left subclavian artery. The defect is outside the heart and pericardium, so cardiopulmonary bypass is unnecessary.

Residual hypertension following surgery seems to be related to the age of the child at the time of repair, so elective surgery should be performed within the first two years of life. The prognosis is good, with less than 5% mortality in children with no other defects.

Tetralogy of Fallot

As the name implies, this disorder involves four separate defects. These defects include pulmonic stenosis, ventricular septal defect, overriding aorta, and right ventricular hypertrophy. Infants with Tetralogy of Fallot (TOF) might have a history of acute cyanosis and heart murmur at birth that worsens over the first year of life. Acute episodes of cyanosis and anoxia, referred to as *blue spells* or *tet attacks*, occur during crying or feeding because the infant's oxygen demands are greater than the blood supply. Children with TOF have noticeable cyanosis, clubbing of the fingers, and growth retardation. When oxygenation is compromised, the child with TOF assumes a squatting position. Children with TOF are at risk for developing emboli, seizures, loss of consciousness, or sudden death following an anoxic episode.

CAUTION

Nursing care for the infant or child with a tet attack involves placing the child in knee chest position and providing supplemental oxygen.

Surgical treatment for TOF involves a palliative shunt (Blalock-Taussig procedure) to increase blood flow to the lungs thereby providing for better oxygenation. Complete elective repair, involving correction of each of the four defects, is usually performed in the first year of life. Surgical repair requires the child to be placed on cardiopulmonary bypass. The operative mortality is less than 5% for total correction of TOF.

NOTE

The movie *Something the Lord Made* (2004) gives an account of the first surgery performed on a child with Tetralogy of Fallot.

Inborn Errors of Metabolism

This refers to inherited diseases caused by the absence or deficiency of a substance, usually an enzyme that is essential to cellular metabolism. Most inborn errors in metabolism involve abnormal metabolism of protein, carbohydrate, or fat. Although many diseases are included in this category, we will focus on two of the most common: phenylketonuria and galactosemia.

Phenylketonuria

Phenylketonuria (PKU) is a genetic disorder in which the child is unable to metabolize phenylalanine into tyrosine. Tyrosine is essential to the formation of melanin (responsible for hair, skin, and eye color) and the hormones epinephrine and thyroxine. Accumulation of phenylalanine affects the normal development of the brain and central nervous system. Without early detection and treatment, the child with PKU develops irreversible brain damage.

Clinical manifestations of PKU include irritability, frequent vomiting, failure to thrive, and seizures. Older children with PKU have bizarre behaviors such as head banging, screaming, arm biting, and other psychotic behaviors.

The most commonly used screening test for PKU is the Guthrie blood test. All newborns are screened for PKU before discharge or within the first week of life because early detection and treatment are necessary to prevent mental retardation.

> **CAUTION**
>
> The Guthrie test is obtained from a heel stick. Remember to stick the newborn on the side of the heel to avoid nerve damage. The test is most reliable if the newborn has ingested a source of protein. If the specimen is obtained before the newborn is 24 hours old, a subsequent sample should be obtained before the newborn is two weeks old.

The treatment for PKU consists of instituting a low-phenylalanine diet begun as soon as possible after diagnosis and continued through adolescence. Specially prepared formulas include Lophenalac and ProPhree Total. Partial breast feeding can be allowed if phenylalanine levels are closely monitored. Solid foods such as cereal, fruits, and vegetables are added according to the recommended schedule. Most high-protein foods are either eliminated or restricted to small amounts. Artificial sweeteners containing aspartame should be avoided because they are converted to phenylalanine.

Galactosemia

Galactosemia is a genetic disorder in which one of the three enzymes necessary to covert galactose to glucose is missing. The infant with galactosemia appears normal at birth, but within a few days of ingesting a formula containing lactose, she begins to vomit and lose weight. Additional symptoms arise from accumulations of galactose, which target the major organs.

Damage done to the liver and spleen results in jaundice, cirrhosis, and portal hypertension. Cataracts—opacities in the lens of the eyes—are usually evident by 1–2 months of age. Lethargy and hypotonia associated with brain damage are evident soon afterward.

Newborn screening for galactosemia is required in most states. Diagnosis is based on history, physical exam, and increased levels of serum galactose. The treatment of galactosemia is aimed at eliminating all milk- and lactose-containing foods, including breast milk. Instead, the infant is fed a soy-protein formula.

> **CAUTION**
>
> Medications that contain lactose should also be avoided.

Respiratory Disorders

These disorders include infections of the upper airway and lower airway and as well as infections of the ears. Three points should be made about respiratory disorders in children. First, respiratory disorders are more common, and often more serious, in infants and children than adults. Some infections, such as otitis media, occur with greater frequency because of anatomical differences. Second, although all children are at risk, certain children are more vulnerable to respiratory disorders. This includes premature and low-birth weight infants and children with AIDS. Finally, children with respiratory disorders are more likely than adults to develop gastrointestinal symptoms such as vomiting and diarrhea, which increase the risk of dehydration and acidosis. This section focuses on the care of children with the most common pediatric respiratory disorders.

Acute Otitis Media

Acute otitis media (AOM) is one of the most common respiratory diseases in childhood. The incidence is highest in children six months to three years of age. Otitis media is more prevalent in the young child because the eustachian tube is straighter, shorter, and wider than in older children or adults. Other factors that contribute to AOM are passive smoking, enlarged adenoids, attendance at day care, and supine positioning with bottle feeding. In AOM the child develops a high fever (103°–104° F), anorexia, vomiting, and pain. The infant or young child might be seen rubbing or pulling at the affected ear or rolling her head from side to side. Increasing pressure can rupture the eardrum. If rupture occurs, pain and fever subside.

The organism responsible for AOM is usually *H. influenza*, although other organisms (such as *S. pneumoniae* and *M. catarrhalis*) can also produce an acute infection. Treatment of AOM involves the use of antibiotics, including oral amoxicillin, sulfonamides, erythromycin, or cephalosporins. Antipyretics such as ibuprofen or acetaminophen can be given to reduce fever and pain.

> **CAUTION**
>
> Oral suspensions are usually administered for 7–10 days. It is important that parents comply by giving the medication for the full course of treatment. Single-dose injections of an appropriate antibiotic can be used if the child has poor absorption of the drug, the child refuses to take the medication, or the parents fail to comply with oral therapy.

Complications of AOM include mastoiditis, meningitis, and hearing loss. Hearing evaluation is recommended for a child who has bilateral OM for a total of three months. Children with AOM should be seen after antibiotic therapy to check for any residual infection and to identify potential complications.

> **NOTE**
>
> More information on otitis media, including myringotomy and insertion of PE tubes, is included in Chapter 8, "Caring for the Client with Sensorineural Disorders."

Tonsillitis

This problem often accompanies pharyngitis and is a major cause of illness in young children. The tissue referred to as *tonsils* is actually made up of several pairs of lymphoid tissue:

▶ Adenoids

▶ Lingual tonsils

▶ Palatine tonsils

▶ Pharyngeal tonsils

Symptoms of tonsillitis include

▶ Difficulty swallowing and breathing

▶ Enlargement of the tonsils

▶ Inability to smell and taste

▶ Mouth breathing

▶ Snoring

The condition can be viral or bacterial in origin.

Viral infections are usually self-limited, and management is aimed at relieving the symptoms of soreness and dryness of the throat.

Tonsillitis is usually caused by a virus; therefore, management focuses on the relief of symptoms. However, if the infection is caused by Group A beta hemolytic streptococcus, antibiotic therapy is ordered. A *tonsillectomy*—surgical removal of the palatine tonsils—is indicated if tonsillar enlargement interferes with eating or breathing, if there is a recurrent history of frequent streptococcal infection, or if there is a history of peritonsillar abscesses. An *adenoidectomy*—surgical removal of the adenoids—is recommended if enlarged adenoids block breathing. In most cases, the tonsils are not removed before three years of age because of the possible complications associated with blood loss in very young children and the possibility of the regrowth of lymphoid tissue.

Preoperative nursing care includes obtaining a detailed history (including a history of unusual bleeding), assessing for signs of upper respiratory infection, and noting whether any teeth are loose. Routine vital signs are obtained to serve as a baseline for postoperative comparison, and a bleeding and clotting time are requested.

Postoperatively the child should be closely observed for continual swallowing, which is an indication of bleeding. An ice collar can be applied to the throat to increase comfort, and analgesics can be given intravenously or rectally for the first 24 hours to decrease pain and promote rest.

When the child is awake and responsive, ice chips and cool, clear liquids are given. Citrus foods, hot foods, and foods with rough textures should be avoided as well as foods that are red, orange, or brown in color. Upon discharge, the parents should be instructed to keep the child out of crowds for 1–2 weeks and to report any signs of new bleeding, which is most likely 7–10 days after surgery. The doctor should be notified immediately if bleeding occurs after discharge.

Laryngotracheobronchitis

This is the most common form of croup in hospitalized children and is a viral infection of the upper airway. It is most common in children between three months and eight years of age. Unlike acute spasmodic croup, which appears suddenly at night, the onset of laryngotracheo-bronchitis (LTB) begins with an upper respiratory infection and low-grade fever. The child is restless and irritable, with noticeable hoarseness and a brassy cough.

The goal of care is to maintain the airway and ensure adequate oxygenation. The child with mild croup is often managed at home and treated symptomatically. The symptoms of hoarseness, cough, and inspiratory stridor can be relieved by providing high humidity with cool mist. The child should be frequently offered fluids to maintain adequate hydration.

> **CAUTION**
>
> Immediate medical attention should be sought if the child develops labored respirations, continuous stridor, or intercostal retractions or refuses to take oral fluids.

If the respiratory condition worsens, treatment includes withholding oral intake and administering IV fluids until the respiratory condition improves. Other measures include cool mist vaporizers, supplemental oxygen, and the administration of antibiotics to treat coexisting infections and steroids or epinephrine to reduce bronchial swelling.

Acute Epiglottitis

This is an upper airway infection that primarily affects children 2–5 years of age, but it can also occur at any age from infancy to adulthood. The primary cause of acute epiglottitis is *H. influenza*.

> **NOTE**
>
> The American Academy of Pediatrics recommends that all children receive the *H. influenza* B conjugate vaccine beginning at two months of age as part of the routine childhood immunization series. This can account for the decline in the incidence of epiglottitis.

The child with epiglottitis is much sicker than symptoms suggest. Typically, the child goes to bed with no symptoms but awakens complaining of a sore throat and pain on swallowing. Additional symptoms include drooling, muffled phonation, inspiratory stridor, and sitting in a tripod position. Upon examination, the physician notes the appearance of a cherry red epiglottis.

> **CAUTION**
>
> Remember that only the physician should assess the child's throat because visualization can precipitate immediate airway obstruction. A tracheostomy set or endotracheal intubation set should be readily available because emergency intervention might be necessary to support respiratory efforts.

Endotracheal intubation or tracheostomy is usually performed if the child has *H. influenza* epiglottitis. These procedures, as well as initiation of intravenous fluids and antibiotics, are usually carried out in the operating room. Even if intubation and assisted ventilation are unnecessary, the child should be maintained in an intensive care area for continual observation for at least 24 hours. Dramatic improvement occurs in 24 hours with antibiotic therapy, and the epiglottis is almost normal within 2–3 days.

Bronchiolitis

This is a lower airway infection that occurs most often in infants and children under two years of age. The respiratory Syncytial Virus (RSV) accounts for most cases of bronchiolitis; however, the condition is also caused by adenoviruses, parainfluenza viruses, and *M. pneumoniae*. Outbreaks occur most commonly in the winter and spring months with peak incidence from November to March.

Symptoms of bronchiolitis include dyspnea, nonproductive cough, wheezing, nasal flaring, intercostal and sternal retractions, and emphysema.

Management of the client with bronchiolitis depends on the age and presenting symptoms. Older children with bronchiolitis can be treated at home, but infants are more likely to need hospitalization. Treatment is aimed at maintaining the respiratory status, decreasing the chance of aspiration, treating the infection, and maintaining acid/base balance. Nursing care includes careful assessment of the vital signs and respiratory status as well as attention to intake and output. Oral fluids might be withheld until respiratory function improves. Additional measures include the use of cool mist vaporizers with or without supplemental oxygen and respiratory therapy with Virazole (ribavirin).

CAUTION

To be effective, ribavirin should be administered within three days of the infection. Healthcare workers who are pregnant should avoid direct care of the client receiving aerosolized Virazole (ribavirin) because the medication can cause birth defects or death of the fetus. Surgical masks do not provide adequate filtration of the Virazole particles.

NOTE

RSV-IGIV (Respigam), which was previously administered to high-risk (premature or low-birth weight) infants is no longer recommended for use in the United States since it interferes with the administration of the MMR and varicella vaccines. Palivizumab (Synagis) is preferred for use because it does not interfere with administration of the MMR vaccine or varicella vaccine. Synagis is given IM as a monthly injection for a total of five injections

Cystic Fibrosis (Mucoviscidosis)

This is inherited as an autosomal recessive gene. The disease affects the exocrine system and produces abnormalities in the lungs, pancreas, and sweat glands. Although cystic fibrosis affects these systems, the prognosis depends on the degree of lung involvement. Lung function has been greatly improved with the use of Pulmozyme (dornase alpha), an enzyme that improves respiratory function.

Symptoms of cystic fibrosis include meconium ileus, frequent upper respiratory infections, malabsorption, failure to gain weight, and heat prostration. Additional health problems include reoccurring nasal polyps and rectal prolapse.

The diagnosis of cystic fibrosis is made by the sweat test, which reveals elevated sodium and chloride levels. The absence of pancreatic enzymes results in malabsorption and steatorrhea or undigested fat in stools. Chest x-ray reveals emphysematous changes in lungs.

The treatment of cystic fibrosis includes the use of antibiotics to treat respiratory infections and pancreatic enzyme replacement to improve absorption and decrease weight loss. The client's diet should be high in carbohydrate, high in protein, and moderate in fat. Extra salt is allowed, and the diet is supplemented with water-soluble preparations of vitamins A, D, E, and K.

TIP

Pancreatic enzyme replacement is based on the client's age and the consistency of the stools. These enzymes, which are given with each meal and snack, are best tolerated when given in applesauce because it disguises the taste.

Gastrointestinal Disorders

Gastrointestinal disorders include infections, malformations, and structural changes that affect the digestion and absorption of nutrients. When we think of the GI tract, and we seldom do unless there is a problem, we typically only think of its role in digestion and elimination. However, the GI tract plays a key role in maintaining fluid and electrolyte balance through its interaction with the kidneys and lungs. Gastrointestinal disorders are considered to be more severe in the infant and young child because of the danger of dehydration and metabolic acidosis.

Gastroenteritis

Gastroenteritis, or acute diarrheal disease, can be caused by an infection with rotavirus, salmonella, or another organism, or it can accompany another illness such as an upper respiratory or urinary tract infection. Additional causes include ingestion of sorbitol or fructose in juices. Regardless of the cause, acute diarrhea is a more severe illness in infants and very young children because they develop dehydration more quickly than adults. Untreated, the condition can quickly progress to a life-threatening situation.

Treatment focuses on determining the cause of the illness, assessing for signs of fluid and electrolyte imbalance, ensuring adequate hydration, and reintroducing an adequate diet. Stool and urine cultures are ordered in addition to the routine lab studies.

Oral rehydration solutions such as Pedialyte and Infalyte replace formula feedings in the child with mild dehydration. Intravenous fluids with electrolytes are started on children with severe dehydration and shock. When symptoms improve, the child can begin to have clear liquids with progression to the BRAT diet (bananas, rice, applesauce, and toast). Although the BRAT diet may still be used, its therapeutic effects have been questioned since it is nutritionally deficient and the increased sugar may encourage diarrhea. Infants can begin formula progression as follows: half-strength soy formula, full-strength soy formula, and (if tolerated) a return to regular formula.

> **CAUTION**
>
> Potassium replacement should be instituted only after assessing for the presence of urinary output.

Pyloric Stenosis

This problem involves a narrowing of the sphincter at the outlet of the stomach, and it occurs most often in firstborn males. The signs and symptoms of pyloric stenosis include projectile vomiting and a palpable olive-shaped mass in the right upper quadrant of the abdomen. X-ray confirms the presences of hypertrophy and an elongation of the pylorus. The disorder is corrected surgically by a procedure known as a *pyloromyotomy* or *Fredet-Ramstedt* procedure. The prognosis following surgery is excellent.

Intussusception

This problem involves an invagination or telescoping of one portion of the bowel into another. The most common site for intussusception is the ileocecal valve or the point where the large and small intestines join. Symptoms associated with intussusception include colicky abdominal pain, the presence of a sausage-shaped mass in the abdomen, and the passage of "currant jelly" stools by an otherwise healthy child. The use of air pressure or water-soluble contrast can be used to diagnose and reduce the intussusception. If conservative measures fail, surgical intervention is required to restore normal bowel function.

Celiac (Gluten-Induced Enteropathy, Celiac Sprue)

This issue is a malabsorptive disorder of the proximal small intestine caused by an intolerance to gluten. Gluten is found in the grain of wheat, oats, barley, and rye. Digestive problems most often appear between the ages of one and five years when the child begins to ingest various foods containing gluten. Symptoms vary but generally include malabsorption, steatorrhea, abdominal distention, and muscle wasting (particularly in the buttocks and extremities). Diagnosis is based on jejunal biopsy, which reveals changes in the intestinal mucosa. The treatment of celiac involves the replacement of gluten-containing grains with corn, rice, and millet as well as avoiding hidden sources of gluten. Hydrolyzed vegetable protein, a common ingredient in many commercially prepared foods, contains gluten and can cause an exacerbation of symptoms. Associated problems include deficiencies in iron, folic acid, and fat-soluble vitamins that are treated with vitamin and mineral supplements.

> **CAUTION**
>
> Strict adherence to dietary restrictions can help minimize the development of small intestine lymphoma, one of the most serious complications of celiac.

Cardiovascular Disorders

These are divided into two groups: *acquired heart disorders* and *congenital heart disorders*, which are sometimes referred to as *congenital heart disease*. Congenital heart disease, which exists at the time of birth, was discussed earlier in this chapter. Acquired heart disease refers to disease processes that occur after birth and can be found in those with a normal heart and cardiovascular system. Two examples of acquired heart disease are rheumatic fever and Kawasaki's disease.

Rheumatic Fever

This is an autoimmune response to Group A beta hemolytic streptococcal infection. The disease, which is self-limiting, affects the skin, joints, brain, serous surfaces, and heart. The most serious complication of rheumatic fever is damage to the valves of the heart, and the valve most often affected is the mitral valve.

The major clinical manifestations of rheumatic fever are the result of inflammation and the appearance of hemorrhagic lesions (Aschoff bodies) that are found in all the affected tissues. The symptoms associated with each of the major manifestations are

▶ **Carditis (heart)**—Includes the presence of an apical systolic murmur, aortic regurgitation, tachycardia, cardiomegaly, complaints of chest pain, and development of mitral stenosis.

▶ **Polymigratory arthritis (joints)**—Includes the presence of red, swollen, painful joints, particularly the larger joints (knees, elbows, hips, shoulders, and wrists). The symptoms move from one joint to another and are most common during the acute phase of illness.

▶ **Erythema marginatum (skin)**—Includes the presence of a distinct red macule with a clear center found on the trunk and on proximal extremities.

▶ **Subcutaneous nodules (serous surfaces)**—Includes the presence of small, painless swellings located over the bony prominences of the feet, hands, elbows, vertebrae, scalp, and scapulae.

▶ **Syndeham's chorea (brain)**— Includes the presence of aimless, jerking movements of the extremities; involuntary facial grimacing; speech disturbances; emotional lability; and muscle weakness.

In addition to the major manifestations, the client with rheumatic fever has minor manifestations that include fever, arthralgia, elevated erythrocyte sedimentation rate, and positive C-reactive protein. Supporting evidence of a preceding Group A beta hemolytic streptococcal infection includes a positive throat culture and a positive antistreptolysin-O (ASLO) titer.

The goals of treatment are eradicating the hemolytic streptococcal infection, preventing permanent cardiac damage, making the child more comfortable, and preventing recurrences of Group A beta hemolytic infection. Nursing interventions include administering prescribed medications (such as penicillin, salicylates, and steroids), promoting rest and proper nutrition, providing emotional support for the child and the family, and teaching regarding the need for periodic follow-up with the physician. In addition, the nurse plays a key role in emphasizing the need for good dental hygiene and regular dental visits.

Kawasaki's Disease (Mucocutaneous Lymph Node Syndrome)

This is an acute systemic vasculitis. The exact cause remains unknown, although it appears to be a problem with the immune system. The disease mainly affects children under five years of age with the peak incidence occurring in toddlers. The disease is best known for the damage done to the heart; however, it involves all the small- and medium-size blood vessels. The most common sequela of Kawasaki's disease (KD) is the dilation of coronary arteries, which results in aneurysm formation. Infants under one year of age and those over five years of age appear to be at the greatest risk for developing coronary problems. KD is one of the major causes of acquired heart disease in children in the United States.

The child with KD develops a high fever that lasts five or more days and fails to respond to antipyretics or antibiotics. Other symptoms include redness of the bulbar conjunctiva, inflammation of the pharynx and oral mucosa, red cracked lips, "strawberry tongue," and swelling of the cervical lymph nodes. One of the most notable symptoms is desquamation that begins at the fingertips and toes and gradually spreads, leaving the soles and palms red and swollen. Swelling is also noted in the weight-bearing joints. Additional findings include increased platelet counts and increased coagulation.

> **NOTE**
>
> Most cases of KD are reported in the winter and early spring. There is also an increased incidence in children who are exposed to recently cleaned carpet, which suggests there is perhaps an immune response.

There is no specific test for KD. The diagnosis is based on the presence of symptoms and supporting lab work that reveals a decreased number of RBC, an increased number of immature WBC, and an increased erythrocyte sedimentation rate. Medical management includes the use of IV immunoglobulin and aspirin.

The nursing care of the child with KD focuses on relieving symptoms, providing emotional support, administering medications, and educating the family. The nurse should carefully monitor the vital signs and assess for signs of cardiac complications, which include congestive heart failure and myocardial infarction.

> **NOTE**
>
> Signs of myocardial infarction in the infant or young child include abdominal pain, vomiting, restlessness, inconsolable crying, pallor, and shock. Signs of congestive heart failure include respiratory distress, tachycardia, and decreased urinary output.

Nursing interventions during the acute phase focus on the relief of symptoms. Inflammation of the skin and mucous membranes accounts for much of the child's discomfort during the acute phase. The nurse can help minimize discomfort by applying soothing, unscented lotions to the skin. Mouth care with a soft-bristled toothbrush is followed by the application of lubricating ointment to the lips. Acetaminophen can be given for fever and to relieve joint pain. The child should be placed in a quiet environment to promote rest.

The administration of intravenous gamma globulin requires that the nurse carefully assess vital signs and observe for signs of an allergic reaction, which include chills, fever, dyspnea, and flank pain.

CAUTION

The nurse must ensure patency of the IV line before administering gamma globulin because extravasation can result in tissue damage.

The child with KD might be discharged on high doses of aspirin for an extended period of time. The nurse should teach parents the side effect signs and symptoms of aspirin toxicity, including tinnitus, dizziness, headache, and confusion. Low-dose aspirin can be continued indefinitely if the child has coronary abnormalities. The child with coronary abnormalities should avoid contact sports.

CAUTION

The nurse should instruct the parents to discontinue the aspirin and notify the physician if the child is exposed to influenza or chickenpox.

Musculoskeletal Disorders

These disorders involve alterations in bones, joints, muscles, or cartilaginous tissues. Musculoskeletal disorders, like fractures, are the result of trauma (refer to Chapter 11, "Caring for the Client with Disorders of the Musculoskeletal System"). Disorders such as congenital hip dysplasia and clubfoot involve prenatal or genetic factors. Other musculoskeletal disorders include scoliosis, Legg-Calve Perthes disease, and muscular dystrophy.

Scoliosis

Scoliosis refers to a lateral curvature of the spine with rotation of the vertebrae. It is the most common spinal deformity and is associated with physiological alterations in the spine, chest, and pelvis. Idiopathic scoliosis is more prevalent in adolescent females, and there is some evidence that it might be genetically transmitted as an autosomal dominant trait. Routine scoliosis screening is often a part of the adolescent physical exam.

> **NOTE**
>
> The Adams position is used to screen for scoliosis. With the examiner standing behind, the child is asked to bend from the waist while allowing the arms to hang freely. When viewed from behind, the child with scoliosis is noted to have a primary and compensatory curvature of the spine.

Conservative treatment includes the use of either the Milwaukee brace or Boston brace and exercise. Surgical correction consists of realignment and straightening the spine with internal fixation. Two surgical methods that can be used are Harrington rods and Luque wires. The Cotrel-Dubousset approach uses both Harrington rods and Luque wires.

Postoperative nursing care includes assessment of vital signs, medication administration for pain, assessment of operative site, and providing emotional support to the client and family.

Logrolling technique should be used when turning the client with Harrington rods.

Legg-Calve-Perthes Disease (Coxa Plana)

This disease is a self-limiting disorder in which there is an aseptic necrosis of the head of the femur. Although the exact cause is unknown, it occurs most often in males 4–8 years of age.

Symptoms include soreness, aching, stiffness, and the appearance of a limp on the affected side. Pain and joint dysfunction are most evident on arising or at the end of the day.

The goal of treatment is to keep the head of the femur within the acetabulum and to prevent microfractures of the epiphysis. Initial measures include bed rest and non-weight-bearing activity. An abduction brace, leg casts, or leather harness sling can be used to prevent weight bearing. Conservative therapy is continued for 2–4 years. Although the condition is self-limiting, the ultimate outcome depends on early recognition and effective treatment.

Muscular Dystrophies

Muscular dystrophies refer to a group of inherited degenerative diseases that affect the cells of specific muscle groups resulting in muscle atrophy and weakness. The most common type, Duchenne muscular dystrophy, is inherited as a sex-linked disorder; therefore, it affects only males. Clinical manifestations of muscular dystrophy include delayed walking; wide-based waddling gait; lordosis; weak, hypertrophied leg muscles; and the use of Gower's maneuver to stand erect. Children with Duchenne muscular dystrophy lose the ability to walk by 9–12 years of age.

> **NOTE**
>
> With Gower's maneuver, the child places his hands on his knees and moves his hands up his legs until he's standing erect.

The goal of treatment is aimed at maintaining mobility and independence for as long as possible. Nursing interventions include dietary teaching to prevent obesity and complications associated with limited mobility, coordinating healthcare services provided by physical therapy, and providing emotional support to the child and family.

Childhood Cancer

Childhood cancer is a leading cause of death in children under 15 years of age. Although survival has increased for most types of cancer, few diagnoses present a greater challenge for the nurse as she cares for the child and his family. Refer to Chapter 9, "Caring for the Client with Cancer," for a detailed review of cancer, treatment modalities, and nursing care. This section briefly reviews the key points of the following childhood cancers: Wilms tumor, leukemia, and osteosarcoma.

Wilms Tumor (Nephroblastoma)

This is the most common type of renal cancer. Parents usually find the tumor while diapering or bathing the infant. The tumor, which is confined to one side, is characteristically firm and nontender. The tumor is also usually encapsulated, so it is responsive to chemotherapy. Survival rates for Wilms tumor are the highest of all childhood cancers.

> **CAUTION**
>
> The nurse should post a DO NOT PALPATE THE ABDOMEN sign on the bed of the child suspected of having Wilms tumor.

Leukemia

Leukemia, a cancer of the blood-forming elements of the bone marrow, is the most common form of childhood cancer. Pathological changes are related to the rapid proliferation of immature white blood cells, and symptoms include anemia; fatigue; lethargy; fever; joint and bone pain; pallor; petechiae; and enlargement of the spleen, liver, and kidneys. Acute lymphoid leukemia, the most common form, is more prevalent in males 1–5 years of age.

Treatment involves a combination of cytotoxic drugs and possible bone marrow transplantation. Nursing interventions include preparing the child and family for diagnostic procedures, administering chemotherapy, observing for signs of infection, and providing continuous emotional support.

Osteogenic Sarcoma (Osteosarcoma)

This cancer type is the most common bone cancer found in children. Most of those affected are males, ages of 10–25. The most common site is the epiphyseal plate of long bones, particularly the femur. Traditional management involves amputation of the affected extremity and intensive chemotherapy. Nursing interventions are the same as those for the child with other forms of cancer.

Ingestion of Hazardous Substances

Injuries and death related to accidental poisoning have declined over the past three decades. This is largely due to the Poison Prevention Packaging Act of 1970, which requires that potentially hazardous drugs and household products be sold in child-resistant containers. Still, poisoning remains a significant health concern for children under six years of age. Common sources of household poisoning are plants, cosmetics and perfumes, cleaning products, and petroleum distillates. Over-the-counter medications such as cough and cold remedies, laxatives, and dietary supplements are also frequently ingested by children.

> **CAUTION**
> Consultation with the physician or poison control center should be done before administering any antidote.

Salicylate Overdose

Salicylate, or aspirin overdose, results in an acid/base imbalance. Symptoms include nausea, vomiting, dehydration, tinnitus, hyperpnea, hyperpyrexia, bleeding, convulsions, and coma. Treatment is aimed at removal through emesis, lavage, or the use of activated charcoal. Additional measures are sodium bicarbonate transfusions to correct metabolic acidosis, vitamin K to control bleeding, and diazepam to control seizures. Hemodialysis might be needed in the most severe cases.

Acetaminophen (Tylenol) Overdose

This results in severe and sometimes fatal damage to the liver. Initial drug levels for are drawn four hours after the drug is ingested, but treatment should begin before the lab results are obtained. Tylenol overdose is treated with IV acetylcysteine. Plasma levels of 300 mcg/ml occurring 4 hours after ingestion or 50 mcg/ml occurring 12 hours after ingestion are associated with hepatotoxicity. In spite of treatment, there can be continuing hepatic damage that makes liver transplantation a necessity.

Lead (Plumbism)

This poisoning results in irreversible damage to the brain. Sources of lead include lead-based paint, lead crystal, ceramic wares, dyes, playground equipment, stained glass, and collectible toys. Lead poisoning affects the hematopoietic, renal, and neurological systems. With low-dose exposure, the child might experience symptoms of impulsivity, hyperactivity, and distractibility. With higher-dose exposure, the child can experience mental retardation, paralysis, blindness, convulsions, and death.

Chelation therapy is used to remove lead from the circulating blood. Commonly used chelation agents include calcium disodium edetate (EDTA), calcium disodium versenate (Versenate), British anti-Lewisite (BAL/Dimercaprol), and Succimer (which can be given orally).

Nursing care includes the administration of medication, which is often painful. If renal function is adequate, Versenate can be given intravenously; otherwise, it is given by injection. The nurse should assess the client receiving Versenate for signs of cerebral edema. Cerebral edema is treated with intravenous mannitol or dexamethasone. The side effects of heavy metal antidotes include malaise, paresthesia, nausea, and vomiting.

> **NOTE**
>
> Houses constructed before 1950 are more likely to have leaded paint. Lead-based paints were officially banned for use in 1978.

Iron Poisoning

This poisoning is usually the result of ingesting vitamins or iron-containing medications intended for adults. Initial symptoms of iron poisoning include vomiting of blood and blood in the stools. If the condition is left untreated, the victim becomes restless, hypotensive, tachypneic, and cyanotic. Hepatic injury, coma, and death can occur within 48–96 hours after ingestion. The treatment of iron poisoning includes emesis or gastric lavage. In cases of severe intoxication, chelation therapy with deferoxamine is necessary.

Diagnostic Tests for Review

The following are routine tests done on most all hospital admissions. Specific tests are ordered to confirm or rule out a particular illness. For example, an erythrocyte sedimentation rate and antistreptolysin titer are ordered for the client with symptoms of rheumatic fever. Positive results on these tests indicate inflammation caused by a preceding infection with Group A beta hemolytic streptococcus. It is helpful if you have a text of laboratory and diagnostic tests with nursing implications as a reference while you review. The routine tests are as follows:

▶ CBC

▶ Urinalysis

▶ Chest x-ray

Pharmacology Categories for Review

The following drug classifications are most commonly ordered for the pediatric client. However, some situations require the nurse to know about drugs rarely given. It is helpful to have a pharmacology text with nursing implications available as you review. The following are the drug classifications most commonly ordered:

▶ Antibiotics

▶ Antipyretics

▶ Analgesics

▶ Vitamin supplements

Exam Prep Questions

1. Assessment findings the nurse could expect to find in the infant with biliary atresia are:

   ○ **A.** Excessive drooling that requires frequent suctioning

   ○ **B.** Pale, frothy stools and poor weight gain

   ○ **C.** Poor tissue turgor and weight loss

   ○ **D.** Clay-colored stools and abdominal distention

2. The mother of a child with cystic fibrosis asks the nurse for information about the disease. The nurse's teaching is based on the knowledge that cystic fibrosis:

   ○ **A.** Produces multiple cysts in the lungs

   ○ **B.** Affects the exocrine glands

   ○ **C.** Is an autosomal dominant disorder

   ○ **D.** Affects the endocrine glands

3. A three-year-old with coarctation of the aorta is scheduled for corrective surgery. Which preoperative lab result should be reported to the physician?

   ○ **A.** HCT 48%

   ○ **B.** WBC 14,000

   ○ **C.** Platelet count 200,000

   ○ **D.** RBC 5.3

4. Which play activity is most appropriate for a 15-month-old with a cyanotic heart defect?

   ○ **A.** Push-pull toy

   ○ **B.** Mobile

   ○ **C.** Shape sorter

   ○ **D.** Pounding board

5. A nine-year-old is admitted with suspected rheumatic fever. Which finding is suggestive of Syndeham's chorea?

   ○ **A.** Irregular movements of the arms and legs and facial grimacing

   ○ **B.** Painless swellings over the surface of the joints

   ○ **C.** Faint areas of red demarcation over the back

   ○ **D.** Swelling and inflammation of the joints

6. The nurse observes that a child with muscular dystrophy has a positive Gower's sign. The nurse documents that the child:

   ○ **A.** Has weak deep tendon reflexes

   ○ **B.** Must use his hands to rise from the floor

   ○ **C.** Has increased spinal reflexes

   ○ **D.** Rocks back and forth in rhythmical fashion

7. The nurse is caring for a child with celiac disease. The nurse's discharge teaching plan should include:

   ○ **A.** Dietary instructions and a list of foods to be avoided

   ○ **B.** Hand-washing instructions to prevent disease transmission

   ○ **C.** Instructions to continue antibiotics for one week

   ○ **D.** Explaining that one attack confers immunity

8. Which play activity is most appropriate for a three-year-old with a hip spica cast?

   ○ **A.** Barbie doll and accessories

   ○ **B.** Toy telephone

   ○ **C.** Coloring book and crayons

   ○ **D.** Puzzle

9. During morning rounds, the nurse notices blood spots on the pillowcase of a child with acute lymphoid leukemia. The nurse should be most concerned about the client's:

   ○ **A.** Red blood cell count

   ○ **B.** White blood cell count

   ○ **C.** Platelet count

   ○ **D.** Reticulocyte count

10. A four-year-old has a right nephrectomy to remove a Wilms tumor. The nurse knows that it is essential to:

   ○ **A.** Request a low-salt diet

   ○ **B.** Restrict fluids

   ○ **C.** Educate the family regarding renal transplants

   ○ **D.** Prevent urinary tract infections

Answer Rationales

1. Answer D is correct. Symptoms of biliary atresia include jaundice, dark urine, clay-colored stools, and liver enlargement. Answer A describes symptoms of esophageal atresia, so it's incorrect. Answer B describes symptoms of cystic fibrosis, so it's incorrect. Answer C describes symptoms of dehydration, so it is incorrect.

2. Answer B is correct. Cystic fibrosis is a chronic disorder that affects the exocrine system or mucous-secreting glands of the body. It is inherited as an autosomal recessive disorder. Answers A, C, and D do not relate to cystic fibrosis, so they are incorrect.

3. Answer B is correct. The WBC is elevated, indicating possible infection. Answers A, C, and D are within normal range, so they are incorrect.

4. Answer C is correct. The shape sorter is most developmentally appropriate for the 15-month-old. Answers A and D require too much energy expenditure for the child with a cyanotic heart defect, so they are incorrect. Answer B is suitable for the infant but not for a 15-month-old, so it's incorrect.

5. Answer A is correct. The child with Syndeham's chorea has facial grimacing, jerking movements of the extremities, and rapidly changing mood. Answer B describes subcutaneous nodules, so it's incorrect. Answer C describes erythema marginatum, so it's incorrect. Answer D describes polymigratory arthritis, so it is incorrect.

6. Answer B is correct. Muscular dystrophy results in hypertrophied weak muscles of the legs and pelvis, which causes the child to use his hands to rise to standing position. Answers A and C have nothing to do with Gower's sign, so they are incorrect. Answer D refers to the movement of the child with autism, so it's incorrect.

7. Answer A is correct. Celiac disease is related to the ingestion of gluten-containing grains. The client should avoid oats, wheat, barley, and rye as well as foods containing those grains. Answers B and C are incorrect. They do not apply to celiac disease because it is not bacterial or viral in origin. Answer D is incorrect because ingestion of substances containing gluten will produce symptoms again.

8. Answer B is correct. The toy telephone is large enough that it cannot be placed beneath the cast, and it promotes social and language development. Answers A, C, and D contain small pieces that can be placed beneath the cast, so they are incorrect.

9. Answer C is correct. Depressed platelet count indicates a potential for bleeding and hemorrhage. Although answers A, B, and D are important, they do not relate to the finding of blood spots on the pillowcase. Therefore, they are incorrect.

10. Answer D is correct. Because the child has only one remaining kidney, it is important to prevent urinary tract infections. Answers A, B, and C are not necessary, so they are incorrect.

Suggested Reading and Resources

▶ Hockenberry, M. and Wilson, D., *Wong's Essentials of Pediatric Nursing.* 8th ed. St. Louis: Elsevier, 2009.

▶ Ball, J., and Bindler, R. *Pediatric Nursing: Caring for Children.* 4th ed. Upper Saddle River, NJ: Pearson Prentice Hall, 2008.

▶ www.aaai.org—American Academy of Allergy, Asthma, and Immunology

▶ www.cdc.gov—Centers for Disease Control

▶ www.lungusa.org—The American Lung Association

▶ www.aafp.org—The American Academy of Family Practice

▶ www.pathguy.com—Dr. Ed Friedlander, pathologist

▶ www.cff.org—Cystic Fibrosis Foundation

▶ www.candlelighters.org—Candlelighters Childhood Cancer Foundation

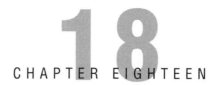

CHAPTER EIGHTEEN

Emergency Nursing

Terms you'll need to understand

✓ Biological weapons

✓ Chemical agent

✓ Emergent

✓ Non-urgent

✓ Urgent

Nursing skills you'll need to master

✓ Performing a head-to-toe assessment

✓ Performing cardiopulmonary resuscitation

✓ Administering medication

✓ Administering intravenous fluids

✓ Administering blood

✓ Applying splints and manual traction

✓ Performing dressing changes

Nursing in the emergency department can be thought of as nursing in the fast lane. Unlike the routine of unit nursing, emergency nursing requires the nurse to respond to diverse conditions with much versatility. Many emergency situations confront the client and his family with fears of death or disability. Therefore, the ER nurse must assist with stabilizing the client's physical condition while providing emotional support to both the client and his family during a time of crisis. Faced with life and death on a daily basis, emergency nursing is not for everyone.

A primary principle in providing emergency care is *triage*, or the sorting of clients into one of three categories:

▶ Emergent

▶ Urgent

▶ Non-urgent

Using this system, the clients with the most life-threatening conditions are cared for first. This is different from the triage applied in disasters or in field situations where scarce resources are allocated to care for the greatest number.

In this chapter you will review some of the most common conditions cared for in the emergency department. You will not spend time on the conditions covered in previous chapters; however, you might want to refer to those chapters after you complete this section. These conditions include burns (see Chapter 7, "Caring for the Client with Burns"), fractures (see Chapter 11, "Caring for the Client with Disorders of the Musculoskeletal System"), ketoacidosis and insulin shock (see Chapter 12, "Caring for the Client with Disorders of the Endocrine System"), myocardial infarction (see Chapter 13, "Caring for the Client with Disorders of the Cardiovascular System"), and seizures and increased intracranial pressure (see Chapter 14, "Caring for the Client with Disorders of the Neurological System"). Instead, you will focus on the ABCDs of emergency care and the treatment of trauma, poisonings, and poisonous bites. Finally, you will review the care of clients who are victims of radiation accidents as well as chemical agents and biological weapons.

The ABCDs of Emergency Care

Initial management of the client in the emergency department is based the ABCD assessment: airway, breathing, circulation, and deficits. Airway obstruction, whether complete or partial, requires prompt intervention. In the case of complete obstruction, appropriate intervention is needed to prevent permanent brain damage or even death. After the airway has been secured, the nurse assesses the client's breathing to determine whether the client's respiratory effort is sufficient or whether assisted ventilation and oxygen will be needed. Evaluation of the client's circulation and control of bleeding are next in the order of trauma assessment. Only relief of airway obstruction and care of sucking chest wounds take priority over the immediate control of bleeding. With airway, breathing, and circulation under control, the nurse turns her attention to assessing for deficits. These include additional injuries such as fractures, burns, wounds, and neurological injuries. Each of these areas is covered in greater detail as they form the basis for trauma interventions.

Airway

The first consideration is to find out whether the airway is patent. Are there signs of partial obstruction or complete obstruction? Signs of partial obstruction include noisy breathing and coughing, and signs of complete obstruction include inability to breathe, inability to talk, inability to cough, and clutching the throat. Death from complete airway obstruction can result in as little as 3–5 minutes due to hypoxia.

Clients who need airway management include those with scores of less than 8 on the Glasgow coma scale, those with maxiofacial injuries, those who have aspirated, and those with inhalation injuries from burns. More information on inhalation injuries from burns can be found in Chapter 7.

Interventions are aimed at maintaining a patent airway. A client with partial obstruction of the airway should be encouraged to cough forcefully. In the event that the airway is completely obstructed, it can be opened using the head-tilt chin lift maneuver or the jaw-thrust maneuver.

After the airway is open, it will be maintained by an oropharyngeal or nasopharyngeal airway or an endotracheal tube.

> **NOTE**
> You might want to refer to the nursing textbooks for guidelines for managing a foreign body airway obstruction and performing cardiopulmonary resuscitation.

> **CAUTION**
> Always provide C spine immobilization before opening the airway of any client with undetermined or suspected neck injuries. The jaw-thrust maneuver should be used for a victim with suspected neck injury because it can be done without extending the neck.

Breathing

The next consideration is to find out whether the rate and depth of respirations are adequate. The normal respiratory rate for adults is 12–20 breaths per minute; for children it's 15–30 breaths per minute; and for infants it's 28–50 breaths per minute. Lung sounds should be clear and equal bilaterally.

Inadequate breathing in the adult is evident in slowed (fewer than 8 breaths per minute) or rapid (greater than 24 breaths per minute) respirations. Other signs of inadequate respirations are labored breathing, intercostal and suprasternal retractions, changes in lung sounds, asymmetry of the chest wall, and cyanosis.

Interventions for ineffective breathing patterns are aimed at providing relief of symptoms. These interventions include maintaining a patent airway and providing supplemental oxygen. High-concentration oxygen is used in any cardiac or respiratory arrest situation.

Circulation

Next you must find out whether circulation is adequate. Are there signs of bleeding? The nurse should assess the rate, rhythm, and strength of the pulse and obtain an admission blood pressure. If the radial pulse can be felt, the systolic blood pressure is usually above 80mm Hg. The nurse should check for capillary refill. If capillary refill is adequate, the area being assessed will return to normal color within 2–3 seconds after blanching. If the area remains white or blue, the area is not receiving adequate circulation.

Circulation is obviously affected by blood loss. The nurse can assess for external bleeding by doing a blood sweep. This is carried out by running a gloved hand from head to toe, pausing periodically to see whether the glove is bloody.

External bleeding can be controlled by applying direct pressure to the area, elevating or immobilizing the affected extremities, or applying direct pressure over arterial pressure points. In most cases bleeding can be stopped by direct pressure over the artery, unless a major artery has been severed. Tourniquets or inflated blood pressure cuffs are applied to an extremity only if hemorrhage cannot be controlled by direct pressure. The tourniquet should be applied just proximal to the wound and only tight enough to control arterial blood loss. The tourniquet should be loosened periodically to prevent neurovascular damage. If there is no further arterial bleeding, the tourniquet should be removed and a pressure dressing applied.

Interventions for inadequate circulation and hypovolemic shock are aimed at restoring adequate circulation and maintaining the blood pressure within normal limits. Infusions of warmed Lactated Ringers are started in at least two veins using a large-bore catheter (14- or 16-guage). IV access, using the upper and lower extremities, is necessary if there is bleeding from a major vessel in the chest or abdomen. Infusion of Lactated Ringers solution helps restore circulation and allows time for blood typing and screening. The restoration of circulating blood volume depends on blood replacement.

Additional interventions for a client with hypovolemic shock include the insertion of a CVP line, insertion of an indwelling urinary catheter, monitoring of arterial blood gases, monitoring of vital signs, maintaining normal body temperature, and treating acid base disturbances. Lactic acidosis, a common side effect of hemorrhage and injury, is associated with poor cardiac function.

Resuscitative efforts continue until the client has a serum lactic acid lower than 2.5 mmol/L within 24 hours after the injury and there are no further signs of hemorrhage.

Deficits

Lastly, you need to ascertain the client's mental status. Are there changes in the client's level of consciousness? Deficits in these areas can reflect neurological injury.

The nurse can test for deficits by assessing the client's responsiveness and orientation. These assessments can be done quickly. To test for responsiveness, the nurse notes the following key points, which are sometimes referred to as *AVPU*:

▶ **Alertness**—Is the client aware of his surroundings and circumstances? Does the client know his name? Is he able to state the year, month, and day? Does he know what happened and where he is?

▶ **Verbal stimuli**—Does the client respond to questions asked by the examiner? Can he state his name? Can he identify common objects? Can he respond to simple requests? If the client can respond appropriately to what he is asked, he is said to be alert and oriented.

▶ **Pain**—Is the client aware of painful stimuli? Can he identify where pain is located? Can he describe the pain? Can he assess the pain using a pain scale?

▶ **Unresponsiveness**—Does the client respond to any stimuli?

The nurse can test the client's orientation by checking the client's awareness of person, place, time, common objects, and event. Questions about his name; where he is; day, month, and year; and what happened help establish that the client is oriented. If the client can answer all these questions and is alert, he is determined to be alert and fully oriented.

After checking for responsiveness and orientation, the nurse assesses the pupils for size, shape, equality, and reaction to light. Pupillary changes should be reported immediately because they indicate changes in neurological status.

Obtaining Client Information

After airway, breathing, circulation, and deficits have been assessed and stabilized, the nurse focuses on obtaining a history of the current condition as well as significant information regarding medications, allergies, and past medical history. The emergency room staff then focuses on the client's reason for seeking treatment.

Trauma

Trauma is defined as unintentional or intentional injury to the body, and it is the number one cause of death in persons under 44 years of age. Most traumatic injuries are the result of motor vehicle accidents (MVAs). Areas affected most often in MVAs are the head, chest, and abdomen. Other traumatic injuries include suicides, homicides, and physical assaults.

After performing the ABCD interventions, the nurse assesses for signs of traumatic injury. Rapid trauma assessment, using a head-to-toe approach, can be done using the mnemonic DCAP—BTLS. The nurse assesses the client for the presence of

▶ Deformities

▶ Contusions

▶ Abrasions

▶ Punctures or penetrations

▶ Burns

▶ Tenderness

▶ Lacerations

▶ Swelling

Head Injuries

Head injuries account for more than one third of the injuries sustained in MVAs. Other sources of head injury include falls and sports injuries. Head injuries are classified as *primary brain injuries* (open or closed head trauma) and *secondary brain injuries* (the result of the primary injury). Examples of primary brain injuries are fracture and penetrating injury. Examples of secondary brain injuries are increased intracranial pressure, hemorrhage, and loss of autoregulation. Interventions are focused on assessing and managing increased intracranial pressure, assessing the level of consciousness using the Glasgow coma scale, controlling seizures, and minimizing neurological deficits. These points are covered in Chapter 14.

NOTE

Coup and injuries affect different portions of the brain. *Coup* (site of impact) injuries occur in the frontal area of the brain. *Contrecoup* injuries occur away from the site of impact. Areas of contrecoup injury include the frontal and temporal areas of the brain.

CAUTION

The use of opiates is contraindicated for a client with a head injury because they cause central nervous system depression.

Chest Injuries

Chest injuries account for about one fourth of the injuries sustained in motor vehicle accidents. Trauma to the head and chest is drastically reduced by the proper use of seat belts and air bags as well as child safety restraints. Chest injuries include pulmonary and cardiac contusions, pericardial tamponade, fractured ribs, flail chest, pneumothorax, hemothorax, and ruptured diaphragm. Interventions include maintaining adequate respirations, controlling hemorrhage, and treatment of the specific injury. For example, pneumothorax and hemothorax are treated with the insertion of chest tubes and closed chest drainage.

CAUTION

Flail chest should be suspected in clients with multiple rib fractures, scapular fractures, and pulmonary contusion. Unequal chest movement characterizes flail chest.

Abdominal Injuries

Abdominal injuries account for about one fourth of the injuries sustained in MVAs. Abdominal injuries can be blunt injuries (such as from seat belts) or penetrating injuries (such as from gunshots or stab wounds). Penetrating injuries can damage hollow structures, particularly the small bowel, or solid organs. The most frequently damaged solid organ is the liver.

The major cause of death from abdominal trauma is hemorrhage. An assessment for abdominal injury should include inspection of the anterior abdomen, flanks, back, genitalia, and rectum. In the case of intra-abdominal injury, blood tends to collect in these areas. Rectal and vaginal examination is performed to determine injuries that might have occurred to the pelvis, bladder, or intestines.

Assessment of abdominal injury begins with obtaining a history of the mechanism of injury. Was the injury penetrating, as in the case of a gunshot, or was it blunt, as in the case of a blow to the abdomen? The abdomen is then inspected for obvious signs of injury. Entrance and exit wounds are noted, as are bruises and characteristic markings such as those left by seatbelts. The examiner auscultates for the presence of bowel sounds and records findings for comparison with later assessments. Areas of progressive distention, involuntary guarding, and tenderness are noted. The nurse should assess the chest for signs of injury that might accompany abdominal trauma.

The incidence of complications from blunt abdominal trauma is greater than from penetrating injuries. This is especially true when there is blunt injury to the liver, kidneys, spleen, or blood vessels, which can result in massive blood loss that can go undetected for some time.

> **CAUTION**
>
> The nurse should be familiar with indications of intra-abdominal bleeding. Ecchymosis around the umbilicus (Cullen's sign) and ecchymosis on either flank (Turner's sign) indicate retroperitoneal bleeding into the abdominal wall.
>
> The nurse should be familiar with indications of damage to the spleen. With the client lying on the left side, the right flank is percussed. Resonance over the right flank (Ballance's sign) indicates rupture of the spleen. Pain in the left shoulder (Kehr's sign) is seen in a client with a ruptured spleen; pain in the right shoulder indicates lacerations of the liver.

Additional indications of abdominal trauma include the absence of bowel sounds, progressive abdominal distention, abdominal pain and tenderness, and evisceration.

> **CAUTION**
>
> Cover abdominal contents with sterile normal saline-soaked gauze. Do not try to return the abdominal contents to the abdominal cavity.

Interventions for the client with abdominal injuries include the insertion of two large-bore IV catheters for delivering fluid and blood replacement, cardiopulmonary monitoring, insertion of an indwelling urinary catheter, and insertion of a nasogastric tube.

> **CAUTION**
>
> You should not insert a nasogastric tube if there is a suspected skull fracture.
>
> The use of opiates for pain control is contraindicated because they can mask important signs and symptoms.

Documenting and Protecting Forensic Evidence

It is essential that the nurse provide accurate documentation and protection of forensic evidence when caring for trauma clients. When removing clothing, the nurse should avoid cutting through any tears, holes, blood stains, or dirt that might be used as evidence. Each piece of clothing should be labeled and placed in an individual paper bag before giving it to the police. The name of the officer, the date, and the time should be documented in the client's chart. Valuables should be placed in the hospital safe or given to a family member with appropriate documentation.

If homicide is suspected, the body of the deceased will be examined by the medical examiner or coroner. All tubes and lines should remain in place. The client's hands should be covered with paper bags to protect evidence that might be on the hands or under the nails. Swabs will be used to obtain tissue samples from beneath the nails. The client's wounds and clothing will also be photographed.

Procedures for protecting forensic evidence are the same for physical and sexual assault.

> **CAUTION**
>
> In cases of suspected sexual assault, the client is instructed not to shower, bathe, or change clothing. A rape trauma kit is used to collect forensic evidence. Swabs are used to obtain tissue specimens from the hands and fingernails. Specimens should be carefully labeled and protected as potential evidence. Photographs of wounds and clothing should include one with a reference ruler and one without a ruler.

Poisoning

Poisoning results from the ingestion, inhalation, or absorption of agents that cause chemical actions that injure the body. Emergency management of the client includes

- Removing or inactivating the poison
- Providing supportive care to maintain vital organ systems
- Administering specific antidotes
- Initiating treatment to facilitate the excretion of the absorbed poison

> **NOTE**
>
> The American Association of Poison Control Centers has a website at www.aapcc.org for further information.

> **CAUTION**
>
> Vomiting is never induced in a client who has ingested corrosive or petroleum distillates.
> Psychiatric consultation should be obtained if the poisoning is determined to be a suicide attempt.

Management of clients with poisonings related to lead, iron, aspirin, and acetaminophen were covered in Chapter 17, "Caring for the Pediatric Client." Treatment of clients with chemical injuries and those with carbon monoxide poisoning was covered in Chapter 7, and interventions for food poisoning were covered in Chapter 10. Treatment of drug overdoses such as narcotics and barbiturates were covered in Chapter 15, "Caring for the Client with Psychiatric Disorders." You might want to review those chapters for comparison with the overall management of poisoning.

Poisonous Stings and Bites

These are mainly produced by hymenopterans (bees, yellow jackets, wasps, hornets, and fire ants) or by venomous snakes (pit vipers). Injected poisons result in clinical manifestations that range from generalized redness, itching, and anxiety to bronchospasm, shock, and death. Snake venom can affect multiple organ systems—especially the cardiovascular, respiratory, and neurological systems.

Management of a client with a sting includes removing the stinger and washing the area with soap and water. The client should be discouraged from scratching the affected area because scratching releases histamine. Oral antihistamines and analgesics lessen pain and itching.

In cases of anaphylaxis or severe allergic reaction, aqueous epinephrine is administered subcutaneously and the injection site is massaged to speed drug absorption. Additional interventions focus on maintaining the client's respiratory and cardiovascular function. Desensitization is recommended for clients with a history of significant local or systemic reactions to stings.

The management of venomous snake bites is a medical emergency. The client should be instructed to lie down. Constricting items such as rings are removed, and the affected area is immobilized below the level of the heart.

> **NOTE**
> If the snake is dead, it should be brought to the emergency room to help identify the species.

Interventions include determining the severity of poisonous effects; obtaining vital signs; measuring the circumference of the affected extremity; and obtaining laboratory specimens for complete blood count, urinalysis, and clotting studies. In cases of *envenomation*—the injection of venom—antivenin is administered. Antivenin is most effective when given within 12 hours of the snake bite.

> **CAUTION**
> Corticosteroids are contraindicated in the first 6–8 hours after the bite because they can interfere with the action of the antivenin.

A test dose of antivenin, using the skin test or eye test, should be done before administering the medication.

The most common cause of allergic reaction to antivenin is too-rapid infusion. Allergic reactions include feelings of facial fullness, itching, rash, and apprehension. These symptoms can be followed by tachycardia, dyspnea, hypotension, and shock. In case of allergic reaction, the antivenin should be discontinued immediately, followed by the intravenous administration of diphenhydramine.

Bioterrorism

The threat of bioterrorism has brought with it new concerns and challenges for emergency personnel. Acts of bioterrorism are carried out using biological and chemical agents that are capable of disabling or killing thousands of people in a relatively short period of time. The unique nature of biological and chemical weapons is extremely frightening. These substances can be liquid or dry; dispensed in food and water supplies; vaporized for inhalation; spread by direct contact; and spread by vectors, including animals, insects, and persons.

Two biological agents most likely to be used as weapons are anthrax and smallpox.

Chemical and Biological Agents

Chemical agents produce effects that are more apparent and occur more quickly than biological agents. Chemical agents are classified as nerve agents, blood agents, vesicants, and pulmonary agents. Some chemical agents, such as chlorine, phosgene, and cyanide, are widely used in industry; therefore, they are widely accessible. Table 18.1 provides information on the symptoms and treatment of various chemical and biological agents.

TABLE 18.1   Chemical and Biological Agents Symptoms and Treatments

Chemical Agent	Symptoms	Treatment
Nerve agents (Tabun; Sarin; Soman; VX)	Salivation; lacrimation; urination; defecation; gastric emptying; pinpoint pupils (everything looks dark); seizures.	Atropine. The initial dose is 2 mg. Additional doses are given until symptoms are resolved (will not reverse miosis). Pralidoxime Chloride: 1 gram IV over 20–30 minutes. Benzodiazepines are given for seizure control or to prevent seizures in severely intoxicated patients.

(continues)

TABLE 18.1 *Continued*

Chemical Agent	Symptoms	Treatment
Cyanides (hydrogen cyanide; cyanogen chloride)	Nonspecific symptoms, including anxiety, hyperventilation, and respiratory distress. Cherry-red skin, although classic, is seldom seen. Lactic acidosis and increased concentration of venous oxygen.	A cyanide antidote kit is used. An amyl nitrite ampule is given and first aid is used until an IV is established. Crush and place the ampule inside the mask of a BVM resuscitator (15 seconds of inhalation; then a 15-second break; repeat until IV is established). Sodium nitrite: 300 mg over two to four minutes. Sodium thoisulfate: 12.5 g over five minutes.
Vesicants (mustard; lewisite)	Redness and blisters; inhalation injury can result in respiratory distress; leukopenia; pancytopenia.	Topical antibiotics. Systemic analgesics. Fluid balance (do not overhydrate because it's not a thermal burn). Bronchodilators and steroids for pulmonary symptoms—only if lewisite is the poison—then British anti-lewisite (BAL) is the antidote.
Pulmonary intoxicants (chlorine; phosgene)	Delayed onset of noncardiogenic pulmonary edema.	Treat hypertension with fluid; no diuretics. Ventilate with PEEP. Use bronchodilators.
Riot control agents	Ear, nose, mouth, and eye irritation.	Irrigate. Treat bronchospasm with bronchodilators and steroids, as needed.

Biological Agent	Symptoms	Treatment
Anthrax	I: 1–6d. FLS; a possibly widened mediastinum; gram stain (gram od) of blood and blood culture (late).	TBI: Treatment can be delayed 24 hours until cultures from incident site are available. PEP (only if instructed by government officials); ciprofloxacin or doxycycline po 8 weeks. In severe cases, ciprofloxacin, doxycycline, or penicillin IV is given.
Cholera	I: 4h–5d. Severe gastroenteritis with rice water diarrhea.	Oral rehydration with WHO solution or IV hydration. Tetracycline, doxycycline (dosage as below or 300 mg one time) po for three days. Ciprofloxacin or norfloxacin po for three days if it's a resistant strain.
Plague	I:2–3d. FLS; CXR: patchy infiltrates or consolidation; gram stain of lymph node aspirate, sputum, or CSP (gram negative, non–spore-forming rods).	Isolation. PEP: Doxycycline or cirprofloxacin for 7 days. Symptomatic: Gentamicin or doxycycline IV for 10–14 days. Meningitis: chloramphenicol.
Tularemia	I: 2–10d. FLS.	Gentamicin for 10–14 days.
Q fever	I: 10–40d. FLS.	Most cases are selflimited. Tetracycline or doxycycline po for five to seven days.

TABLE 18.1 *Continued*

Biological Agent	Symptoms	Treatment
Smallpox	I: 7–17d (average is 12). FLS. Later, an erythematous rash develops that progresses to pustular vesicles. Electron or light microscopy of pustular scrapings. PCR.	Isolation. PEP: Vaccinia vaccine scarification and vaccinia immune globulin IM.
Viral encephalitides	I: 1–6d. FLS. Immunoassay.	Supportive.
Viral hemorrhagic fevers	I: 4–21d. FLS. Easy bleeding and petechiae; enzyme immunoassay.	Isolation and supportive care. Some clients respond to ribavirin.
Botulism	I: 1–5d. Descending bulbar, muscular, and respiratory weakness.	Supportive. PEP: Toxoid. Symptomatic: anti-toxin.
Staphylococcus enterotoxin B	I: 3–12h. FLS.	Supportive.
Ricin	I: 18–24h. FLS, pulmonary edema, and severe respiratory distress.	Supportive
T-2 mycotoxins	I: 2–4h. Skin, respiratory, and GI symptoms.	Supportive

Abbreviation	Meaning	Dosages
CSF	Cerebro-spinal fluid	Chloramphenicol: 50–75 mg/kg/d, divided q 6 hrs.
CXR	Chest x-ray	Ciprofloxacin: po: 500 mg q 12 h; IV: 400 mg q 8–12 h
d	Days	Doxycycline: po: 100 mg q 12 h; IV: 200 mg initially then 100 mg q 12h
h	Hours	Erythromycin: po: 500 mg q 6 h
FLS	Flu-like symptoms	Gentamicin: 3–5 mg/kg/d
GLI	Gastrointestinal	Norfloxacin: po: 400 ml
I	Incubation period	Penicillin: IV: 2 million units q 2 h
PCR	Polymerase chain reaction	Tetracycline: po: 500 mg q 6 h
PEP	Post-exposure prophylaxis	Streptomycin: IM: 15 mg/kg/BID
TBI	Threatened biologic incident	Vaccinia immune globulin: IM: 0.6 ml/kg
WHO	World Health Organization	WHO solution: 3.5g NaCl, 2.5g NaHCO3, 1.5g KCl, and 20g glucose per liter of water

Compiled by Richard N. Bradley, MD, Assistant Medical Director, Houston Fire Department, EMS Division. Permission to use the above charts granted by *The Drop* magazine, published by the Special Forces Association of Fort Bragg, North Carolina; Winter 2001 issue.

Nuclear Warfare

Another source of terrorist activity involves the threat of nuclear warfare. Radioactive material includes not only nuclear weapons, but also radioactive samples of plutonium and uranium as well as medical supplies such as those used in cancer treatments. Exposure of a large number of people could be accomplished by placing this radioactive material in a public place.

The following list highlights three types of radiation injury that can occur:

▶ **External irradiation**—The client does not require special isolation or decontamination.

▶ **Contamination**—The client requires immediate medical management to prevent incorporation.

▶ **Incorporation**—The client requires immediate medical management because the cells, tissues, and susceptible organs (kidneys, bones, liver, and thyroid) have taken up the radioactive material.

Management of the client follows the hospital and countrywide guidelines for radiation disasters. These guidelines are very specific regarding decontamination and treatment of the injured. Staff is required to wear protective clothing, including two pairs of gloves, masks, caps, goggles, and booties. Dosimetry badges should be worn by all caregivers participating in the client's care.

Decontamination should take place outside the hospital whenever possible. Clothing should be removed, double bagged, and placed in a plastic container outside the facility. In a case where decontamination is delayed until hospital arrival, the client should be assessed with the radiation survey meter to determine external contamination. The client is taken to an area away from the ER equipped with a shower, collection pool, tarp, and collection containers for clothing and personal items. Additional washings should continue until the client is free from contamination.

Internal contamination or incorporation requires the use of cathartics and gastric lavage with chelating agents. These agents bind with the radioactive substances, which are then excreted in the urine, feces, and vomitus. Samples are obtained to determine the effectiveness of internal decontamination.

Acute radiation syndrome (ARS) can occur after a radiation injury. The development of ARS is dependent on the dose of radiation rather than the source, and symptoms vary according to the body system. Effects on the hematopoietic system are evident in the decreased number of white blood cells, red blood cells, and platelets that make the client vulnerable to infection and bleeding. Neurological effects include headache, nausea, and vomiting. Radiation of the skin produces redness, desquamation, and (in some instances) necrosis.

Triage Categories for Disaster Victims

A final point should be made regarding the care of clients in disasters such as those posed by terrorist acts or nuclear accidents. In disasters, the rules of hospital triage no longer apply. Faced with hundreds and possibly thousands of casualties, caregivers must use the color-coding system developed by the North Atlantic Treaty Organization (NATO). Triage categories for disaster situations are detailed in Table 18.2.

TABLE 18.2   NATO Triage Color Codings

Category	Color
Minimal—injuries are minor and treatment can be delayed	Green
Immediate—injuries are life-threatening but survivable with minimal care	Red
Delayed—injuries are significant and require medical care	Yellow
Expectant—injuries are extreme, and survival is unlikely	Black

Diagnostic Tests for Review

Diagnostic tests carried out for clients in the ER are mostly the same as those used for hospitalized clients. In some instances, such as poisonings, more specific tests such as toxicology screens might be ordered. The nurse should be familiar with the tests and diagnostic procedures routinely performed in the ER. These tests include

▶ Bleeding tests (PT, PTT, INR)

▶ CBC

▶ Chest x-ray

▶ Complete metabolic panel

▶ CT scan

▶ Liver profile

▶ MRI

▶ Urinalysis

Pharmacology Categories for Review

Categories of medications administered in the ER are much the same as for clients admitted to medical surgical units. These categories include

- Analgesics
- Antiarrhythmics
- Antibiotics
- Anticonvulsants
- Antiemetics
- Antihistamines
- Anxiolytics
- Bronchodilators
- Cardiotonics
- Emetics
- Local anesthetics
- Vasoconstrictors

Exam Prep Questions

1. The nurse is triaging four clients injured in a train derailment. Which client should receive priority treatment?

   ○ **A.** A 42-year-old with dyspnea and chest asymmetry

   ○ **B.** A 17-year-old with a fractured arm

   ○ **C.** A 4-year-old with facial lacerations

   ○ **D.** A 30-year-old with blunt abdominal trauma

2. Direct pressure to a deep laceration on the client's lower leg has failed to stop the bleeding. The nurse's next action should be to:

   ○ **A.** Place a tourniquet proximal to the laceration.

   ○ **B.** Elevate the leg above the level of the heart.

   ○ **C.** Cover the laceration and apply an ice compress.

   ○ **D.** Apply pressure to the femoral artery.

3. A pediatric client is admitted after ingesting a bottle of vitamins with iron. Emergency care would include treatment with:

   ○ **A.** Acetylcysteine

   ○ **B.** Deferoxamine

   ○ **C.** Calcium disodium acetate

   ○ **D.** British antilewisite

4. The nurse is preparing to administer Ringer's Lactate to a client with hypovolemic shock. Which intervention is important in helping to stabilize the client's condition?

   ○ **A.** Warming the intravenous fluids

   ○ **B.** Determining whether the client can take oral fluids

   ○ **C.** Checking for the strength of pedal pulses

   ○ **D.** Obtaining the specific gravity of the urine

5. The emergency room staff is practicing for its annual disaster drill. According to disaster triage, which of the following four clients would be cared for last?

   ○ **A.** A client with a pneumothorax

   ○ **B.** A client with 70% TBSA full thickness burns

   ○ **C.** A client with fractures of the tibia and fibula

   ○ **D.** A client with smoke inhalation injuries

6. An unresponsive client is admitted to the emergency room with a history of diabetes mellitus. The client's skin is cold and clammy, and the blood pressure reading is 82/56. The first step in emergency treatment of the client's symptoms would be:

   ○ **A.** Checking the client's blood sugar

   ○ **B.** Administering intravenous dextrose

   ○ **C.** Intubation and ventilator support

   ○ **D.** Administering regular insulin

7. A client with a history of severe depression has been brought to the emergency room with an overdose of barbiturates. The nurse should pay careful attention to the client's:

   ○ **A.** Urinary output

   ○ **B.** Respirations

   ○ **C.** Temperature

   ○ **D.** Verbal responsiveness

8. A client is to receive antivenin following a snake bite. Before administering the antivenin, the nurse should give priority to:

   ○ **A.** Administering a local anesthetic

   ○ **B.** Checking for an allergic response

   ○ **C.** Administering an anxiolytic

   ○ **D.** Withholding fluids for 6–8 hours

9. The nurse is caring for a client following a radiation accident. The client is determined to have incorporation. The nurse knows that the client will:

   ○ **A.** Not need any medical treatment for radiation exposure

   ○ **B.** Have damage to the bones, kidneys, liver, and thyroid

   ○ **C.** Experience only erythema and desquamation

   ○ **D.** Not be radioactive because the radiation passes through the body

10. The emergency staff has undergone intensive training in the care of clients with suspected anthrax. The staff understands that the suggested drug for treating anthrax is:

   ○ **A.** Ancef (cefazolin sodium)

   ○ **B.** Cipro (ciprofloxacin)

   ○ **C.** Kantrex (kanamycin)

   ○ **D.** Garamycin (gentamicin)

Answer Rationales

1. Answer A is correct. Following the ABCDs of basic emergency care, the client with dyspnea and asymmetrical chest should be cared for first because these symptoms are associated with flail chest. Answer D is incorrect because he should be cared for second because of the likelihood of organ damage and bleeding. Answer B is incorrect because he should be cared for after the client with abdominal trauma. Answer C is incorrect because he should receive care last because his injuries are less severe.

2. Answer B is correct. If bleeding does not subside with direct pressure, the nurse should elevate the extremity above the level of the heart. Answers A and D are done only if other measures are ineffective, so they are incorrect. Answer C would slow the bleeding but will not stop it, so it's incorrect.

3. Answer B is correct. Deferoxamine is the antidote for iron poisoning. Answer A is the antidote for acetaminophen overdose, making it wrong. Answers C and D are antidotes for lead poisoning, so they are wrong.

4. Answer A is correct. Warming the intravenous fluid helps to prevent further stress on the vascular system. Thirst is a sign of hypovolemia; however, oral fluids alone will not meet the fluid needs of the client in hypovolemic shock, so answer B is incorrect. Answers C and D are wrong because they can be used for baseline information but will not help stabilize the client.

5. Answer B is correct. The client with 70% TBSA burns would be classified as an emergent client. In disaster triage, emergent clients, code black, are cared for last because they require the greatest expenditure of resources. Answers A and D are examples of immediate clients and are assigned as code red, so they are wrong. These clients are cared for first because they can survive with limited interventions. Answer C is wrong because it is an example of a delayed client, code yellow. These clients have significant injuries that require medical care.

6. Answer A is correct. The client has symptoms of insulin shock and the first step is to check the client's blood sugar. If indicated, the client should be treated with intravenous dextrose. Answer B is wrong because it is not the first step the nurse should take. Answer C is wrong because it does not apply to the client's symptoms. Answer D is wrong because it would be used for diabetic ketoacidosis, not insulin shock.

7. Answer B is correct. Barbiturate overdose results in central nervous system depression, which leads to respiratory failure. Answers A and C are important to the client's overall condition but are not specific to the question, so they are incorrect. The use of barbiturates results in slow, slurred speech, so answer D is expected, and therefore incorrect.

8. Answer B is correct. The nurse should perform the skin or eye test before administering antivenin. Answers A and D are unnecessary and therefore incorrect. Answer C would help calm the client but is not a priority before giving the antivenin, making it incorrect.

9. Answer B is correct. The client with incorporation radiation injuries requires immediate medical treatment. Most of the damage occurs to the bones, kidneys, liver, and thyroid. Answers A, C, and D refer to external irradiation, so they are wrong.

10. Answer B is correct. Cipro (ciprofloxacin) is the drug of choice for treating anthrax. Answers A, C, and D are not used to treat anthrax, so they are incorrect.

Suggested Reading and Resources

▶ Ignatavicius, D., and Workman, S. *Medical Surgical Nursing: Critical Thinking for Collaborative Care.* 6th ed. Philadelphia: Elsevier, 2008.

▶ Brunner, L., and Suddarth, D. *Textbook of Medical Surgical Nursing.* 12th ed. Philadelphia: Lippincott Williams & Wilkins, 2009.

▶ LeMone, P., and Burke, K. in *Medical Surgical Nursing: Critical Thinking in Client Care.* 4th ed. Upper Saddle River, NJ Pearson Prentice Hall, 2008.

▶ Lewis, S., Heitkemper, M., Dirksen, S., O'Brien, P., and Bucher, L. *Medical Surgical Nursing: Assessment and Management of Clinical Problems.* 7th ed. Philadelphia: Elsevier, 2007.

▶ Lehne, R. *Pharmacology for Nursing Care.* 7th ed. Philadelphia: Elsevier, 2009.

CHAPTER NINETEEN

Cultural Practices Influencing Nursing Care

Terms you'll need to understand

- ✓ Culture
- ✓ Ethnicity
- ✓ Heritage
- ✓ Religion
- ✓ Time Orientation
- ✓ Tradition
- ✓ Values

Nursing skills you'll need to master

- ✓ Communication skills

Cultural practices and beliefs are passed down from generation to generation. The United States has always been a melting pot of varying cultural groups. Today more than ever, nurses must be aware of traditional medicine practices and cultural beliefs that influence healthcare. Migration trends indicate that one in three Americans is an ethnic minority. Understanding your own views and those of the client, while avoiding stereotyping the client, are an integral part of client care. The NCLEX exam has changed to reflect these differences in client populations. This chapter explores cultural differences including environmental, social, religious, communication, space, and time differences among varying populations. The chapter covers these differences as they affect healthcare practices and discusses how you as a nurse can utilize knowledge of these beliefs in nursing practice.

Cultural Assessment

The nurse must be able to assess the client for differences in beliefs and utilize the knowledge gained to plan care for the client. It is critical that you know about your client's beliefs and culture in order to effectively treat him and not engage in acts that might be considered offensive to him.

Understanding Client Beliefs

As you assess the cultural background and beliefs of your client, you should remember that beliefs can be considered beneficial, maladaptive, or neutral. An example of a *beneficial belief*, or one that is helpful to the nurse, in planning care for the client would be a Hispanic client who believes in the use of garlic with his antihypertensive medication to lower blood pressure. Because garlic has been linked to lowering cholesterol and triglyceride levels, this is beneficial. If, however, he refuses his blood pressure medication and uses only the garlic, this would be a *maladaptive* consideration. A *neutral* consideration is one that is neither helpful nor harmful to the client.

Folk medicine, used by many groups, involves the use of nonprofessional healthcare providers such as medicine men and midwives. These practitioners often use remedies that are not found in the local pharmacy. Herbs and potions are often used to treat fevers, pain, and upset stomach. The nurse should teach the client that although not inherently harmful, some natural substances can interact with medications and ultimately either alter the effect of the medication or cause an adverse reaction.

Working with Clients Who Speak Different Languages

The nurse might not be able to speak the language of the client he or she is trying to help. For this reason, it is useful to be able to use other techniques to communicate during teaching sessions. The following are 10 tips to use if you do not speak the client's language:

1. Sit down next to the client. Regardless of language differences, the client will understand a calm, caring tone in your voice.

2. Respect the client's personal space and watch his body language for cues that you are getting too close or touching him inappropriately.

3. If a client is from a culture different from your own, don't treat her differently from other clients because she does not speak English. Do not talk to her as if she were deaf. Speaking loudly will not help her understand you.

4. Use an interpreter when one is available. Many hospitals have individuals employed in other areas of the hospital who can help with translation. Investigate these possibilities before the client arrives for the visit.

NOTE

Literature should be given to the client in his own language when available. Many hospitals and healthcare facilities provide interpreters when needed.

---

5. Explain medical and nursing terms simply and clearly. Ask the client to demonstrate when possible. Remember that demonstration is the best indicator that the client understands your teaching.

6. Involve the extended family when possible. In most cultures, family is an important part of the client's healthcare.

7. Be careful not to offend members of the family by asking them to perform duties that are not allowed or preferred in their culture. For example, in Hispanic culture, the father might not want to bathe his child. When you are unsure, always ask—and do not assume.

8. Be careful if you do not have a thorough knowledge of the language. Many words have an entirely different meaning when pronounced incorrectly.

9. Use the title Mr. or Mrs. unless you know the person well. Not using these titles is often seen as disrespectful.

10. Do not assume that the client is angry if she speaks more loudly. Do not assume that the client is disinterested if she does not make eye contact.

Healthcare of Hispanics/Latinos

The fastest growing minority in the United States is the Hispanic/Latino population. Some Hispanic people believe that disease is caused by an imbalance in hot and cold. They also believe that health is maintained by preventing exposure to extreme temperatures. A "hot" disease is treated with a "cold" remedy. Some examples of "hot" conditions are diabetes, hypertension, pregnancy, and indigestion. These problems are treated with cold compresses and cold liquids. Some examples of "cold" conditions are menstrual cramps, colic, and pneumonia. These problems should be treated with hot liquids such as broths, hot tea, or hot coffee. Warm baths can also help relieve these conditions.

Food is an important part of socialization in the Hispanic/Latino population. Use of grains and spices is prevalent in food preparation. Cheese, eggs, milk, and lard are used to prepare many of their dishes. The nurse should be aware of these practices particularly when teaching the client about dietary modification for the client with hypertension and hypercholesterolemia.

Hispanics/Latinos use herbs to treat most illnesses and maintain health. Examples of the use of herbs are garlic to treat hypertension and cough; chamomile to treat nausea and anxiety; and a laxative tea combined with stomach massage to cure anorexia, stomach pains, and diarrhea. Peppermint is also used to treat dyspepsia. Manzanilla is another herb used as a tea to treat stomach and intestinal pain, and anise (a star-shaped seed) is used to treat nausea and colic and to increase breast milk.

A healer is often used to provide herbal remedies or to deliver babies. These *santero/santera* are well-respected in the community and should be considered part of the health team. Several differences that you should be aware of exist between the modern American healthcare provider and the traditional healer. Table 19.1 highlights some of these differences.

TABLE 19.1   Comparison of Hispanic/Latino Traditional Healers to Modern Medicine

Traditional Healers	Modern Medicine
Informal and know the entire family.	It's formal, and the visit is with the client and not the family unit.
Make house calls.	Doctor's visits occur only in the clinic and often only by appointment.
The male is considered the head of the household. Always discuss any decisions with the husband or father.	Information is released to the client only. Healthcare providers comply with laws in regard to confidentiality.
Bartering is used as payment and the cost is very low.	It's often very expensive.
Involves spirituality with healing.	Often the healthcare provider is a specialist who deals with only the system involved in the illness.
Most of the time the healer is a part of the community where the client and family live.	The physician or nurse practitioner might be located many miles away.

Modified from Spector R.E. *Cultural Diversity in Health and Illness*, 6th ed., Prentice Hall, 2003.

The "evil eye" (*mal de ojo*) is thought to cause fever, crying, and vomiting in the infant. It is believed to be brought on by a person with a strong eye who looks at the baby in an admiring manner. The treatment for the evil eye is to sweep the body with eggs, lemons, and bay leaves.

Susto, or fright sickness, is brought on by an emotional trauma. Any traumatic event can bring on a susto. The result is a fever, vomiting, or diarrhea. The treatment involves brushing the body with *ruda*, a rough object, for nine consecutive nights.

Bilis is a disease of the intestinal tract brought on by anger. If untreated, bilis can cause acute nervous tension and chronic illness.

Empacho is a disease that can affect children. It is caused by food particles being trapped in the intestine. To manage this illness, the client lies face down with his back bare. The healer pinches a piece of skin at the waist, listening for a snap as the skin is released. This is repeated several times to dislodge the material. Prayer should accompany these rituals. Many Puerto Rican parents believe that an amulet pinned to the baby's shirt will protect her from evil. *Jabon de la mano milagrosa* is a soap used by a miracle man to clean and protect a person from evil spirits. Many also believe that candles should be burned to ward off evil spirits. The nurse should consider the strong religious beliefs of many in the Hispanic culture. Often a priest is the spiritual advisor and should be notified in the case of birth, illness, or death.

Time Considerations

The Hispanic population often views time differently from Americans. Time is viewed in generalities, so the nurse must be aware that the client might view time as present, past, or future. This difference can also affect the teaching plan. If the nurse tells the client to take the medication two times per day, the client might not understand the need to take the medication every 12 hours

Use of Nonverbal/Verbal Communication

Most Hispanics speak Spanish or a dialect of it as their primary language. They also might speak English. It is an untrue assumption that if the client does not speak English, he is less intelligent. Many drug companies now provide written material in both Spanish and English. The nurse should use a translator when needed and should allow time for the client to respond to teaching. Eye contact is often avoided out of respect. The nurse should not assume that the client is disinterested or bored if he avoids eye contact. A handshake is often used to communicate agreement or understanding. Intimate zones are reserved for family and close friends. A distance of approximately 1 1/2'—4' should be reserved for personal distance, and a distance of 4'—12' should be observed for social distance. The nurse should respect this spatial territory when providing healthcare.

Childbirth and Pain Response

It is very important for the nurse to be aware that the Hispanic client might not complain of pain. Watching the client's nonverbal cues will help to prevent complications. During labor, the woman might remain stoic. She will often not ask for pain medication until late in the labor process, if at all. Female relatives are often present for the birth of the infant.

Hispanic women might go into a 40-day period of rest after the birth of the infant. During this time the woman might be confined to the home with limited activity. An abdominal binder might be used to prevent air from entering the uterus and to promote healing. Filipino and Pacific Islanders might also perform this practice. Many in the Hispanic culture practice baptism of the infant by sprinkling with water. These clients do not believe that colostrum is good for the infant, so the nurse should consult with the mother and father before placing the baby to the breast in the delivery room. Modesty must be maintained during breast feeding.

Healthcare of Native Americans and Alaskan Natives

Native Americans are considered those whose ancestors inhabited North America and Alaska. There are 170 North American tribes, and Inuit are also included in this group. These groups identify themselves in families or tribes. In order to work effectively with this group, the nurse must form a working relationship with the tribe leader.

Native Americans believe in the need to be one with nature and hold in reverence animals such as the eagle, buffalo, and deer. This group, like the Hispanic population, uses medicine men. In Native American culture, this person is called a *shaman*. Native Americans believe that evil spirits and devils are responsible for illness, so masks are worn to hide from the devil. An amulet called a *thunderbird* is worn for good luck and protection. Navajo medicine men are often called on to use sand painting to diagnose ailments. Some Native Americans conduct sacred ceremonies that rely on having visions and using plants and objects that symbolize the individual or the illness that is being treated. Chanting, prayer, and dancing are also used to treat illness and drive off the evil spirits. Sweat lodges are used by some groups to help in the treatment of fever. Herbs, corn meal, and medicine bundles are used in the Indian population to treat most illness.

Although herbs are used, most Native Americans will take medications prescribed by the physician. Decisions regarding healthcare should be directed to the male members of the family.

Time Considerations

Most Native Americans and Inuit are relaxed in their view of time and view life in the present. An appointment time for a clinic visit might be ignored or the client might arrive late. The nurse should consider this factor when making clinic appointments.

Use of Nonverbal/Verbal Communication

Many Native Americans and Inuit speak English as their primary language. However, some still speak the native language of their forefathers, especially when communicating with one another. The nurse might have difficulty understanding the native language because several dialects exist. The nurse might have problems understanding the client because he will probably speak in a low tone. These clients expect the listener to be very attentive during the discussion. The need for listening is compounded by the fact that eye contact often is considered disrespectful. In order to insure adequate communication, the nurse should limit discussion to multiple parties at the same time and eliminate external noise when possible.

Childbirth and Pain Response

Native Americans tend to be very quiet. The nurse must be aware of nonverbal cues that indicate understanding of teaching. Some nonverbal clues are nodding positively or negatively or the client complying with the nurse's request. The client might be in a great deal of pain before the nurse realizes that she needs medication.

The family is extremely important to the well-being of the client during childbirth; the extended family typically attends the birth. Use of village women to assist with childbirth is also a part of their culture. Women might not complain of pain during the labor and birth. In Navajo culture, the umbilical cord is given to the family after the birth of the child to be buried near a tree so that the child will grow strong and wise.

Healthcare of Asian-Americans

Asian-Americans have come to the United States from more than 20 countries and speak more than 100 languages. Since 1965, their population in the United States has grown from 1 million to more than 10.9 million. The nurse dealing with this large minority must consider the variations in healthcare beliefs to promote the well-being of the client and family. The client who is Asian-American is respectful of those in authority. For this reason, he might not disagree with the nurse or doctor, though he does not hold the same thoughts or values. The client might nod in agreement rather than pointing out questions or concerns. This can lead to confusion and error in client treatment. Observation of the client performing skills that the nurse has presented can help to ensure that the client understands. Many in this group self-medicate. This practice can lead to complications and prevent early diagnoses of disease. Asian medicine includes therapies such as acupuncture, acupressure, herbs, and dietary supplements. Clients might be reluctant to use herbs because they fear that Western doctors or nurses will disapprove of traditional remedies. Asian clients often believe in the yin (cold) and yang (hot) theory. They believe that illness is caused by a disruption in this environment. "Hot" foods include beef, chicken, eggs, fried foods, red foods, and foods served hot. "Cold" foods include pork, most vegetables, boiled foods, foods served cold, and white foods. Noodles and soft rice are considered neither cold nor hot. To maintain fluid balance, Chinese-Americans prefer hot tea to ice water.

Some Chinese believe that illness is a result of moral retribution by the gods, and rituals must be performed to satisfy the gods and restore balance. A poor combination of the stars with the birth order can also lead to disharmony.

Some Cambodians practice cupping, pinching, coining, or rubbing an ill person's skin to treat illnesses. Usually the forehead or abdomen is used, depending on the type and location of the illness. With the practice of *cupping*, a hot cup is placed on the skin. As it cools, the cup contracts and the skin is pulled into the cup, leaving a circular mark or blister on the skin. It is believed that this practice draws the evil spirit into the cup. *Pinching* is the practice of pinching the skin between the thumb and index finger to the point of producing a contusion on the chest, on the neck, on the back, at the base of the nose, or between the eyes. *Coining* is the rubbing of the skin with the side of a coin, causing bruising. The nurse should be careful not to assume child abuse if she witnesses this practice. However, teaching regarding the dangers to the infant should be included in the plan of care.

If the client is Hindu, Sikh, or Buddhist, he might have beliefs that affect medical treatment. Hinduism accepts modern medicine but believes that illness is caused by past sins. Because life and death are part of an unending cycle, efforts to prolong life are discouraged and CPR might be forbidden. Sikhism clients might accept healthcare, but refuse certain aspects of treatment. Female clients often refuse examination by a male, and removing the undergarments might be very traumatic for the client.

Buddhist clients will probably refuse treatment on holy days. They believe that spirits invading the body cause illness and will ask for a priest in times of birth and death. They also believe the body should pass into eternity whole, which forbids organ donation and performance of an autopsy. When death is imminent, the priest is called. He will tie a thread around the neck or wrist to ensure that the person will pass into eternity in peace—the nurse should not remove this string. The priest will then pour water in the client's mouth and place the dying client on the floor. After death, the family washes the body before cremation. Some Buddhists might refuse to move the body because they believe that it takes time for the spirit to leave. In the Shinto religion, the body is wrapped in a white kimono and straw shoes are applied. Because reincarnation is a primary belief of this group, materials containing gelatin and insulin produced from beef are forbidden.

Time Considerations

Asian-Americans live in the present. Many of them believe in reincarnation and that, if they die, they go immediately to paradise. For this reason the nurse might encounter difficulty in teaching regarding preventive care.

Use of Nonverbal/Verbal Communication

For some Asian-Americans, direct eye contact is considered a sign of disrespect. The nurse should be aware of this difference in communication and should not consider a lack of eye contact as a sign of a lack of interest or difficulty hearing. The client might nod as a sign of compliance or understanding and respect. Shaking hands with a person of the opposite sex is considered forward and inappropriate.

Childbirth and Pain Response

Asian clients will probably be stoic and not complain of pain until it becomes unbearable. Childbirth is a time of celebration for the Asian-American family. The extended family is present and usually takes the infant after delivery, especially if the mother has had a Cesarean section. This allows the mother to rest and recover. This time is considered a "hot" time.

After the birth, the postpartum period is considered a "cold" time because the uterus is more open. The client might therefore refuse to shower or do peri-care in the traditional American manner; however, she might allow a heat lamp to be used to improve healing. The postpartal period is much longer in most Asian cultures: A length of 30–40 days is thought to provide time for healing. The family stays close during this time to provide emotional and physical support.

Most Chinese prefer to give birth side-lying because this position is thought to be less traumatic to the infant. Many in the Hindu religion believe that placing honey in the mouth of the infant ensures a sweet life. However, this practice is discouraged by healthcare providers in the United States because honey can carry botulism. Many in the Chinese culture believe that colostrum is not good for the baby. The mother is often given hot rice water to drink to restore the balance between the body and nature.

Healthcare of Arab-Americans

The term *Arab* is associated with people from a region of the Middle East extending from Northern Africa to the Arabian Gulf. The large majority of Arabs are members of the Islamic (Muslim) religion. Their cultural and religious beliefs direct most of their beliefs regarding healthcare. Prayer and fasting are a major part of the Muslim client's day. Nurses should be willing to accommodate the client's desire to pray, and the bed should be positioned facing toward Mecca. So, if the client is in the mainland United States, the bed should face southeast. A sick client who is unable to fully kneel and touch his head to the floor might be allowed by his religious leaders to sit up while praying. During Ramadan, Muslims must fast from sunrise to sunset. If the client has a life-threatening condition, accommodations can be made, but this fasting does pertain to IV therapy and most injections.

Cleanliness is very important to the Arab-American client. The left hand is used for toileting; therefore, the client will avoid using the left hand to eat or touch others. Food should be kept clean and free of odors. Because alcohol is forbidden, medications and liquids containing alcohol should be avoided.

Most Arab-Americans prefer to be treated by a healthcare worker of the same sex. When prescribing medications, pills and injections are preferred—suppositories should be avoided if possible.

In some countries, secluding women from men and restricting movement outside the home is practiced. Covering of women in public is practiced and harsh treatment of women is allowed.

The dying client must confess his sins to be taken to heaven. The body is washed and wrapped in a white cloth and the head is turned to the right shoulder. The body of the client who has died should be positioned facing east. A prayer called a *Kalima* is said.

Time Considerations

Arab-Americans live in the present, so many do not plan for retirement or save for future needs. Preventive medicine is a concept that is difficult for them to understand. This group, like many others, might be less aware of appointment times. Scheduling of office visits should allow for this cultural difference.

Use of Nonverbal/Verbal Communication

As with other cultures, nonverbal communication is used frequently in Arab cultures. Women are particularly prone to speaking softly and might not voice health concerns, especially to a male healthcare provider.

Childbirth and Pain Response

Response to pain differs with each individual. Some clients in this group will be stoic, but some might respond to pain by crying or moaning. It is generally believed that an injection of pain-killing medication works better than a pill. The nurse should assess changes in vital signs and other cues such as grimacing to be able to provide pain medication as needed. During childbirth, group prayer is used to strengthen the mother, and women assist the client during childbirth. At the time of birth, a prayer is said into the baby's ear. The mother is then secluded from the group for a period of time to allow for cleansing. Because blood is considered a pollutant, a ritual bath is performed before the woman can resume relations with her husband. In some African cultures, such as in Ghana and Sierra Leone, some women will not resume sexual relations with their husbands until after the baby is weaned.

Nursing Plan Dietary Considerations Across Cultures

Dietary considerations play a part in the nursing plan of care for all cultural populations. See Table 19.2 for information regarding variations in dietary management.

TABLE 19.2   Dietary Practices of Various Cultural Groups

Culture	Grains	Fruits	Vegetables	Meats	Milk
Hispanic	Prefer potatoes and corn.	Prefer most fruits.	Prefer spicy vegetables such as chili peppers, tomatoes, onions, beets, and cabbage.	Prefer eggs, pinto beans, and most meats (all are allowed).	Cheese is preferred, and milk is seldom consumed because lactose intolerance is common in this group.
Chinese	Consume starchy grains such as rice.	All fruits are eaten by this group.	Prefer Chinese vegetables such as water chestnuts and bean sprouts. These are used in cooking.	All meats are consumed.	They eat ice cream, but few other milk products.
Chinese (to include Buddhist)	All grains are allowed.	All fruits are allowed.	All vegetables are allowed.	Devout Buddhists restrict meats and do not eat beef.	Cheese and milk products are allowed.
Japanese	Prefer rice.	They do not consume most fruits.	All vegetables are consumed.	All meats are consumed.	There is a high incidence of lactose intolerance, and little milk is consumed.

(continues)

TABLE 19.2 *Continued*

Culture	Grains	Fruits	Vegetables	Meats	Milk
Europeans (to include persons of the Jewish faith)	Most grains are allowed, but must be prepared using Kosher standards. Leavened bread and cakes are forbidden during Passover.	All fruits are consumed.	All vegetables are consumed	Pork is forbidden, as are fish without scales. All meats must be prepared according to Biblical ordinances, and blood is forbidden.	Milk products should not be eaten at the same meal that contains meat and meat products.
Arab-Americans (to include the Islamic religion)	All grains are allowed.	All fruits are allowed.	All vegetables are allowed.	Beef, pork, and some fowl are restricted; all meat must be slaughtered according to a ritual letting of blood.	Milk is allowed.

TIP

Do not assume that because a person is a member of a particular group that she will behave like others. The nurse must get to know the person.

Religious Beliefs and Refusal of Care Considerations

Various religious beliefs affect how the client is treated and can lead to a refusal of some traditional medicines. It is important for the nurse to understand these differences to assist the client with healthcare and teaching. Table 19.3 breaks down some religions, the treatments their practitioners might refuse, and how prayer plays a role in their medicinal views.

TABLE 19.3 **Religious Beliefs Affecting Healthcare and Death**

Religion	Treatment Considerations	Role of Prayer
Buddhism	Treatment is accepted, but beef and beef products are not allowed.	A priest is called for last rites to be performed.

TABLE 19.3 Religious Beliefs Affecting Healthcare and Death

Religion	Treatment Considerations	Role of Prayer
Christian (Catholic)	They eat no meat on Fridays during Lent. They might want to attend mass during hospitalization on Friday, Saturday, or Sunday.	At the time of death, a priest is called for last rites.
Christian (Protestant)	All treatments are allowed to preserve life.	Practices vary in respect to death and burial.
Church of Jesus Christ of Latter-day Saints (Mormon)	Most treatments are allowed.	At the time of death, the religious leader is called for last rites. Burial is preferred to cremation.
Hindu	A priest is called for consultation prior to treatments. Believe in reincarnation, so the body should be preserved. Amputations of limbs or removal of diseased body parts might be refused.	Believe in prayers and rituals.
Judaism	Orthodox Jew interpret dietary laws stringently. There are three key characteristics of kosher food preparation: only designated animals can be eaten. Pork is not allowed, some animals must be ritualistically killed, dairy products and meats are not eaten at the same meal. Passover is a time of fasting. This practice can lead to dehydration in the elderly and sick. Matzoh, an unleavened bread, can result in constipation. The infant is circumcised on the eighth day of life.	At the time of death, the rabbi is called for last rites, the body is washed, and someone remains with the body until burial.
Jehovah's Witness	Might refuse blood transfusions and surgery or treatments.	Believe prayer will save.
Russian Orthodox Church	All treatments are allowed. Most followers observe fast days, and on Wednesdays and Fridays, most eat no meat. During Lent, all animal products (including dairy products) are forbidden.	At the time of death, the religious leader is called for last rites.
Sikhism	Treatment is accepted. After death, the client will receive the five Ks: kesh (uncut hair), kangna (wooden comb), kara (wrist band), kirpan (sword), and kach (shorts) .	The priest is called to perform ritualistic last rites.

(continues)

CAUTION

Be sure that you do not assume that a client understands your teaching. The best indicator of understanding is demonstration.

Case Study

1. Juanita is a recent immigrant from Mexico. She is admitted to the labor and delivery unit in active labor. Although she is very cooperative, she appears frightened and hesitant to follow instructions. Upon investigation, the nurse realizes that Juanita does not speak English. Which action by the nurse would help to calm Juanita and establish a therapeutic relationship?

2. Juanita's husband is present and speaks some English. During a brief discussion with Juanita's husband, the nurse finds that this is Juanita's third pregnancy. The nurse should realize that the husband should be included in signing permits because:

3. As Juanita's labor progresses the nurse notices that she does not ask for pain medication. The nurse is aware that:

4. After delivery, the nurse asks Juanita whether she is planning to breast feed. When might Juanita initiate breast feeding?

5. After delivery, the nurse notices that Juanita does not get out of bed unless she is encouraged and does not actively help with the care of the infant. The nurse is aware that the reason for Juanita's actions might be:

Answers to Case Study

1. The first action by the nurse should be to assess the best method of communication. If the nurse does not speak Spanish, finding a translator that the client feels comfortable with would be an excellent beginning.

2. Juanita should sign her permits, but her husband should be included in the client's care because in many Hispanic families, the husband makes the decisions. If Juanita is unable to sign, her husband can sign the permit for her.

3. Some clients of Hispanic decent might not complain of pain. Ask the client if she would like to have pain medication and administer the medication as ordered.

4. Some clients of Hispanic decent do not believe that colostrum is good for the baby. The nurse should ask the client rather that assuming that she will want to breast feed in the delivery room.

5. Many clients of Hispanic decent practice a 40-day period of rest after delivery. The nurse should encourage Juanita to exercise to prevent emboli while respecting her cultural differences.

Exam Prep Questions

1. The client is a practicing Hindu. Which food should be removed from the client's tray?

    ○ **A.** Bread

    ○ **B.** Cabbage

    ○ **C.** Steak

    ○ **D.** Apple

2. A Korean client is admitted to the postpartum unit following the delivery of a 9 lb. infant. Although the client does not refuse to shower, the nurse notices that she stands in the shower, but does not allow the water to touch her. Which of the following should be the next action by the nurse?

    ○ **A.** Ask the client why she refuses to shower.

    ○ **B.** Call the doctor and report the client's refusal to shower.

    ○ **C.** Tell the client that the nurse will obtain a heat lamp to assist in healing the perineum.

    ○ **D.** Turn the shower so that the water sprays on the client.

3. An infant is admitted with a volvulus and scheduled for surgery. The parents are Jehovah's Witnesses and refuse to sign the permit. Which action by the nurse is most appropriate?

    ○ **A.** Obtain a court order.

    ○ **B.** Call the doctor.

    ○ **C.** Tell them that the surgery is optional.

    ○ **D.** Monitor the situation.

4. Which medication will most likely be refused by a Muslim client?

    ○ **A.** Insulin

    ○ **B.** Cough syrup

    ○ **C.** NSAIDs

    ○ **D.** Antacids

5. The condition of an Arab client who is terminally ill deteriorates and death seems imminent. If the client is hospitalized in the mainland United States, the nurse should position the bed facing which direction?

   ○ **A.** Northeast

   ○ **B.** Southeast

   ○ **C.** West

   ○ **D.** South

6. An 88-year-old female Jewish client is admitted to the hospital and diagnosed with diabetes. Which type of insulin is refused by this client?

   ○ **A.** Beef

   ○ **B.** Pork

   ○ **C.** Synthetic

   ○ **D.** Fish

7. The nurse observes that a Hispanic client and his family have been late for their appointment the last three times. Which of the following is the best explanation for this behavior?

   ○ **A.** A lack of concern for the health of the client.

   ○ **B.** An attempt to avoid talking to the nurse.

   ○ **C.** The client probably forgot the appointment time.

   ○ **D.** The client and family view time differently than does the nurse.

8. A 90-year-old client from Thailand is diagnosed with terminal cancer. The family seems unconcerned and, although they do not refuse treatment for the client, they do not assist with treatment. Which of the following is the nurse's likely assessment of this behavior?

   ○ **A.** The family believes in the cycle of life and that death is a step into the next cycle.

   ○ **B.** The family is in denial concerning the diagnosis and needs further teaching.

   ○ **C.** The family is planning to get another opinion regarding the diagnosis.

   ○ **D.** The family is not concerned with the treatment and care of the client.

9. The nurse is assisting a client from Iraq with her bath. The nurse notices that the client uses only her left hand to bathe her genital area. Which of the following is the correct assessment of this behavior?

    ○ **A.** The client's dominant hand is her left one.

    ○ **B.** The client is using her nondominant hand to more easily cleanse the perineum.

    ○ **C.** The client believes that the right hand is reserved for eating and touching others and that the left hand is the dirty hand.

    ○ **D.** The client has in some way injured her right hand, making it difficult to use it.

10. A Japanese client refuses to eat the ice cream or drink the milk on his tray. Which action by the nurse would indicate an understanding of the client's needs?

    ○ **A.** She obtains yogurt for the client instead.

    ○ **B.** She obtains an order for Lactaid dietary supplement.

    ○ **C.** She removes the milk from the tray and says nothing to the client.

    ○ **D.** She asks the client why he will not drink the milk.

Answer Rationales

1. Answer C is correct. In the Hindu religion, beef is prohibited. All breads, vegetables, and fruits are allowed, so answers A, B, and D are incorrect.

2. Answer C is correct. Many in Asian cultures believe that the postpartal period is a "cold" time when the body is open. This is treated with heat, and a shower is thought to be a cold therapy that allows illness to enter the body. The nurse should comply with the client's wish not to shower at this time. A heat lamp might be accepted because it is a hot therapy and will assist with healing.

3. Answer B is correct. A volvulus is an emergency situation in which the bowel is twisted. Refusal of treatment can lead to death, so the next action to take is to call the doctor. It might require a court order to get a permit for the surgery or the court might comply with the parent's wishes, so answer A is incorrect. The surgery is not optional, so answer C is incorrect. Volvulus is an emergency situation and action must be taken if the child is to survive. Monitoring only waste precious time, so answer D is incorrect.

4. Answer B is correct. Most cough syrups contain alcohol, which is forbidden in the Islamic religion. Attempts should be made to obtain a cough suppressant that does not contain alcohol. The client will most likely take insulin, nonsteroidal anti-inflammatory drugs, and antacids, so answers A, C, and D are incorrect.

5. Answer B is correct. At the time of death, the Muslim client will wish to be positioned facing Mecca, which is to the southeast of the United States. Answers A, C, and D are therefore incorrect.

6. Answer B is correct. Pork is not allowed in the diet or medications of Jewish clients. Both synthetic and beef insulins are allowed, so answers A and C are incorrect. There is no such thing as a fish insulin, so answer D is incorrect.

7. Answer D is correct. If the client misses an appointment or is late for the appointment, it is not necessarily true that the client is disinterested or forgot. Many in the Hispanic culture see time as a relative thing and live in the present.

8. Answer A is correct. Clients who practice the Hindu religion believe that death is part of the cycle of life. There is no data to support answers B, C, or D as an answer.

9. Answer C is correct. In the Islamic religion, the left hand is reserved for toileting. The right hand is considered clean and is used to eat and touch others. There is no data to support that the client is left handed or that the right hand might be injured, so answers A, B, and D are incorrect.

10. Answer B is correct. Many of Japanese descent are lactose intolerant—it is not that milk is not allowed in their culture. Yogurt also causes gas and bloating, so answer A is incorrect. Removing the items from the tray does not provide the needed calcium in the diet, so answer C is incorrect. It is inappropriate to ask "why" in most cultures, so answer D is incorrect.

Suggested Reading and Resources

▶ Brink, P. *Transcultural Nursing: A Book of Readings*. Engelwood Cliff, NJ: Prentice Hall, 1976.

▶ Potter, P., and Perry, A. *Basic Nursing, A Critical Approach*. St. Louis: Mosby, 1998.

▶ Fernandez, V., and Fernandez, K. *Transcultural Nursing: Basic Concepts and Case Studies*: http://www.culturaldiversity.org/2006.

▶ Geiger, J., and Davidhizar, R. *Transcultural Nursing: Assessment in Intervention*. St. Louis: Mosby, 1991.

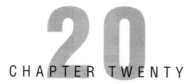

CHAPTER TWENTY

Legal Issues in Nursing Practice

Terms you'll need to understand

- ✓ Assault
- ✓ Battery
- ✓ Civil laws
- ✓ Common laws
- ✓ Consent
- ✓ Criminal laws
- ✓ Ethics
- ✓ Felony
- ✓ Incident report
- ✓ Informed consent
- ✓ Intentional torts
- ✓ Invasion of privacy
- ✓ Licensure
- ✓ Malpractice
- ✓ Malpractice insurance
- ✓ Misdemeanor
- ✓ Negligence
- ✓ Nursing Practice Act
- ✓ Patient's Bill of Rights
- ✓ Regulatory laws
- ✓ Restraints
- ✓ Tort

Safe nursing practice requires knowledge of the practice and legal boundaries of the registered nurse, the licensed practical nurse, and the nursing assistant.

The state boards of nursing are responsible for ensuring that those licensed to practice nursing are safe practitioners and that they abide by approved standards of nursing practice. Practicing nurses, physicians, consumers, as well as an attorney and an executive officer appointed by the governor of the state generally make up the state boards of nursing. In addition, the directors of nursing from nursing schools within the state make up some boards of nursing. The state boards of nursing also have the ability to suspend, restrict, and revoke the license of a nurse convicted of a felony or misdemeanor. In the case of alcohol and drug addiction, the state boards of nursing can require the nurse to enter a recovering nurse program under the direction of the board.

Nursing or Nurse Practice Acts define the authority of the board of nursing, define the boundaries of scope of nursing practice, state the requirements for licensure, identify the grounds for disciplinary action, and identify the titles and types of licensure. The purpose of the Nursing Practice Act is to protect the public from unsafe practitioners, and to promote competence and quality in nursing practice.

No matter which state you have a license to practice in, the Nursing Practice Act of that state will bind you. Nursing Practice Acts vary from state to state, but they are all very much the same in many ways. Boards of Nursing have authorization to take legal action against a nurse or a group of nurses found to be in violation of the state's nursing practice standards as set out by the legislature.

This chapter explores the laws that impact your nursing practice. It also defines and discusses issues affecting your nursing practice and some questions included on the NCLEX exam in relation to legal and ethical issues.

> **CAUTION**
>
> If asked to perform any activity or skill that is out of your scope of practice by a physician, a supervisor, an administrator, or any other person in direct authority over you, you have the right and the obligation to refuse. If asked to perform a skill that you learned in school but have never performed, ask for help. If asked to operate a type of equipment that you are unfamiliar with, ask for help. Remember that the law and the National Council of State Boards of Nursing expect you to ensure the safety of the client, and you are responsible if harm comes to the client because of your care or lack of care.

Types of Laws

Several types of laws govern nursing practice: statutory/regulatory, civil, criminal, and common law. The nurse is responsible for abiding by each type of law.

Statutory Laws/Regulatory Laws

Statutory laws are those created by elected officials within the legislative body. An example of this type of law is the Nursing Practice Act. These laws and their implementing rules and regulations set forth which activities the nurse can perform. It is imperative that a newly licensed nurse be aware of these and abide by them in daily practice. Often, as a nurse, you might be asked to perform duties that you do not feel comfortable performing. Remember that if your nursing school did not teach you a task or skill, it probably is out of your scope of practice. Professional organizations, such as the National League for Nursing, American Association of Colleges of Nursing and others, routinely review and approve nursing curriculums. So, you can be fairly certain that if you did not learn a task in school, it is within your rights to refuse to perform that task.

Civil Laws

Civil laws are laws passed to protect the civil and private rights of individuals and provide civil remedies as opposed to criminal laws. This type of law usually involves the violation of one's right against another and ensures equal treatment for all clients without regard to race, social status, ability to pay for services, or country of origin. If a violation of civil law is found, federal or state funds can be withheld or suit can be brought against the doctor, the nurse, or the facility for which they work. Damages usually involve money and sanctions. If the nurse is found to have caused harm to the client because of a lack of care, further action can be filed.

Criminal Laws

A *felony* is a crime of a serious nature that is punishable by jail time and loss of the nurse's license. A *misdemeanor*, on the other hand, is a lesser crime that can result in imprisonment for less than one year or a fine. An example of a misdemeanor is the use of a controlled substance. A felony example is the possession of large quantities of drugs with the intent to sell them. Many other types of actions are also criminal, such as stealing from a client or abusing a client. These involve the police and the board of nursing taking action. Even if the nurse is not caring for clients at the time the crime is committed, the state board of nursing can take action against the nurse. Action taken by the board can include suspension or loss of the license to practice nursing.

Common Law

Common law is a non-statutory body of law that has evolved from court decisions and case law. Common law has provided the right to consent for services that need to be rendered when the client is unable to give consent herself or to provide for the right to refuse consent. The Patient's Bill of Rights describes these concepts, which are listed here:

As a client you have the right to

▶ Receive respectful treatment that will be helpful in the course of your recovery.

▶ Refuse a treatment or to end treatment without harassment by the healthcare community. This is often a problem because physicians want the client to survive. However, the client and family might be more concerned with death and dignity while dying. Hospice care can help during this time.

▶ A safe environment that is free from fear of physical, emotional, or sexual abuse or neglect. This includes cleanliness of the facility and the healthcare providers.

▶ Refuse electronic recording of your conversations with healthcare workers. You can also request that conversations be recorded.

▶ Have written information regarding any care that is being provided or that the physician proposes. You also have the right to a written statement of all fees and services and the cost of each. You also have the right to see the licensure, educational training, and experience of your healthcare provider. You can also ask to see to which professional organizations your healthcare providers belong and any limitations that have been placed on her by her regulatory organization.

▶ Report unethical or illegal behavior that you observe and to ask questions about your care.

▶ Refuse to answer questions or to disclose any information you choose not to share.

▶ Confidentiality. You can take legal action if the healthcare worker does not abide by the Health Information Protection Privacy Act (HIPPA).

▶ Receive a second opinion from another healthcare worker, physician, counselor, or nurse practitioner.

▶ See your files and receive a photocopy of your chart.

▶ Request that the doctor, counselor, or nurse inform you of your progress or lack of progress during your treatment.

▶ Know who will know about you and be able to see your chart.

Code of Ethical Behavior in Nursing Practice

Ethics are the principles that guide nursing decisions and conduct as they pertain to what is right or wrong. They also involve moral behavior. The nurse is expected to behave in a way that maintains the integrity of the client and family. Situations often arise that require the nurse to make a judgment, and a dilemma results when the nurse's values differ from those of the client and family. The nurse must remember that clients have the right to make decisions for themselves without the expressed opinion of the nurse. In 2001, the American Nurses Association released the Code of Ethics for Nursing. This code discusses the obligation and duties of the nurse. The following list describes the Code of Ethics for Nursing:

▶ The nurse practices with compassion and respect for the dignity, worth, and uniqueness of the individual, unrestricted by social or economic status, personal attributes, or the nature of the disease. For example, the nurse might not be comfortable caring for the alcoholic client, but is ethically obligated to provide the best and most compassionate care possible.

▶ The nurse is committed to the client, whether the client is an individual, a family, or a community. The home health nurse might be asked to care not only for the client, but also the family and or the whole community. In some cultures, the family and community are included in decision making. The nurse must respect the client's wishes in this matter.

▶ The nurse is expected to serve as an advocate for the client. The nurse also is responsible for protecting the health, safety, and rights of the client.

▶ The nurse is responsible and accountable for delegating tasks consistent with optimal client care. The nurse is expected to be aware of the roles and responsibilities of other healthcare workers.

▶ The nurse is expected to preserve one's own integrity and safety, to maintain competence, and to continue personal and professional growth. This basically means that in states where continuing education units are required, the nurse will abide by these regulations to keep a current license.

▶ The nurse participates in activities that establish, maintain, and improve the conditions of the work environment. The nurse is responsible for promoting activities that foster ethical values in nursing.

▶ The nurse participates in the advancement of the profession through education, research, and development of nursing knowledge.

> ▶ The nurse collaborates with others in the health community to meet client needs.

> ▶ The nurse is responsible for maintaining the integrity of nursing and its practice, and for shaping social policy through professional organizations.

Legal Theories That Affect Nursing Practice

Standards of care apply to the practice of nursing and all professions. Because legal action can be taken against the nurse for failure to follow the standard of care, it is important for the nurse to be familiar with legal terminology. The following sections discuss several legal theories affecting nursing practice. These include negligence, malpractice, assault and battery, tort, and fraud. These are the most common causes of action brought against the nurse, so the sections that follow cover each in detail.

Negligence

First, *negligence* is defined as a lack of reasonable conduct and care. Negligence involves omitting an act expected of a person with knowledge or performing an act that a reasonable person would not perform. If the nurse fails to perform an act, such as putting the side rail up on a bed, and the client falls out of bed, resulting in injury, the nurse can be charged with negligence. It is reasonable for the client to expect the nurse to know that the side rail should be used to prevent injury. Other examples of negligence are the failure to administer medications ordered by the physician.

Malpractice

Malpractice is professional negligence, misconduct, or unreasonable lack of skill that results in injury or loss of professional services. A nurse can be accused of negligence and malpractice in the same context. If the nurse fails to take the vital signs, and the client's condition deteriorates and the client eventually dies, the nurse can be accused of both negligence and malpractice. Although malpractice is often thought of as more severe than negligence, both can result in harm to the client. Other examples of malpractice include medication errors, carelessness with application of heat and cold, and failure to assess symptoms such as shock and respiratory distress.

Witnessing Consent for Care

The nurse is responsible for witnessing informed consent. The nurse is not responsible for obtaining informed consent, even though the nurse might get the client to sign the form before surgery or blood administration. The legal responsibility for obtaining informed consent, resides with the person providing the treatment. This individual is often the physician. The nurse documents and communicates information regarding client care to the doctor.

Tort

A *tort* is a legal wrong against a person or his property. If a psychiatric nurse is given the responsibility of searching the belongings of a client admitted to the unit and, during the search of the client's luggage, the clothes are torn and the property destroyed, the nurse can be alleged to have committed a tort. In this example, the tort was unintentional; however, a tort can be either intentional or unintentional. Other examples of a tort are assault, battery, or slander because they are wrongful acts carried out with the intent to do harm.

Assault and Battery

Assault is the unjustifiable threat or attempt to touch or injure another person. *Battery* is the actual touching of another without consent. An example is a nurse on the psychiatric unit who uses undue power to restrain a client during an altercation. In such a situation, the nurse can be charged with assault and battery.

Fraud

Fraud is the intent to mislead in any form. Examples of fraud are the recording of vital signs that were not taken and the recording of blood glucose levels that were not obtained.

Managing Client Care

A portion of the NCLEX exam, called *Safe Effective Care*, includes the management and delegation of client care. The nurse is responsible for delegating client assignments. Delegation is the handing over of a task to another person. The usual team of healthcare workers includes the registered nurses, the licensed practical nurses/licensed vocational nurses, and the nursing assistants (UAP; *unlicensed assistive personnel*). The National Council of State Boards of Nursing (NCSBN) and state boards of nursing are responsible for ensuring the safety of clients. They work with the American Hospital Association to formulate rules and regulations that govern the nursing practice of these workers. The nurse must utilize Maslow's Hierarchy of Needs when delegating care to others. The most critical clients should be assigned to the most educated and experienced nurse, whereas the most stable clients should be assigned to the care of the lesser-qualified personnel. The registered nurse coordinates the healthcare and makes assignments to other workers. When the client is admitted to the unit, the registered nurse should see the client first. A client being discharged home or to another unit must be seen by the registered nurse before discharge, as well.

The licensed practical nurse should be assigned to care for the client who needs skilled nursing care but is stable. Care of central venous infusions, blood transfusions, intravenous infusion of chemotherapy agents, and unstable clients are duties that should be assigned to the registered nurse. Administering medications orally or by injection, changing sterile dressing, and inserting nasogastric tubes are examples of duties that can be performed by the licensed practical nurse. The nursing assistant can perform activities of daily living, such as feeding and bathing the client. The nursing assistant can also be assigned to take the vital signs of the stable client. Your healthcare facility might have more strict or different policies, so be certain to know your hospital's policies. The following list provides examples of activities that can be performed by the registered nurse and activities that licensed practical nurses can perform:

▶ **Ambulating the client**: The nurse (RN/LPN) can measure the client for crutches, assist the client to ambulate using crutches, and teach him regarding the correct methods of ambulation with crutches. The nurse (RN/LPN) can ambulate the client, but the nursing assistant can only ambulate the stable client.

The nurse (RN/LPN) can measure the client for a walker, ambulate the client with a walker, and teach him how to use the walker.

The nurse (RN/LPN) can measure the client for a cane, ambulate the client with a cane, and teach him how to use the cane.

▶ **Applying heat and cold**: The nurse (RN/LPN) can apply heat lamps, heating pads, and warm, moist soaks. The nurse (RN/LPN) can also apply cold applications.

▶ **Applying restraints of all types**: The RN and the physician are the only two personnel who can place the client in seclusion on the psychiatric unit.

▶ **Bathing the client**: The nurse (RN/LPN/UAP) can bathe the client and assist the client with performing the activities of daily living.

▶ **Central venous pressure monitoring**: The nurse (RN/LPN) can check the central venous pressure and assist the doctor with inserting a central catheter. Even though both the RN and LPN have knowledge of the hemodynamics of the heart, the best nurse to assign to interpreting central venous pressures is the registered nurse.

▶ **Collecting specimens**: The nurse (RN/LPN) can collect specimens such as sputum, wound, urine, and stool.

▶ **Electrocardiogram interpretations**: The nurse (RN/LPN) can interpret the ECG monitor and should know the life-threatening arrhythmias and the management of each.

▶ **IV therapy**: The registered nurse can start, manage, and discontinue intravenous infusions. The licensed practical nurse can maintain, regulate, and discontinue IV infusions according to written protocol. The LPN is not authorized to start IV therapy unless the licensed vocational nurse (LVN) or LPN is certified to perform this task.

The RN can insert peripherally inserted central venous catheters (PICCs) with certification. The LPN, however, is not authorized to perform this skill.

The RN can hang and monitor blood transfusions. The LPN can take the vital signs of the client receiving the blood transfusion, but should not be the primary nurse responsible for this client.

▶ **Medication administration**: The nurse (RN/LPN) can insert vaginal and rectal suppositories. The registered nurse can administer IV medications, an IV push, and IV piggyback medications. The licensed practical nurse should not be assigned to this task unless he is IV certified. Intravenous push medications are not usually included in this certification. The nurse (RN/LPN) can administer oral medications, topical medications, intramuscular medications, intradermal medications, and subcutaneous medications.

▶ **Nasogastric tubes**: The nurse (RN/LPN) can insert nasogastric tubes for Levin suction or gavage feeding. The nurse (RN/LPN) can insert medications through nasogastric feeding tubes and percutaneous esophagoscopy gavage feeding tubes (PEG tubes). The RN and LPN can discontinue nasogastric tubes.

▶ **Teaching**: The RN is responsible for teaching the client prior to discharge. The LPN is part of the health team and supports the RN in the teaching plan.

▶ **Tracheostomy care/endotracheal care**: The nurse (RN/LPN) can suction and provide ventilator support (the nurse is expected to know how to manage the client on the ventilator). The RN and LPN can clean the tracheostomy and provide oxygenation.

▶ **Traction**: The nurse (RN/LPN) can set up and maintain skin traction, but cannot implement skeletal traction.

▶ **Urinary catheters**: The nurse (RN/LPN) can insert Foley and French catheters. The RN and LPN can irrigate Foley catheters with a physician's order. Both can discontinue Foley and French catheters, as well.

▶ **Vital signs**: The nurse (RN/LPN) can perform the task of taking the vital signs and evaluating them. The nursing assistant can take the vital signs of the stable client.

▶ **Wound care (sterile)**: The nurse (RN/LPN) can perform decubitus care, cast care, and sterile dressing changes.

NOTE

Nursing or Nurse Practice Acts vary from state to state. The nurse is responsible for knowing the laws in the state where he/she will practice. It is the responsibility of the nurse to contact the board of nursing to obtain a copy of the Nursing Practice Act. The state board of nursing has been authorized to take action against a nurse found guilty of failure to comply with rules and regulations set forth by the law. These examples are not a comprehensive list of all the skills registered nurses/licensed practical nurse can do.

CAUTION

Do not assign a nursing assistant to calculate hourly intake and output, take post-operative vital signs, or care for an unstable client. A registered nurse or licensed practical nurse should be assigned to these tasks.

The nurse must be aware of infection control and isolation needs. If the client has an infection, he should not be assigned to share a room with a client who is immune-suppressed or has had surgery. A pregnant client should not be assigned to share a room with a client with teratogenic infections or who is receiving medications that can be harmful to the fetus. A pregnant nurse should not be assigned to care for a client who has a radium implant or one who is receiving chemotherapy or other medication that can harm the baby.

Another responsibility of the registered nurse and the licensed practical nurse is to serve as a client advocate. She must ensure that referrals are made and that facility policies are maintained. The registered nurse helps with formulating the policies and often serves as the head nurse, supervisor, or director of nursing. Often the registered nurse is the one assigned to call social services, dietary, and other services, although the licensed practical nurse can assist with these responsibilities. As the charge nurse, the RN also might be called on to counsel co-workers and settle differences that arise among personnel.

Case Study

1. Amy, a recently licensed nurse, has been assigned to the critical care unit. On the third day of orientation, her preceptor tells her that she has been doing an excellent job and that she has decided to assign her six patients for the day. Amy feels unsure about this assignment. What should she do?

2. Amy is asked to perform a skill that she has never done. Which action would be best to ensure the safety of the client?

3. Amy's client asked for medication for a headache. After checking the chart she finds that there is no order for pain medication. Amy decides to give two Tylenol (acetaminophen) for pain. If harm comes to the client, what can Amy can be charged with?

4. If harm comes to the client as a result of Amy's action, Amy can be charged with:

5. If Amy decides to chart medication that she did not give, with what can she be charged?

Answers to Case Study

1. Amy is a newly licensed nurse that has been on the unit for three days. Because she feels unsure of herself, she should explain this to the preceptor. If she is not comfortable with the tasks assigned to her, she should refuse the assignment and immediately contact the nurse in charge.

2. Amy should ask the preceptor to allow her to watch the skill performed and then perform the task herself with the preceptor watching. This action would allow her time and orientation to the task and ensure the safety of the client.

3. Amy can be charged with administering medication without an order by the state board of nursing.

4. Amy can be accused of malpractice if harm comes to the client.

5. Amy can be charged with fraud and falsifying documents.

Exam Prep Questions

1. The nurse is making assignments for the day. Which client should be assigned to the pregnant nurse?

   - ○ **A.** The client receiving radium linear accelerator radiation therapy for cancer
   - ○ **B.** The client with a radium implant for vaginal cancer
   - ○ **C.** The client who has just been administered radioactive isotopes for cancer
   - ○ **D.** The client who returned from placement of iridium seeds for prostate cancer

2. The nurse is planning room assignments for the day. Which client should be assigned to the only private room?

   - ○ **A.** The client with Cushing's disease
   - ○ **B.** The client with diabetes
   - ○ **C.** The client with acromegaly
   - ○ **D.** The client with myxedema

3. The charge nurse witnesses the nursing assistant being abusive to a client in the nursing home facility. The nursing assistant can be charged with which of the following?

   - ○ **A.** Negligence
   - ○ **B.** Tort
   - ○ **C.** Assault
   - ○ **D.** Malpractice

4. Which assignment is outside the realm of nursing practice for the licensed practical nurse?

   - ○ **A.** Inserting a Foley catheter
   - ○ **B.** Discontinuing a nasogastric tube
   - ○ **C.** Obtaining a sputum specimen
   - ○ **D.** Starting a blood transfusion

5. The client returns to the unit from surgery with a blood pressure of 100/50, pulse 122, and respirations 30. Which action by the nurse should receive priority?

   - ○ **A.** Continue to monitor the vital signs.
   - ○ **B.** Contact the physician.
   - ○ **C.** Ask the client how he feels.
   - ○ **D.** Ask the LPN to continue the post-op care.

6. Which nurse should be assigned to care for the client with preeclampsia?

   ○ **A.** The RN with 2 weeks experience on postpartum

   ○ **B.** The RN with 3 years experience in labor and delivery

   ○ **C.** The RN with 10 years experience in surgery

   ○ **D.** The RN with 1 year experience in the neonatal intensive care unit

7. Which information should be reported to the state board of nursing?

   ○ **A.** The facility fails to provide literature in both Spanish and English.

   ○ **B.** The narcotic count has been incorrect on the unit for the past three days.

   ○ **C.** The client fails to receive an itemized account of his bills and services received during his hospital stay.

   ○ **D.** The nursing assistant assigned to the client with hepatitis fails to feed the client and give him a bath.

8. The nurse is found to have charted blood glucose results without actually performing the procedure. After talking to the nurse, the charge nurse should do which of the following?

   ○ **A.** Call the board of nursing

   ○ **B.** File a formal reprimand and monitor the nurse

   ○ **C.** Terminate the nurse

   ○ **D.** Charge the nurse with a tort

9. The home health nurse is planning for the day's visits. Which client should be seen first?

   ○ **A.** The 78-year-old who had a gastrectomy three weeks ago with a PEG tube

   ○ **B.** The five-month-old discharged one week ago with pneumonia who is being treated with amoxicillin liquid suspension

   ○ **C.** The 50-year-old with MRSA being treated with vancomycin via a PICC line

   ○ **D.** The 30-year-old with an exacerbation of multiple sclerosis being treated with cortisone via a centrally placed venous catheter

10. The emergency room is flooded with clients injured in a tornado. Which clients can be assigned to share a room in the emergency department during the disaster?

   ○ **A.** A schizophrenic client having visual and auditory hallucinations and the client with ulcerative colitis

   ○ **B.** The client who is six months pregnant with abdominal pain and the client with facial lacerations and a broken arm

   ○ **C.** A child whose pupils are fixed and dilated and his parents and a client with a frontal head injury

   ○ **D.** The client who arrives with a large puncture wound to the abdomen and the client with chest pain

Answers to Exam Questions

1. Answer A is correct. The pregnant nurse should not be assigned to any client with radioactivity present. The client receiving linear accelerator therapy travels to the radium department for therapy, and the radiation stays in the department. Thus, the client is not radioactive. The client in answer B poses a risk to the pregnant client, so answer B is incorrect. Answer C is incorrect because the client is radioactive in very small doses. For approximately 72 hours, the client should dispose of urine and feces in special containers and use plastic spoons and forks. The client in answer D is also radioactive in small amounts, especially upon return from the procedure, so answer D is incorrect.

2. Answer A is correct. The client with Cushing's disease has adrenocortical hypersecretion. This increase in the level of cortisone causes the client to be immune-suppressed. The client with diabetes poses no risk to other clients and is not immunosuppressed, so answer B is incorrect. The client in answer C has an increase in growth hormone and poses no risk to himself or others, so the answer is incorrect. The client in answer D has hyperthyroidism, or myxedema, and poses no risk to others or himself, so it is incorrect.

3. Answer C is correct. Assault is defined as striking or touching the client inappropriately. Negligence is failing to perform care for the client, so answer A is incorrect. A tort is a wrongful act committed on the client or his belongings, so answer B is incorrect. Malpractice is failing to perform an act that the nurse knows should be done or doing something wrong that causes harm to the client, so answer D is incorrect.

4. Answer D is correct. The LPN can be assigned to insert Foley and French urinary catheters, discontinue Levin and gavage gastric tubes, and obtain all types of specimens.

5. Answer B is correct. The vital signs are abnormal and should be reported immediately. Continuing to monitor the vital signs can result in deterioration of the client's condition, so answer A is incorrect. Asking the client how he feels would supply only subjective data, so answer C is incorrect. The LPN is not the best nurse to be assigned to this client because he is unstable, so answer D is incorrect.

6. Answer B is correct. The nurse in answer B has the most experience in knowing the possible complications involved with preeclampsia. The nurse in answer A is a new nurse to this unit, so the answer is incorrect. The nurse in answer C has no experience with the postpartal client, so the answer is incorrect. The nurse in answer D also has no experience with postpartal clients, so the answer is incorrect.

7. Answer B is correct. The Joint Commission on Accreditation of Hospitals will probably be interested in the problems in answers A and C, so they are incorrect. The failure of the nursing assistant to assist the client with hepatitis should be reported to the charge nurse. If the behavior continues, termination can result, but it doesn't need to be reported to the board, so answer D is incorrect.

8. Answer B is correct. The next action after discussing the problem with the nurse is to document the incident. If the behavior continues or if harm has resulted to the client, the nurse might be terminated and reported to the board of nursing, so answers A and C are incorrect. A tort is a wrongful act to the client or her belongings, so answer D is incorrect.

9. Answer D is correct. The client who should receive priority is the client with multiple sclerosis being treated with cortisone via the central line because this client is at highest risk for complications. The clients described in A and B are stable at the time of the assigned visit. They can be seen later. The client in C has methicillin-resistant staphylococcus aureus (MRSA). Vancomycin is the drug of choice and can be administered later, but it must be scheduled at specific times of the day to maintain a therapeutic level, so answer C is incorrect.

10. Answer B is correct. Out of all these clients, it is best to hold the pregnant client and the client with a broken arm and facial lacerations in the same room. The other clients need to be placed in separate rooms, so answers A, C, and D are incorrect.

Suggested Reading and Resources

▶ National Council of State Boards of Nursing: http://www.ncsbn.org/

▶ Tappen, R., Weiss, S., and Whitehead, D. *Essential Nursing Leadership and Management.* 4th ed. Philadelphia: F.A. Davis, 2006.

▶ State boards of nursing for respective states: http://www.allnursingschools.com/faqs/boards.php

Practice Exam I

NCLEX-RN Exam Cram, Third Edition

1. The physician has ordered a urine specimen for vanillymandelic acid (VMA) levels in a client with severe uncontrolled hypertension. Which foods would interfere with VMA test results?

   ○ **A.** Whole grain breads and cereals

   ○ **B.** Chocolate pudding and gelatins

   ○ **C.** Spinach and kale

   ○ **D.** Beef and beef products

2. The nurse has just received the change of shift report. Which client should the nurse assess first?

   ○ **A.** A client two hours post lobectomy with 150 mls drainage in the past hour

   ○ **B.** A client two days post gastrectomy with scant drainage

   ○ **C.** A client with pneumonia with an oral temperature of 102°

   ○ **D.** A client with a fractured hip in Buck's traction

3. A client with pernicious anemia has been receiving B12 injections for the past six weeks. Which laboratory finding indicates that the medication is having the desired effect?

   ○ **A.** Neutrophil count of 60%

   ○ **B.** Basophil count of 0.5%

   ○ **C.** Monocyte count of 2%

   ○ **D.** Reticulocyte count of 1%

4. The nurse is providing discharge teaching for a client taking phenelazine. The nurse should instruct the client to avoid eating:

○ **A.** Peanuts, dates, and raisins

○ **B.** Figs, chocolate, and eggplant

○ **C.** Cracked wheat, peas, and beef

○ **D.** Milk, cottage cheese, and ice cream

5. A client recovering from a stroke exhibits signs of unilateral neglect. Which behavior is suggestive of unilateral neglect?

○ **A.** The client is observed leaning to the left, although he believes he is sitting upright.

○ **B.** The client is unable to distinguish between two tactile stimuli presented simultaneously.

○ **C.** The client is unable to complete a range of vision without turning his head from side to side.

○ **D.** The client is unable to carry out cognitive and motor activities at the same time.

6. A client with acute lymphocytic leukemia develops severe neutropenia following chemotherapy. In addition to the institution of reverse isolation, the nurse should:

○ **A.** Request that foods be served with disposable utensils.

○ **B.** Ask the client to wear a mask when visitors are present.

○ **C.** Prep IV sites with mild soap and water.

○ **D.** Provide foods in sealed single-serving packages.

7. A new nursing graduate indicates in charting entries that he is a licensed registered nurse, although he has not yet received the results of the licensing exam. The graduate's action can result in a charge of:

○ **A.** Fraud

○ **B.** Tort

○ **C.** Malpractice

○ **D.** Negligence

8. The nurse is assigning staff for the day. Which client should be assigned to the nursing assistant?

   ○ **A.** A six-month-old with bronchiolitis

   ○ **B.** An eight-year-old two days post appendectomy

   ○ **C.** A two-year-old with periorbital cellulites

   ○ **D.** A one-year-old with a fractured tibia

9. During the change of shift, the oncoming nurse notes a discrepancy in the number of meperidine ampules listed and the number present in the narcotic drawer. The nurse should:

   ○ **A.** Notify the hospital pharmacist.

   ○ **B.** Notify the nursing supervisor.

   ○ **C.** Notify the board of nursing.

   ○ **D.** Notify the director of nursing.

10. Due to a high census, a number of clients have had to be transferred to other units within the hospital. Which client should be transferred to the postpartum unit?

   ○ **A.** A 76-year-old female with a total knee replacement

   ○ **B.** A 45-year-old male with a herniated lumbar disc

   ○ **C.** A 20-year-old female with severe depression

   ○ **D.** A 28-year-old male with ulcerative colitis

11. A client with nephrotic syndrome is placed on a low-sodium diet. Which of the following snacks is suitable for a client with sodium restriction?

   ○ **A.** Peanut butter cookies

   ○ **B.** A grilled cheese sandwich

   ○ **C.** Cottage cheese and fruit

   ○ **D.** A fresh orange

12. A home health nurse is making preparations for her morning visits. Which one of the following clients should the nurse visit first?

   ○ **A.** A client with CVA with tube feedings

   ○ **B.** A client with emphysema who complains of nighttime dyspnea

   ○ **C.** A client who has had a mastectomy

   ○ **D.** A client with Parkinson's disease

13. A client with Sjogren syndrome develops xerostomia. The nurse can help alleviate the discomfort associated with xerostomia by:

   ○ **A.** Instilling artificial tears

   ○ **B.** Administering analgesic meds

   ○ **C.** Splinting the affected joints

   ○ **D.** Providing a saliva substitute

14. The nurse is making assignments for the day. The staff consists of an RN, an LPN, and a nursing assistant. Which client should be assigned to the nursing assistant?

   ○ **A.** A client with laparoscopic cholecystectomy

   ○ **B.** A client with bacterial pneumonia

   ○ **C.** A client with suspected ectopic pregnancy

   ○ **D.** A client with transient ischemic attacks

15. The nurse is caring for a client with cerebral palsy, athetoid type. The nurse should provide frequent rest periods because:

   ○ **A.** Grimacing and writhing movements decrease with relaxation and rest.

   ○ **B.** Hypoactive deep tendon reflexes become more active with rest.

   ○ **C.** Stretch reflexes are increased with rest.

   ○ **D.** Fine motor movements are improved with rest.

16. The physician has ordered a culture from a child suspected of having pertussis. The nurse should obtain a culture of:

   ○ **A.** Blood

   ○ **B.** Nasopharyngeal secretions

   ○ **C.** Stool

   ○ **D.** Urine

17. Which of the following preoperative diets is the most appropriate for a client scheduled for a hemorrhoidectomy?

   ○ **A.** High fiber

   ○ **B.** Low residue

   ○ **C.** Bland

   ○ **D.** Clear liquid

18. An effective means of managing discomfort in a post-hemorrhoidectomy client is:

   ○ **A.** Medicated suppository

   ○ **B.** Aspirin

   ○ **C.** Sitz baths

   ○ **D.** Ice packs

19. To assist a blind client with ambulation, the nurse should walk:

   ○ **A.** To the side and slightly in front of the client while the client holds onto the nurse's arm

   ○ **B.** To the front of the client while the client holds onto the nurse's arm

   ○ **C.** To the front of the client while the nurse holds onto the client's arm

   ○ **D.** To the side of the client while the nurse holds onto the client's arm

20. A client is receiving blood. Which of the following findings should be reported immediately?

   ○ **A.** Pedal edema

   ○ **B.** Temperature of 99.2°

   ○ **C.** Blood pressure of 100/52

   ○ **D.** Adventitious breath sounds

21. Following renal transplantation, the client is started on oral doses of cyclosporine. Which of the following instructions should be included for a client receiving cyclosporine?

   ○ **A.** The diet should be supplemented with additional sources of iron.

   ○ **B.** Dilute the solution in chocolate milk and drink it immediately.

   ○ **C.** Store the medication in the refrigerator to preserve its effectiveness.

   ○ **D.** The medication will be gradually tapered off and discontinued after three months.

22. A client with chronic renal failure is placed on a low-protein diet. The nurse explains that a low-protein diet is best for those with renal disease because:

   ○ **A.** Protein breaks down into waste products that increase the workload of the kidneys.

   ○ **B.** Protein increases the amount of sodium and potassium to be regulated by the kidneys.

   ○ **C.** Protein decreases the amount of serum albumin and promotes edema formation.

   ○ **D.** Protein decreases serum calcium and phosphorus levels.

23. A client admitted with burn injury is determined to have second-degree partial thickness burns. Which of the following describes the client's burns?

   ○ **A.** Reddened areas, dry texture

   ○ **B.** Brownish areas, dull appearance

   ○ **C.** Blackened area, not painful

   ○ **D.** Erythematous, moist area, painful

24. Which of the following clients would not be a candidate for therapy with imipramine (Tofranil)?

   ○ **A.** A client with a history of myocardial infarction

   ○ **B.** A client with a history of hepatitis

   ○ **C.** A client with a history of enuresis

   ○ **D.** A client with a history of gastric ulcers

25. An 18-month-old is hospitalized with intussusception. Which of the following observations best indicates that he is adequately hydrated?

   ○ **A.** The drainage from his nasogastric tube is gradually decreasing.

   ○ **B.** His IV is infusing at the prescribed rate.

   ○ **C.** He wets a diaper at least every 4 hours.

   ○ **D.** His urinary specific gravity is 1.012.

26. A client with depression fails to show improvement with amitriptyline (Elavil) and is started on a monoamine oxidase inhibitor. Which of the following symptoms can occur as a result of MAO food reaction?

   ○ **A.** Petechiae

   ○ **B.** Nausea

   ○ **C.** Headache

   ○ **D.** Dystonia

27. An 11-year-old client with a fractured femur returns from surgery with a Steinmann pin through her lower femur and skeletal traction. Which of the following findings indicate that the traction is ineffective?

   ○ **A.** The client uses the trapeze to lift her hips off the bed when using the bedpan.

   ○ **B.** The foot plate is against the end of the bed.

   ○ **C.** The weights are suspended only 18 inches from the floor.

   ○ **D.** The ropes of the traction move freely through the pulley.

28. A four-year-old is admitted to the PICU following surgery to correct a Ventral Septal Defect (VSD). Several hours after surgery, he is noted to be restless and irritable. In the past hour, his pulse rate has increased from 106 to 110, his BP remains unchanged, and his respirations are rapid and shallow. The most likely interpretation of these findings is that:

    ○ **A.** He is developing fluid volume deficit.

    ○ **B.** He has symptoms of impending shock.

    ○ **C.** He is in pain.

    ○ **D.** He is developing heart failure.

29. A 15-year-old male is admitted with a closed head injury following an MVA. He has multiple abrasions, has fractures of the mandible, and was unconscious for several minutes after the accident. Which of the following orders should the nurse discuss with the doctor?

    ○ **A.** Keep the head elevated 30°.

    ○ **B.** Apply Neosporin ointment to the abrasions.

    ○ **C.** IV D5W at 75 ml/hr. for 8 hours.

    ○ **D.** Meperidine 75 mg IM q 3 hrs. PRN pain.

30. A client with a TURP returns from surgery with an indwelling catheter attached to a drainage bag and continuous bladder irrigation. Two hours after surgery, he complains of bladder spasms. The nurse should give priority to:

    ○ **A.** Offering him fluids by mouth

    ○ **B.** Administering the prescribed analgesic

    ○ **C.** Assessing catheter patency

    ○ **D.** Massaging the symphysis pubis

31. Which of the following instructions should be included in the discharge teaching of a client with mandibular wires?

    ○ **A.** Swallow saliva that collects in your mouth to help keep your mouth from becoming dry.

    ○ **B.** Move your lips as little as possible.

    ○ **C.** Clean the wires with saline-moistened cotton swabs.

    ○ **D.** Keep wire cutters with you at all times.

32. Following a cholescystetomy, the client's diet should be:

- ○ **A.** Low residue
- ○ **B.** Low fat
- ○ **C.** Low protein
- ○ **D.** Low sodium

33. Obstructive biliary tract disease and gallbladder disease are often associated with:

- ○ **A.** Hypertension
- ○ **B.** Diabetes
- ○ **C.** Obesity
- ○ **D.** Infertility

34. Which of the following is a sign of osteomyelitis?

- ○ **A.** Fever and tachycardia
- ○ **B.** Nausea and dehydration
- ○ **C.** Erythema distal to the injury site
- ○ **D.** Fatigue and lethargy

35. A client with renal disease should be monitored frequently for complications of her illness. Which of the following is a complication of renal disease?

- ○ **A.** Hepatitis
- ○ **B.** Cardiomegaly
- ○ **C.** Osteoporosis
- ○ **D.** Hypocholesterolemia

36. A client is being monitored for cardiac arrhythmias. While monitoring the client, the nurse recognizes bizarre QRS complexes that are lacking a P wave. The nurse would recognize these beats as:

- ○ **A.** Atrial tachycardia
- ○ **B.** Premature ventricular beats
- ○ **C.** Signs of a heart block
- ○ **D.** Premature atrial beats

37. A client with a diagnosis of trichimonas is treated with metronidazole (Flagyl). Which instruction should the nurse give the client taking Flagyl?

   ○ **A.** Take the medication with juice.

   ○ **B.** Do not drink alcohol while taking Flagyl.

   ○ **C.** Return to the clinic for regular eye exams.

   ○ **D.** Allow six weeks for the drug to be effective.

38. The nurse initiates cardioversion on the client in ventricular fibrillation. Cardioversion is synchronized with which part of the ECG complex?

   ○ **A.** T-wave

   ○ **B.** S-T segment

   ○ **C.** Q-T interval

   ○ **D.** QRS complex

39. An elderly client is experiencing kyphosis. The nurse can help alleviate the pain associated with kyphosis by:

   ○ **A.** Administering a heating pad to the client's back

   ○ **B.** Telling the client about relaxation exercises

   ○ **C.** Administering narcotics routinely

   ○ **D.** Applying ice to the client's extremities

40. A client is scheduled for surgery and has an order for promethezine (Phenergan) to be administered with meperidine (Demerol). The nurse is aware that the promethezine is administered to:

   ○ **A.** Dry secretions

   ○ **B.** Decrease nausea

   ○ **C.** Provide pain relief

   ○ **D.** Prevent infections

41. While caring for a client receiving oxygen, the nurse identifies the odor of cigarette smoke. Which action by the nurse is most appropriate?

   ○ **A.** Tell the client that smoking is allowed only outside the hospital.

   ○ **B.** Ask the client whether he has been smoking.

   ○ **C.** Say nothing because she is unsure about where the smoke is coming from.

   ○ **D.** Call the head nurse and report the finding.

42. The urinary output of a client with a renal calculi in the urethra will most likely be:

   ○ **A.** Increased

   ○ **B.** Decreased

   ○ **C.** Unchanged

   ○ **D.** Dark and foamy

43. The client having a voiding cystogram will be placed in which position?

   ○ **A.** Prone

   ○ **B.** Dorsal recumbent

   ○ **C.** Lithotomy

   ○ **D.** Left Sims'

44. Glomerulonephritis is an example of which of the following types of renal disease?

   ○ **A.** Postrenal disease

   ○ **B.** Intrarenal disease

   ○ **C.** Prerenal disease

   ○ **D.** Extrarenal disease

45. The client has an order for ondansetron (Zofran). The nurse is aware that this medication is given to relieve:

   ○ **A.** Nausea

   ○ **B.** Fever

   ○ **C.** Pain

   ○ **D.** Anxiety

46. The client is admitted with a painless lesion of the perineum. A positive FTA-ABS indicates that the client has syphilis. The medication most often given to treat syphilis is:

   ○ **A.** Dexamethasone (Decadron)

   ○ **B.** Penicillin-G (Penicillin)

   ○ **C.** Acyclovir (Zovirax)

   ○ **D.** Alendronate (Fosamax)

47. Infants with congenital heart defects are predisposed to the development of thrombi. Primary prevention of this complication includes:

   ○ **A.** Frequent change of position

   ○ **B.** Adequate hydration

   ○ **C.** Providing range of motion

   ○ **D.** Prevention of upper respiratory infections

48. A client receiving a thiazide diuretic should be instructed to eat a diet rich in:

   ○ **A.** Calcium

   ○ **B.** Potassium

   ○ **C.** Magnesium

   ○ **D.** Folate

49. A client with Parkinson's disease is visited by the home health nurse. Which of the following environmental factors requires intervention by the nurse?

   ○ **A.** The client has a house cat.

   ○ **B.** The client has a bathroom down the hallway from his bedroom.

   ○ **C.** The client has a gas heater.

   ○ **D.** The client lives alone.

50. When preparing the preschool-aged child for surgery, the nurse should remember that preschoolers:

   ○ **A.** Have little awareness of their environment

   ○ **B.** Fear the loss of body integrity

   ○ **C.** Are able to conceptualize the surgery

   ○ **D.** Will resist any explanation about the surgery

51. Which of the following drugs, if overingested, can result in metabolic alkalosis?

   ○ **A.** Acetaminophen

   ○ **B.** Docusate

   ○ **C.** Aspirin

   ○ **D.** Calcium carbonate

52. An elderly client with Alzheimer's has become belligerent with her daughter because her daughter will not allow her to care for herself. According to Orem's theory of nursing, which of the following actions will best assist the client with nighttime voiding?

- ○ **A.** Ask the client to void before retiring to bed.
- ○ **B.** Leave a night light on.
- ○ **C.** Wake the client periodically during the night.
- ○ **D.** Withhold fluids after 6 p.m.

53. A client is admitted to the chemical dependency unit for treatment of chronic alcoholism. It has been almost 12 hours since his last alcohol intake. On admission, the nurse should give priority to:

- ○ **A.** Obtaining the client's vital signs every two hours
- ○ **B.** Obtaining a complete alcohol and drug history
- ○ **C.** Starting an IV of D5LR
- ○ **D.** Obtaining a CBC and urinalysis

54. Diuretic therapy with furosemide (Lasix) is ordered for a client with congestive heart failure. The nurse compares the admission data obtained three days earlier with today's data. He determines that the medication is having its intended effect because the client's:

- ○ **A.** Appetite has improved.
- ○ **B.** Urinary output has decreased.
- ○ **C.** Breath sounds have improved.
- ○ **D.** Temperature has decreased.

55. The client receiving chlordiazepoxide (Librium) should be taught to avoid:

- ○ **A.** Chocolate
- ○ **B.** Cheese
- ○ **C.** Shellfish
- ○ **D.** Alcohol

56. The definitive diagnosis of benign prostatic hypertrophy is made by:

- ○ **A.** Biopsy
- ○ **B.** Pap smear
- ○ **C.** Rectal exam
- ○ **D.** Serum phosphatase elevations

57. A client with COPD is admitted with respiratory acidosis. The nurse determines that efforts to correct the client's acidosis are effective by observing that:

- ○ **A.** The client's CO_2 level has decreased.
- ○ **B.** The client no longer complains of shortness of breath.
- ○ **C.** The client's blood sugar is within normal limits.
- ○ **D.** The client's ability to concentrate has improved.

58. A client is admitted with thrombophlebitis and started on intravenous heparin. Which diagnostic study will the nurse anticipate?

- ○ **A.** Protime
- ○ **B.** Partial thromboplastin time
- ○ **C.** PT
- ○ **D.** INR

59. Which of the following best indicates that the client understands teaching about stoma care?

- ○ **A.** The client asks questions about skin preparations for the stomal site.
- ○ **B.** The client is able to repeat the stoma care instructions.
- ○ **C.** The client performs proper skin care and applies a stomal bag.
- ○ **D.** The client asks for additional literature regarding management of a stoma.

60. A client scheduled for an arteriogram tells the nurse, "I'm afraid to have that test done." The nurse's best response would be:

- ○ **A.** "You seem upset, I'm sure you will feel better soon."
- ○ **B.** "What about the test causes you fear?"
- ○ **C.** "Are you afraid that you won't wake up?"
- ○ **D.** "You have nothing to be afraid of."

61. The client who is taking warfarin sodium (Coumadin) should be taught:

- ○ **A.** To take the medication on an empty stomach
- ○ **B.** To limit his dietary intake of green, leafy vegetables
- ○ **C.** To report visual halos and blurring of vision
- ○ **D.** To increase his dietary intake of green, leafy vegetables

62. Which of the following selections would be best for a client with gallbladder disease?

- ○ **A.** A peanut butter and jelly sandwich, apple, and milk

- ○ **B.** A roast beef sandwich, pickle spear, and iced tea

- ○ **C.** Sliced chicken breast, cole slaw, fruit gelatin, and coffee

- ○ **D.** Baked fish, peas and carrots, sponge cake, and skim milk

63. Which of the following actions by the client indicates an acceptance of her mastectomy?

- ○ **A.** She verbalizes acceptance of the mastectomy.

- ○ **B.** She looks at the operative site.

- ○ **C.** She asks for information about breast reconstruction.

- ○ **D.** She remains silent during dressing changes.

64. An intramuscular injection of vitamin K (aquamephyton) is ordered to:

- ○ **A.** Prevent hyperbilirubinemia

- ○ **B.** Promote clotting

- ○ **C.** Prevent hypoglycemia

- ○ **D.** Promote respiratory stability

65. Which of the following menus is most appropriate for a client receiving cortisone?

- ○ **A.** A ham sandwich, potato chips, pickle slice, and cola

- ○ **B.** A tuna sandwich, tossed salad with thousand island dressing, and coffee

- ○ **C.** A hamburger on a whole wheat bun, fries, applesauce, and iced tea

- ○ **D.** Sliced turkey breast, roll with butter, green beans, baked potato, and iced tea

66. The nurse has explained to a client scheduled for surgery that he will not be able to eat or drink after midnight. The client asks whether he can smoke after that time. Which of the following responses by the nurse would be most appropriate?

- ○ **A.** "Smoking is not allowed because it will make you more thirsty."

- ○ **B.** "I'll check with your surgeon."

- ○ **C.** "You can smoke because it will suppress your appetite before surgery."

- ○ **D.** "Smoking is not permitted because it stimulates stomach secretions."

67. Which of the following is most important to have on hand during a blood transfusion?

- ○ **A.** An alternative IV line
- ○ **B.** Diphenhydramine
- ○ **C.** Acetaminophen
- ○ **D.** A tourniquet

68. A nurse can best assess edema in an extremity by:

- ○ **A.** Checking the extremity for pitting
- ○ **B.** Weighing the client
- ○ **C.** Measuring the circumference of the extremity
- ○ **D.** Observing the client's output

69. Which of the following nursing interventions best prepares a six-year-old for a craniotomy?

- ○ **A.** Allow him to tour the pediatric intensive care unit.
- ○ **B.** Let him bandage a doll's head.
- ○ **C.** Encourage him to talk about his fear.
- ○ **D.** Allow him to draw a picture.

70. The primary nursing diagnosis for a client with Parkinson's disease is:

- ○ **A.** Alteration in tissue perfusion
- ○ **B.** Alteration in safety
- ○ **C.** Alteration in elimination
- ○ **D.** Alteration in thought processes

71. A client receiving intravenous Garamycin begins to complain of her "ears ringing." The nurse's first action should be to:

- ○ **A.** Slow the IV rate
- ○ **B.** Discontinue the medication
- ○ **C.** Call the doctor
- ○ **D.** Administer Benadryl

72. The nurse knows that a client receiving heparin has reached the therapeutic level when:

    ❍ **A.** The client's level is the same as the control.

    ❍ **B.** The control is twice the client's level.

    ❍ **C.** The client's level is 1 ½–2 times the control.

    ❍ **D.** The control and client's level are the same.

73. A client injured in a motor vehicle accident is placed on mechanical ventilation. A complication of mechanical ventilation is:

    ❍ **A.** Hypercapnia

    ❍ **B.** Hypotension

    ❍ **C.** Hypoperfusion

    ❍ **D.** Hyperthermia

74. Which of the following staff should be assigned to care for a client with a C-section delivery of a 9-pound infant?

    ❍ **A.** A licensed practical nurse with two years experience in labor and delivery

    ❍ **B.** A registered nurse with two weeks experience on the postpartum unit

    ❍ **C.** A registered nurse with six months experience on the postpartum unit

    ❍ **D.** A registered nurse with five years experience in surgical intensive care

75. An obstetric client is admitted with spontaneous rupture of membranes. Exam reveals that the cervix is 8 cm dilated and an erratic fetal heart rate appears during contractions. The nurse should give priority to:

    ❍ **A.** Applying an internal monitor

    ❍ **B.** Turning the client onto her side

    ❍ **C.** Assisting the client to ambulate

    ❍ **D.** Moving the client to the delivery area

76. The primary nursing diagnosis for the client with Cushing's disease is:

    ❍ **A.** Alteration in nutrition

    ❍ **B.** Potential for infection

    ❍ **C.** Alteration in body image

    ❍ **D.** Ineffective individual coping

77. Which of the following pediatric clients should be placed in reverse isolation?

   ○ **A.** A 7-year-old with acute lymphocytic leukemia

   ○ **B.** A 4-year-old with osteomyelitis

   ○ **C.** A 10-year-old with hepatitis A

   ○ **D.** A 6-year-old with spasmodic laryngitis

78. The nurse is taking the vital signs of a moribund client when the client suddenly grabs the nurse's hand. The nurse should:

   ○ **A.** Continue to take the vital signs.

   ○ **B.** Obtain medication for the client's agitation.

   ○ **C.** Talk calmly to the client while continuing to take the vital signs.

   ○ **D.** Cease taking the vital signs because it is making the client more agitated.

79. A client with a history of asthma has an allergy to both aspirin and penicillin. Which of the following medications should be avoided by the client?

   ○ **A.** Acetaminophen

   ○ **B.** Kefzol

   ○ **C.** Erythromycin

   ○ **D.** Tetracycline

80. A pediatric client with sensory hearing loss has received repeated antibiotic therapy for otitis media. Which of the following antibiotics could have contributed to her hearing loss?

   ○ **A.** Keflex

   ○ **B.** Gentamycin

   ○ **C.** Amoxicillin

   ○ **D.** Larotid

81. The client with multiple sclerosis asks the nurse, "Will I have much pain as the disease worsens?" The nurse's best response is:

   ○ **A.** "You can have severe headaches with multiple sclerosis."

   ○ **B.** "The doctor can order analgesics that will help control the pain."

   ○ **C.** "The amount of discomfort you feel will depend on your pain tolerance."

   ○ **D.** "Pain is not a characteristic of multiple sclerosis."

82. A client recuperating from a T-4 spinal injury wants to learn to use a wheelchair. To prepare the client for use of a wheelchair, the nurse should teach her to do:

    ○ **A.** Leg lifts to prevent hip contractures

    ○ **B.** Push-ups to strengthen her arm muscles

    ○ **C.** Balancing exercises to help her maintain equilibrium during transfer

    ○ **D.** Quadriceps setting exercises to maintain muscle tone

83. Which of the following activities would be most therapeutic for a withdrawn hallucinating client?

    ○ **A.** Watching a movie with several other clients

    ○ **B.** Working on a puzzle

    ○ **C.** Playing a game of solitaire

    ○ **D.** Taking a walk with the nurse

84. A client is admitted with a provisional diagnosis of Addison's disease. Which of the following symptoms would the nurse expect to find as he performs the client's physical assessment?

    ○ **A.** Edema

    ○ **B.** Hirsutism

    ○ **C.** Pendulous abdomen

    ○ **D.** Dry skin

85. While caring for a client with Cushing's disease, the nurse notes that the client experiences wide mood swings. The client's emotional lability is most likely due to:

    ○ **A.** Increased glucocorticoid levels

    ○ **B.** Alteration in body image

    ○ **C.** Decreased aldosterone levels

    ○ **D.** Ineffective coping patterns

86. Which client is most likely to experience extreme uterine contractions (afterpains) after delivery?

    ○ **A.** Gravida 1 para 0

    ○ **B.** Gravida 2 para 0

    ○ **C.** Gravida 1 para 1

    ○ **D.** Gravida 3 para 3

87. The nurse observes that a client uses tissues to open all doors and to adjust knobs on the TV. No other staff members have reported the behavior. The nurse should:

  ○ **A.** Ignore the behavior.

  ○ **B.** Provide the client a can of disinfectant.

  ○ **C.** Talk with the client about the behavior.

  ○ **D.** Take the tissues away from the client.

88. The physician orders Rocephin 2 gm in 100 ml to infuse over 45 minutes. The IV is to infuse via a macrodrip (10 gtts per ml). The nurse should set the IV rate at:

  ○ **A.** 12 gtts/min

  ○ **B.** 22 gtts/min

  ○ **C.** 32 gtts/min

  ○ **D.** 42 gtts/min

89. Which of the following pieces of equipment should be kept at the bedside of a client immobilized with Crutchfield tongs?

  ○ **A.** Wire cutters

  ○ **B.** Torque wrench

  ○ **C.** Pliers

  ○ **D.** Flat-head screwdriver

90. Which of the following patterns describes a reassuring fetal heart rate?

  ○ **A.** A fetal heart rate of 160–180 BPM

  ○ **B.** A baseline variability of 20–30 BPM

  ○ **C.** Ominous periodic changes that occur with fetal sleep

  ○ **D.** Acceleration of FHR with fetal movement

91. In evaluating the effectiveness of IV oxytocin for a client with secondary dystocia, the nurse should expect:

  ○ **A.** A precipitous delivery

  ○ **B.** Cervical effacement with delivery

  ○ **C.** Infrequent contractions lasting longer than 90 seconds

  ○ **D.** Progressive cervical dilation with contractions lasting less than 90 seconds

92. A test is scheduled for tomorrow. The student states, "I can't think about that test today." The student is using the defense mechanism known as:

   ○ **A.** Suppression

   ○ **B.** Repression

   ○ **C.** Denial

   ○ **D.** Rationalization

93. A client is admitted for treatment of long-standing substance abuse. During the intake assessment, the client states, "I don't know what everyone is so upset about. I don't have a problem because I can quit anytime I want to." The client's statement is an example of:

   ○ **A.** Displacement

   ○ **B.** Denial

   ○ **C.** Rationalization

   ○ **D.** Reaction formation

94. A client with borderline personality disorder refuses to talk with the staff and demands to see his doctor. He insists that only the doctor knows what is best for him. The client is using the defense mechanism referred to as:

   ○ **A.** Denial

   ○ **B.** Splitting

   ○ **C.** Projection

   ○ **D.** Rationalization

95. A client is admitted for psychiatric evaluation after she attempted to stab her husband. On learning that he plans to visit, she states, "I'm so glad my husband is coming to see me." The client is using the defense mechanism known as:

   ○ **A.** Transference

   ○ **B.** Rationalization

   ○ **C.** Conversion reaction

   ○ **D.** Reaction formation

96. A client admitted with frequent urinary tract infections is scheduled for an IVP. Preparation for an IVP includes:

   ○ **A.** Collection of a 24-hour urine

   ○ **B.** Administration of a laxative

   ○ **C.** A soft, bland diet the evening before the scheduled x-ray

   ○ **D.** Administration of radiopaque tablets the morning of the x-ray

97. A client with suspected renal cancer is admitted with complaints of hematuria. Further assessment of the client would most likely reveal the presence of:

   ○ **A.** Urinary casts

   ○ **B.** Costovertebral mass

   ○ **C.** Suprapubic pain

   ○ **D.** Burning on urination

98. A client with an acute attack of gouty arthritis is started on allopurinol. The client should be instructed to:

   ○ **A.** Take the medication 30 minutes before meals.

   ○ **B.** Increase his fluid intake to 3000 ml per day.

   ○ **C.** Take the medication before going to bed.

   ○ **D.** Rise slowly from a sitting position to prevent dizziness.

99. A client taking Atorvastation (Lipitor) asks the nurse the purpose of the medication. The nurse should tell the client that the medication will:

   ○ **A.** Decrease her blood pressure

   ○ **B.** Improve her appetite

   ○ **C.** Decrease her cholesterol level

   ○ **D.** Improve her bone density

100. A client with renovascular hypertension returns from having a renal arteriogram. The nurse should give priority to:

   ○ **A.** Applying warm wet packs to the insertion site

   ○ **B.** Encouraging the client to flex and extend the procedural leg

   ○ **C.** Withholding PO fluids for 4–6 hours after the procedure

   ○ **D.** Checking the color, temperature, and pulses in the procedural leg

101. Anasarca, a characteristic finding in clients with nephritic syndrome, is due to renal changes that result in:

   ○ **A.** Hypoalbuminemia

   ○ **B.** Hypertension

   ○ **C.** Hyperalbuminemia

   ○ **D.** Hyperthermia

102. Which of the following findings is most typical of a client with a fractured hip?

   ○ **A.** Pain in the hip and affected leg

   ○ **B.** Diminished sensation in the affected leg

   ○ **C.** Absence of pedal and femoral pulses in the affected extremity

   ○ **D.** Disalignment of the affected extremity

103. A client receiving aminophylline complains of nausea and "feeling jittery." The nurse's first action should be to:

   ○ **A.** Administer an antiemetic.

   ○ **B.** Check the client's blood pressure.

   ○ **C.** Request a sedative.

   ○ **D.** Check the aminophylline level.

104. A gravida 2 para 0 is admitted from the ER with spontaneous rupture of membranes. She states that she has seen the doctor only twice during the pregnancy and that she is unsure of her exact due date. Exam reveals the presence of green-tinged fluid in the vaginal vault. The fetus is noted to be in a LOP position with an FHR of 110 BPM. Based on the assessment, the nurse suspects:

   ○ **A.** Fetal distress

   ○ **B.** The presence of an intrauterine infection

   ○ **C.** A post-mature fetus

   ○ **D.** That the fetus has a TE fistula

105. A male client is admitted for evaluation of a sudden hearing loss. No physical cause can be found for his sudden deafness; however, a friend reveals that the client's fiancée recently canceled their engagement, saying that she needed more time to think about the marriage. The client's deafness is an example of:

- ○ **A.** Conversion reaction
- ○ **B.** Hypochondriasis
- ○ **C.** Reaction formation
- ○ **D.** Histrionic personality disorder

106. The best choice for the child following a tonsillectomy is:

- ○ **A.** Fruit punch
- ○ **B.** Strawberry soda
- ○ **C.** Banana Popsicle
- ○ **D.** Ice cream

107. The nurse is monitoring a client receiving an IV of Nipride in D5W. The IV bag has a foil covering, and the nurse notes that the IV fluid has a light brownish tint. The nurse should:

- ○ **A.** Discard the solution.
- ○ **B.** Obtain a bag of normal saline.
- ○ **C.** Cover both the solution bag and the IV tubing with foil.
- ○ **D.** Do nothing because the solution is expected to be light brown in color.

108. A client is admitted to the ER with reported heroin intoxication. Which of the following signs is consistent with opiate use?

- ○ **A.** The client's pupils are dilated.
- ○ **B.** The client's speech is rapid.
- ○ **C.** The client's BP is elevated.
- ○ **D.** The client's pupils are constricted.

109. A client with seizure disorder has an order for Dilantin (phenyltoin) IVP. The nurse knows that Dilantin should:

- ○ **A.** Be administered in a solution of D5W
- ○ **B.** Be administered in a solution of LR
- ○ **C.** Not be administered any faster than 50 mg/minute
- ○ **D.** Not be administered IVP

110. The client with COPD is admitted with a total hip replacement. The best position for the client with a right total hip replacement is:

- ○ **A.** With the right hip flexed 90°
- ○ **B.** With the right hip flexed 35°
- ○ **C.** Supine with pillows supporting the right leg
- ○ **D.** Sims' position with the right leg adducted

111. An 18-month-old has been hospitalized six times for upper airway infections. Diagnostic studies including sweat analysis confirm the diagnosis of cystic fibrosis, an autosomal recessive disorder affecting the exocrine system. Which of the following statements describes the inheritance pattern for autosomal recessive disorders?

- ○ **A.** An affected gene is inherited from both the father and mother, who remain symptom free.
- ○ **B.** Males are affected at twice the rate as females.
- ○ **C.** Autosomal recessive disorders tend to skip generations, so the children of affected parents will have children with the disorder.
- ○ **D.** The disorder is transmitted by an affected gene on one of the six chromosomes.

112. A nine-month-old is seen in the well child clinic. During the nursing assessment, the mother asks, "Shouldn't he be making baby sounds by now? My friend's little boy is the same age and he is already saying *dada*." The nurse reports the mother's concerns to the doctor for follow-up based on the knowledge that infants should be making rudimentary sounds by age:

- ○ **A.** one month
- ○ **B.** two months
- ○ **C.** four months
- ○ **D.** eight months

113. A football player is well paid for his superior athletic ability. Described by his friends as quiet and brooding, on the field he is known for his overly aggressive plays. The client's behavior is an example of:

- ○ **A.** Displacement
- ○ **B.** Conversion
- ○ **C.** Sublimation
- ○ **D.** Repression

114. A 15-month-old continually turns his cup upside down and shakes milk from the spout. The mother is convinced that he does this on purpose and asks the nurse what she should do. The nurse's response should be guided by the knowledge that:

- ○ **A.** Toddlers often misbehave to get the attention of adults.
- ○ **B.** Toddlers are able to use thought processes to experience events and reactions.
- ○ **C.** Negative actions that are not immediately punished will be repeated.
- ○ **D.** Manipulation of objects in their environment enables the toddler to learn about spatial relationships.

115. A father suspected of child abuse tells the nurse, "I shouldn't have grabbed him so hard. I had a really bad day at work and got all stressed out. The kid just wouldn't listen to me." The defense mechanism used by the father is:

- ○ **A.** Projection
- ○ **B.** Displacement
- ○ **C.** Undoing
- ○ **D.** Compensation

116. A female client seen in the health department's STD clinic is diagnosed with chlamydia. Before the client leaves the clinic, the nurse should:

- ○ **A.** Obtain the names and addresses of the client's sexual contacts.
- ○ **B.** Tell the client to avoid alcohol while taking her prescription for Flagyl.
- ○ **C.** Instruct the client to avoid sexual relations until the infection is resolved.
- ○ **D.** Tell the client to douche after sexual intercourse.

117. A client with iron deficiency anemia is started on ferrous sulfate tablets. The nurse has instructed the client on the appropriate way to take her medication. Which of the following statements indicates that the client understands the nurse's teaching?

- ○ **A.** "I can take my iron tablets with a glass of milk."
- ○ **B.** "I need to take my iron tablets daily before breakfast."
- ○ **C.** "Taking my iron tablets before I go to bed will cut down on stomach upset."
- ○ **D.** "Taking my iron tablets with a glass of orange juice will help me absorb more of the medicine.

118. Which of the following infants is in need of additional growth assessment?

   ○ **A.** Baby girl A: age 4 months, BW 7 pounds 6 ounces, present weight 14 pounds 14 ounces

   ○ **B.** Baby girl B: age 2 weeks, BW 6 pounds 10 ounces, present weight 6 pounds 11 ounces

   ○ **C.** Baby girl C: age 6 months, BW 8 pounds 9 ounces, present weight 15 pounds 0 ounces

   ○ **D.** Baby girl D: age 2 months, BW 7 pounds 2 ounces, present weight 9 pounds 10 ounces

119. A client on assisted ventilation develops a right-sided tension pneumothorax. Which of the following signs is associated with a right-sided tension pneumothorax?

   ○ **A.** Diminished breath sounds on the right

   ○ **B.** Left-sided tracheal deviation

   ○ **C.** Right-sided tracheal deviation

   ○ **D.** Presence of bilateral ronchi

120. A client arrives at the emergency room with an HR of 120, an RR of 48, and hemoptysis. The nurse should give priority to:

   ○ **A.** Obtaining a history of the current illness

   ○ **B.** Applying oxygen via mask

   ○ **C.** Obtaining additional vital signs

   ○ **D.** Checking arterial blood gases

121. The nurse is performing a post-op assessment of an elderly client with a total hip repair. Although he has not requested medication for pain, the nurse suspects that the client's discomfort is severe and prepares to administer pain medication. Which of the following signs would not support the nurse's assessment of acute post-op pain?

   ○ **A.** Increased blood pressure

   ○ **B.** Inability to concentrate

   ○ **C.** Dilated pupils

   ○ **D.** Decreased heart rate

122. An obstetrical client elects to have epidural anesthesia with Marcaine. After the epidural anesthesia is given, the nurse should monitor the client for signs of:

  ❍ **A.** Seizure activity

  ❍ **B.** Respiratory depression

  ❍ **C.** Postural hypotension

  ❍ **D.** Hematuria

123. A client in the intensive care unit is overheard telling his wife, "It's impossible to get any sleep in this place with all the noise and lights on all the time." After talking with the client, the nurse determines that the client is bothered by sensory disturbance related to being in the ICU. Which laboratory finding would confirm the nurse's assessment of sensory disturbance?

  ❍ **A.** Increased urine catecholamines

  ❍ **B.** Decreased TSH

  ❍ **C.** Erratic changes in BUN levels

  ❍ **D.** Increased blood glucose levels

124. Immediately after surgery the client with an above-the-knee amputation of the right leg refuses to look at the operative site. The most immediate diagnosis that can be made is:

  ❍ **A.** Self-care deficit

  ❍ **B.** Potential for infection

  ❍ **C.** Disturbance in self-concept

  ❍ **D.** Cognitive deficit

125. Which of the following describes the proximodistal development in the infant?

  ❍ **A.** The infant is able to raise his head before he is able to sit.

  ❍ **B.** The infant can control movements of his arms before he can control movements of his fingers.

  ❍ **C.** The infant responds to pain with his whole body before he can localize pain.

  ❍ **D.** The infant is able to make rudimentary vocalizations before using spoken words.

126. The RN is preparing to administer a transfusion of whole blood. Which action by the nurse predisposes the client to the development of hyperkalemia?

  ○ **A.** Allowing the blood to warm to room temperature

  ○ **B.** Administering blood that is 24 hours old

  ○ **C.** Administering blood with an 18-gauge needle

  ○ **D.** Filling the drip chamber below the level of the filter

127. A client with abdominal surgery is admitted to the recovery room with an NG tube to low suction. Which of the following lab values indicates a complication of NG suction?

  ○ **A.** Hgb 13.0 gm

  ○ **B.** Na 150 mEq/L

  ○ **C.** K 3.4 mEq/L

  ○ **D.** Cl 90 mEq/L

128. Which of the following statements regarding wound healing is correct?

  ○ **A.** Healing occurs within 10 days.

  ○ **B.** Healing by second intention results in excessive scar formation.

  ○ **C.** Third intention healing involves an open wound with healing taking place from the inside out.

  ○ **D.** Healing by third intention is accomplished through immediate wound closure by staples or sutures.

129. The nurse is teaching bladder management to a client with paraplegia. Which of the following statements indicates the client needs further teaching on dietary modifications to accommodate bladder changes?

  ○ **A.** "I need to eat plenty of citrus fruits to prevent bladder infections."

  ○ **B.** "I need to drink at least eight glasses of water a day."

  ○ **C.** "Including cranberry juice in my diet will prevent urinary infections."

  ○ **D.** "I need to avoid milk and milk products."

130. A client with mastoiditis has a left mastoidectomy with tympanoplasty. The nurse should observe the client for signs of damage to the sixth cranial nerve, which include:

- ○ **A.** Inability to chew
- ○ **B.** Inability to look laterally
- ○ **C.** Inability to swallow
- ○ **D.** Loss of scalp sensation

131. The nurse caring for a client with Meniere's syndrome can help minimize attacks by teaching the client to limit her dietary intake of:

- ○ **A.** Fats
- ○ **B.** Carbohydrates
- ○ **C.** Sugars
- ○ **D.** Salt

132. The nurse is caring for a dark-skinned client hospitalized with hepatitis. The nurse can best observe the presence of jaundice in the client by assessing the client's:

- ○ **A.** Palms and soles
- ○ **B.** Nail beds
- ○ **C.** Sclera
- ○ **D.** Hard palate

133. A two-year-old is hospitalized with gastroenteritis and dehydration. Which of the following methods is best for evaluating changes in skin turgor?

- ○ **A.** Pinching the abdominal tissue while the client is supine
- ○ **B.** Pinching the tissue of the forearm while the client is sitting
- ○ **C.** Pressing the skin of the lower extremities while the client is supine
- ○ **D.** Pinching the skin of the lower extremities while the client is sitting

134. Which of the following meals would be best tolerated by the client receiving Leukeran?

- ○ **A.** Peanut butter sandwich, orange juice, and Jell-O
- ○ **B.** Warm pea soup, apricot fruit slush, and ice cream
- ○ **C.** Lasagna with meat sauce, salad, and tea
- ○ **D.** Steak, baked potato, and milk

135. A client with myxedema should be prescribed which diet?

    ○ **A.** Fats

    ○ **B.** Carbohydrates

    ○ **C.** Sugars

    ○ **D.** Low salt

136. The nurse is caring for a client from the Middle East. The nurse is aware that the client will most likely:

    ○ **A.** Want to take time for prayer during the day

    ○ **B.** Ask for specially prepared foods

    ○ **C.** Refuse blood products

    ○ **D.** Want to be treated by a medicine man

137. A 15-year-old hospitalized with a sarcoma is being treated with Adriamycin. Which action by the nurse indicates an understanding of the drug?

    ○ **A.** The nurse asks the client whether she would like to talk about the treatment she's receiving.

    ○ **B.** The nurse implements isolation precautions.

    ○ **C.** The nurse provides the client with a wig.

    ○ **D.** The nurse strains the client's urine.

138. Which of the following activities would be best tolerated by a client with muscular dystrophy?

    ○ **A.** Swimming

    ○ **B.** Riding a bicycle

    ○ **C.** Playing golf

    ○ **D.** Skating

139. A client undergoes cryosurgery for the removal of a basal cell carcinoma on the ear. Which of the following best describes the appearance of the area a few days after surgery?

    ○ **A.** It's dry, crusty, and itchy.

    ○ **B.** It's oozing and painful.

    ○ **C.** It's dry and tender.

    ○ **D.** It's swollen, tender, and blistered.

140. A culture is taken of a lesion suspected of being herpes. The nurse knows that the specimen:

- ○ **A.** Should be packed on ice
- ○ **B.** Should be kept warm
- ○ **C.** Should be double-bagged
- ○ **D.** Requires no special handling

141. A client with AIDS shows symptoms of herpes simplex stomatitis. Which drug therapy can be anticipated for the client?

- ○ **A.** Lypressin
- ○ **B.** Liothyroxine
- ○ **C.** Acyclovir
- ○ **D.** Dexamethasone

142. While assisting a client with AM care, the nurse notes small elevated skin lesions less than 0.5 cm in diameter over the client's back. The nurse should describe the lesions as:

- ○ **A.** Macules
- ○ **B.** Plaques
- ○ **C.** Wheals
- ○ **D.** Papules

143. A six-month-old is brought to the ER by her mother. During the assessment, the nurse finds multiple bruises in different stages of healing and decreased range of motion of the right leg. X-ray confirms a fracture of the right femur. Which statement made by the mother would contribute to a diagnosis of child abuse?

- ○ **A.** "She got her leg caught in the crib and twisted it."
- ○ **B.** "She hurt her leg while she was crawling."
- ○ **C.** "I can't remember her falling or getting hurt."
- ○ **D.** "She fell out of her car seat before I could get the belt fastened."

144. A client with a pyloric obstruction is admitted to the hospital with persistent vomiting. Which of the following blood gases would the nurse expect to see in the client with vomiting?

- ○ **A.** pH 7.33, PCO_2 30 mm Hg
- ○ **B.** pH 7.50, PCO_2 32 mm Hg
- ○ **C.** pH 7.30, PCO_2 50 mm Hg
- ○ **D.** pH 7.47, PCO_2 40 mm Hg

145. The doctor has ordered the insertion of an NG tube to determine the extent of gastric bleeding in a client with a gastric ulcer. To facilitate the insertion of the NG tube, the nurse should:

    ○ **A.** Place the NG tube in warm water prior to insertion.

    ○ **B.** Place the client in a supine position.

    ○ **C.** Ask the client to swallow as the tube is advanced.

    ○ **D.** Ask the client to hyperextend his neck as the nurse begins to insert the tube.

146. A client with acute leukemia has developed oral ulcerations. The nurse can increase the client's comfort by suggesting that he:

    ○ **A.** Avoid brushing his teeth until the ulcers heal

    ○ **B.** Rinse his mouth frequently with normal saline

    ○ **C.** Rinse his mouth frequently with hydrogen peroxide

    ○ **D.** Cleanse his teeth and mouth with lemon and glycerin swabs

147. The parents of a child with cystic fibrosis discuss nutritional requirements and the need for vitamin supplements with the nurse. The nurse explains that it is necessary to give daily supplements of vitamins A, D, E, and K because:

    ○ **A.** Children with cystic fibrosis require vitamin supplements because their metabolism is increased.

    ○ **B.** Children with cystic fibrosis do not eat a well-balanced diet.

    ○ **C.** Children with cystic fibrosis do not absorb fat-soluble vitamins.

    ○ **D.** Children with cystic fibrosis have an increased excretion of water-soluble vitamins.

148. A client with a gastric ulcer is losing a significant amount of blood via the NG tube. The client's pulse is weak and thready, and she is hypotensive. A continuous irrigation of normal saline is ordered. How should the client be positioned?

    ○ **A.** High Fowler's

    ○ **B.** Semi-Fowler's

    ○ **C.** Supine

    ○ **D.** Left-side lying

149. A client with diabetes insipidus will require lifelong therapy with vasopressin. Which of the following should the nurse include in his teaching plan for the client?

- ○ **A.** The client will need to take her medication with meals.
- ○ **B.** The client will need to learn how to check the specific gravity of her urine.
- ○ **C.** The client will need to modify her daily activities.
- ○ **D.** The client will need to learn the proper method of drug administration.

150. Which of the following instructions should be included in the pre-op teaching of a client scheduled for a transphenoidal hypophysectomy for the removal of a pituitary tumor?

- ○ **A.** "It will be necessary to shave some of your hair."
- ○ **B.** "It will be important for you to cough and deep breathe after the surgery."
- ○ **C.** "You will need to lie supine for 24 hours after surgery."
- ○ **D.** "You will not be able to brush your teeth for at least a week after surgery."

151. A 34-year-old male is admitted to the hospital with a possible diagnosis of pheochromocytoma. Which of the following symptoms would the nurse not expect to see during an attack?

- ○ **A.** Hypertension
- ○ **B.** Diaphoresis
- ○ **C.** Apprehension
- ○ **D.** Bradycardia

152. A client with suspected Addison's disease is scheduled for a rapid corticotrophin stimulation test. Which of the following will the nurse include in her teaching?

- ○ **A.** The need to limit fluid intake
- ○ **B.** The need for periodic blood samples
- ○ **C.** The need for collection of a 24-hour urine
- ○ **D.** The need for frequent IV injections

153. Which of the following lab values might the nurse expect to see in a client with Addison's disease?

- ○ **A.** WBC 10,000
- ○ **B.** BUN 22
- ○ **C.** K+ 3.5 mEq/L
- ○ **D.** Na+ 142 mEq/L

154. A 56-year-old male is admitted with a diagnosis of gastroesophageal reflux disease (GERD). The client is most likely to report esophageal discomfort following a meal of:

   ○ **A.** Chicken in lemon sauce, rice, and fruit juice

   ○ **B.** Turkey, salad, and a glass of red wine

   ○ **C.** Poached salmon, mashed potatoes, and milk

   ○ **D.** Hamburger, peas, and cola

155. A 28-year-old client is being treated with acute pelvic inflammatory disease. Which of the following positions will afford the most comfort for this client?

   ○ **A.** Prone

   ○ **B.** Flat, left Sims'

   ○ **C.** Semi-Fowler's

   ○ **D.** Flat, with legs elevated

156. A client with ulcerative colitis is placed on Azulfidine. Which of the following instructions should be included in the nurse's teaching?

   ○ **A.** The client should be instructed to avoid exposure to sunlight because the drug causes sun sensitivity.

   ○ **B.** The client should be instructed to take the medication with meals.

   ○ **C.** The client should be instructed to take the medication even when he is feeling well.

   ○ **D.** The client should be instructed to take the medication as prescribed because it will stop the loss of blood in the stools.

157. A client with a C6 spinal injury begins to complain of a severe headache. When assessing the client, the nurse notes that her BP is 190/100 and she is diaphoretic. Which of the following nursing actions is most appropriate at this time?

   ○ **A.** Increase the rate of IV fluids.

   ○ **B.** Make sure that the Foley catheter is patent.

   ○ **C.** Place the client flat in bed.

   ○ **D.** Administer oxygen.

158. Which of the following lab reports indicates that a client with acute glomerulonephritis is improving?

- ○ **A.** Positive ASO titer
- ○ **B.** Increased C reactive protein
- ○ **C.** Negative eosinophil count
- ○ **D.** Decreased erythrocyte sedimentation rate

159. Which of the following snacks would be permitted for a child with acute renal failure?

- ○ **A.** Peanut butter and jelly sandwich
- ○ **B.** Orange juice and graham crackers
- ○ **C.** Marshmallows
- ○ **D.** Cheese and crackers

160. Which of the following dietary choices should be avoided by a client with a recent bone marrow transplant?

- ○ **A.** Applesauce
- ○ **B.** Apple juice
- ○ **C.** Apple pie
- ○ **D.** Raw apple

161. Which of the following activities is most suitable for a 10-year-old with asthma?

- ○ **A.** Soccer
- ○ **B.** Swimming
- ○ **C.** Basketball
- ○ **D.** Constructing model cars

162. Which of the following musical instruments is best for a teen with asthma?

- ○ **A.** Guitar
- ○ **B.** Piano
- ○ **C.** Drums
- ○ **D.** Clarinet

163. A client returns from surgery after having a suprapubic prostatectomy. On assessing the client, the nurse notes that his urine is bright red with many clots. Which of the following nursing actions is most appropriate?

- ○ **A.** Check the client's vital signs and notify the physician.

- ○ **B.** Check whether the continuous irrigation is working properly.

- ○ **C.** Recognize that this is a normal finding after surgery and continue post-op care.

- ○ **D.** Apply traction on the catheter and notify the physician.

164. Diuretic therapy for hypertension often necessitates the addition of high-potassium foods in the client's diet. Which of the following diuretics does not require the client to increase his intake of potassium?

- ○ **A.** Spironolactone (Aldactone)

- ○ **B.** Furosemide (Lasix)

- ○ **C.** Hydrochlorothiazide (Hydrodiuril)

- ○ **D.** Ethacrynic acid (Edecrin)

165. Which of the following meals provides the lowest amount of potassium?

- ○ **A.** Orange, cream of wheat, bacon

- ○ **B.** Toast, jelly, soft boiled egg

- ○ **C.** Raisin bran, milk, grapefruit

- ○ **D.** Melon, pancakes, milk

166. Which of the following instructions should be included for the client taking calcium supplements?

- ○ **A.** The client should take her calcium with meals.

- ○ **B.** The client should take all her daily calcium supplement at one time.

- ○ **C.** The client should take her calcium supplement after meals to prevent stomach upset.

- ○ **D.** The client can use calcium-based antacids to supplement her diet.

167. When caring for a client with hypocalcemia, the nurse should assess for:

- ○ **A.** A decreased level of consciousness

- ○ **B.** Tetany

- ○ **C.** Bradycardia

- ○ **D.** Respiratory depression

168. A client is admitted to the burn unit with an electrical burn. Which of the following areas probably sustained the greatest degree of injury?

○ **A.** The skin

○ **B.** The intrathoracic

○ **C.** The muscles supporting the long bones

○ **D.** The bones

169. A client with hyperkalemia is to receive an infusion of 250 ml of 20% glucose with 20 units of regular insulin. The rationale for this therapy is:

○ **A.** Potassium elimination is enhanced.

○ **B.** Potassium binds with the glucose and is excreted by the kidneys.

○ **C.** Glucose uptake by the cell drives the potassium into the cell.

○ **D.** Insulin lowers the potassium by lowering blood glucose.

170. Which of the following organs is most likely to suffer permanent damage from hypovolemic shock?

○ **A.** The heart

○ **B.** The skin

○ **C.** The brain

○ **D.** The kidneys

171. A client has sustained second- and third-degree burns over her entire left arm and posterior trunk. Using the Rule of Nines, which percentage of the client's body is burned?

○ **A.** 9%

○ **B.** 18%

○ **C.** 27%

○ **D.** 36%

172. A client who received complete thickness burns at 7:30 a.m. was rushed to the emergency room where IV therapy with lactated Ringer's was begun. He is to receive 8,000 ml of solution in 24 hours. According to the Parkland formula, how much solution should he receive by 11:30 p.m.?

○ **A.** 4,000 ml

○ **B.** 5,000 ml

○ **C.** 6,000 ml

○ **D.** 7,000 ml

173. The drug of choice for managing status epilepticus is:

   ❍ **A.** Carbamazepine (Tegretol)

   ❍ **B.** Diazepam (Valium)

   ❍ **C.** Clonazepam (Klonopin)

   ❍ **D.** Valproic acid (Depakene)

174. Which of the following electrolytes must be maintained in a steady state for a client receiving lithium?

   ❍ **A.** Sodium

   ❍ **B.** Potassium

   ❍ **C.** Chloride

   ❍ **D.** Magnesium

175. The greatest threat during the immediate post-burn period results from burn shock. Which of the following statements best describes why burn shock occurs?

   ❍ **A.** Damaged tissues release histamine and other substances that can result in vasodilatation and increased capillary permeability with a loss of fluid from the vascular compartment to the interstitial space.

   ❍ **B.** Large amounts of fluid are lost from the burn site, which results in a decrease in circulating volume.

   ❍ **C.** Large amounts of epinephrine are released, leading to severe vasoconstriction and shock.

   ❍ **D.** Release of epinephrine leads to tachycardia, ineffective cardiac output, and shock.

176. A client with an acute attack of gout is started on colchicine. She should be instructed to report which of the following symptoms?

   ❍ **A.** Diarrhea

   ❍ **B.** Headache

   ❍ **C.** Itching

   ❍ **D.** Fever

177. A baby girl is born with a meningomyelocele. To prevent trauma to the sac, the nurse should place the infant:

　　○ **A.** Supine and flat

　　○ **B.** Prone with the hips slightly elevated

　　○ **C.** Prone with the head slightly elevated

　　○ **D.** Side lying

178. A client with a cholesterol level of 240 mg is instructed to modify his diet. Which of the following diets provides a low-cholesterol, low-saturated fat breakfast?

　　○ **A.** Oatmeal, skim milk, toast with margarine, orange juice, coffee

　　○ **B.** French toast, margarine, syrup, crisp bacon, coffee

　　○ **C.** Pancake, margarine, syrup, sausage, fresh fruit, tea

　　○ **D.** Toasted bagel, cream cheese, poached egg, coffee

179. While caring for a child who had a revision of a ventriculoperitoneal shunt, the nurse notes clear drainage from the incision. Which of the following actions should the nurse take first?

　　○ **A.** Notify the physician to obtain further orders.

　　○ **B.** Mark the dressing and continue to monitor.

　　○ **C.** Check the dressing for the presence of glucose.

　　○ **D.** No action is necessary because some drainage is expected.

180. Which of the following findings distinguishes a hydrocele from an inguinal hernia?

　　○ **A.** The swelling cannot be reduced and is translucent.

　　○ **B.** The swelling cannot be reduced and is opaque.

　　○ **C.** The swelling can be reduced and is translucent.

　　○ **D.** The swelling can be reduced and is opaque.

181. A client with lung cancer is advised to increase the protein and kilocalorie content of his diet. Which of the following choices will best meet his need for increased protein and calories?

　　○ **A.** Toast, jelly, chicken broth

　　○ **B.** Crackers, butter, fresh vegetables

　　○ **C.** Crackers, fresh fruit, ginger ale

　　○ **D.** Crackers, cheese, fruit yogurt

182. A child at summer camp comes to see the camp nurse 10 minutes after being stung by a bee. The child complains of tingling around her mouth and tightness in her chest. The nurse's first action is to summon help and to:

○ **A.** Administer O_2 at 4L/min by nasal cannula.

○ **B.** Apply a tourniquet proximal to the bee sting and give epinephrine subcutaneously.

○ **C.** Administer O_2 at 6L/min and give Benadryl 25 mg PO.

○ **D.** Reassure the child that she is only excited due to the sting.

183. A 14-month-old is receiving Digoxin and Lasix twice a day. In planning his care, the nurse should assess for which complication?

○ **A.** Hypokalemia

○ **B.** Hyperkalemia

○ **C.** Hypocalcaemia

○ **D.** Hyponatremia

184. The first postpartal bleeding noted by the mother after delivery is:

○ **A.** Lochia rubra

○ **B.** Lochia serosa

○ **C.** Lochia alba

○ **D.** Lochia canta

185. An elderly client has reduced hepatic functioning. Before giving medication, the nurse should be aware that diminished hepatic function will:

○ **A.** Decrease the possibility of drug toxicity

○ **B.** Prevent analgesics from being given

○ **C.** Reduce the blood level of certain drugs

○ **D.** Increase the possibility of drug toxicity

186. A client with seizure disorder is to receive Dilantin (phenytoin) and phenobarbital. The nurse knows that when she administers phenobarbital and phenytoin that:

- ○ **A.** A larger dose of phenobarbital might be required because of an increase in metabolism.

- ○ **B.** A smaller dose of phenobarbital might be required because of a decrease in metabolism.

- ○ **C.** There will be no need to alter the amount of phenobarbital given.

- ○ **D.** The two drugs cannot be given together.

187. While assessing a pre-op client, the nurse learns that the client is allergic to shellfish. How might this data affect the client's surgical experience?

- ○ **A.** The anesthesiologist might need to alter the type of anesthesia used.

- ○ **B.** The physician might need to alter the type of skin preparation used.

- ○ **C.** The physician might need to alter the type of antibiotics ordered post-operatively.

- ○ **D.** The physician might need to monitor the client's thyroid levels post-operatively.

188. The nurse is reviewing a client's pre-op lab values. Which of the following lab results warrants immediate attention?

- ○ **A.** Prothrombin time of 1 minute and 20 seconds

- ○ **B.** Hematocrit 38 ml/dl

- ○ **C.** Hemoglobin 14 g/dl

- ○ **D.** White blood count 6,000/mm

189. Spinal headaches are a common occurrence following spinal anesthesia. Which of the following nursing interventions can help prevent a spinal headache?

- ○ **A.** Placing the client in a quiet room

- ○ **B.** Significantly increasing the client's fluid intake

- ○ **C.** Administering PRN pain medication

- ○ **D.** Raising the head of the bed to 45°

190. A client with a recent spinal cord injury is experiencing dysreflexia and is noted to have a BP of 240/110. The nurse's initial response should be to:

○ **A.** Check the client's pulse and respiratory rate.

○ **B.** Elevate the client's head to a 45° angle.

○ **C.** Place the client flat and supine.

○ **D.** Administer antihypertensive and recheck BP in 15 minutes.

191. Which of the following instructions should be given to a client regarding testicular self-exam?

○ **A.** The testicular exam should be done bimonthly.

○ **B.** The testicular exam should be done while in the shower or tub.

○ **C.** A small penlight should be used to transilluminate the scrotal sac.

○ **D.** The testicular exam should be done yearly.

192. A six-month-old has been hospitalized for the treatment of acute diarrhea. Discharge diet includes the use of Isomil instead of Similac formula until the next clinic appointment. Which of the following statements explains the change in infant formula?

○ **A.** Isomil is less expensive than Similac.

○ **B.** The infant has developed a permanent lactose intolerance.

○ **C.** Isomil is an excellent oral rehydration formula.

○ **D.** Infants commonly have a lactose intolerance after a diarrheal illness.

193. The client has a cast applied following a fracture of the femur. The doctor tells the nurse to petal the cast. The nurse is aware that he intends for her to:

○ **A.** Cut the cast down both sides.

○ **B.** Cut a window in the cast.

○ **C.** Cover the edges with cast batting.

○ **D.** Cut the cast down one side.

194. The client with a colostomy does not feel that the irrigating solution has drained completely. The nurse can enhance the effectiveness of the colostomy irrigation by telling the client to:

○ **A.** Massage the abdomen gently.

○ **B.** Reduce the amount of irrigation solution.

○ **C.** Increase his oral intake.

○ **D.** Place a heating pad on the abdomen.

195. A client with a partial bowel obstruction has a Miller-Abbot tube inserted to decompress the bowel. While the tube is in place, the nurse should give priority to:

○ **A.** Using only normal saline to irrigate the tube every four hours

○ **B.** Advancing the tube 3–4 inches as ordered by the physician

○ **C.** Changing the tape securing the tube to the client's face daily to prevent skin breakdown

○ **D.** Attaching the tube to high constant suction

196. A client is brought to the emergency room with injuries sustained in an auto accident. While performing his assessment, the nurse notes the presence of Cullen's sign. Cullen's sign is suggestive of:

○ **A.** A neurological injury

○ **B.** A ruptured spleen

○ **C.** A bowel perforation

○ **D.** Retroperitoneal bleeding

197. A client with chronic pancreatitis is receiving pancreatin. Which of the following observations is most indicative that the drug treatment is having the desired effect?

○ **A.** The client's appetite is improved.

○ **B.** The client's weight loss is greater than 10 pounds.

○ **C.** The client's stools contain less fat and occur with less frequency.

○ **D.** The client's tissue bruises less easily.

198. A non-stress test has been ordered for a pregnant client with diabetes mellitus. Non-stress testing is a part of the diabetic's prenatal care because:

○ **A.** Fetal movement is adversely affected by diabetes.

○ **B.** Maternal insulin levels can have a negative effect on fetal energy.

○ **C.** Diabetes can adversely affect development of placental vessels.

○ **D.** Fetal lung maturity is most easily determined by non-stress testing.

199. The obstetric client is determined to have oligohydramnios. Which fetal anomaly is associated with oligohydramnios?

○ **A.** Diabetes

○ **B.** Renal agenesis

○ **C.** Tracheo-esophageal fistula

○ **D.** Tracheo-esophageal atresia

200. A client receiving aminophylline IV complains of feeling nervous and shaky. The nurse is aware that these are symptoms of:

  ○ **A.** CNS depression that accompanies xanthine derivatives

  ○ **B.** CNS stimulation that sometimes accompanies xanthine derivatives

  ○ **C.** The anticholinergic effects of aminophylline

  ○ **D.** Cardiovascular depression that can accompany xanthine derivatives

201. The client with herpes zoster will most likely have an order for which category of medication?

  ○ **A.** Antibiotics

  ○ **B.** Antipyretics

  ○ **C.** Antivirals

  ○ **D.** Anticoagulants

202. A client with chronic bronchitis is admitted with complaints of chest pain. Which of the following drug orders should the nurse question?

  ○ **A.** Nitroglycerin

  ○ **B.** Ampicillin

  ○ **C.** Propranolol

  ○ **D.** Verapamil

203. Which of the following instructions should be included in the teaching for the client with arthritis?

  ○ **A.** Avoid exercise because it fatigues the joints.

  ○ **B.** Take prescribed anti-inflammatory medications with meals.

  ○ **C.** Apply hot compresses at night.

  ○ **D.** Avoid weight-bearing activity.

204. An elderly client with a fractured hip is placed in Buck's traction. The primary purpose for Buck's traction for this client is:

  ○ **A.** To decrease muscle spasms

  ○ **B.** To prevent the need for surgery

  ○ **C.** To alleviate the pain associated with the fracture

  ○ **D.** To prevent bleeding associated with hip fractures

205. *Triage* refers to the classification of injury severity during a disaster. Which of the following clients should receive priority during triage?

- ○ **A.** Open fractures of the tibia and fibula
- ○ **B.** Burns of the head and neck
- ○ **C.** Crushing injury of the arm
- ○ **D.** Contusions and lacerations of the head without loss of consciousness

206. The client is admitted to the unit with the following lab values. Which of the following lab values should be reported immediately?

- ○ **A.** BUN 18 mg/dl
- ○ **B.** PO_2 72%
- ○ **C.** Hemoglobin 10 mg/dl
- ○ **D.** White blood cell count of 5500

207. Which of the following findings is consistent with a diagnosis of cardiac overload?

- ○ **A.** Central venous pressure reading of 15
- ○ **B.** Carbon dioxide reading of 30
- ○ **C.** Hemoglobin of 18
- ○ **D.** Potassium level of 5.5

208. A 28-year-old primigravida with pregestational diabetes visits the clinic six weeks gestation. Which of the following statements indicates that she understands the nurse's teaching regarding her insulin needs during pregnancy?

- ○ **A.** "As the baby grows, I will need more insulin because the baby will not be able to make insulin."
- ○ **B.** "Changes in hormone levels will make my body more resistant to insulin, so I will need more insulin as the pregnancy progresses."
- ○ **C.** "As the baby grows, I will need less insulin because the baby uses up any extra glucose."
- ○ **D.** "If I maintain an adequate balance of diet and exercise, my insulin requirements will be the same."

209. Which of the following positions is best for a client with preeclampsia who is in labor?

   ◯ **A.** Left Sims'

   ◯ **B.** High Fowler's

   ◯ **C.** Trendelenberg

   ◯ **D.** Supine

210. A symptom of impending cardiac decompensation in a pregnant client with heart disease is:

   ◯ **A.** Increasing dyspnea

   ◯ **B.** Transient palpitations

   ◯ **C.** Occasional activity intolerance

   ◯ **D.** Periodic shortness of breath

211. A client with acute pancreatitis is experiencing severe abdominal pain. Which of the following orders should be questioned by the nurse?

   ◯ **A.** Meperidine 100 mg IM q 4 hours PRN pain

   ◯ **B.** Mylanta 30 ccs q 4 hours via NG

   ◯ **C.** Cimetadine 300 mg PO q.i.d.

   ◯ **D.** Morphine 8 mg IM q 4 hours PRN pain

212. A client is admitted, and an order for continuous observation is written. The nurse is aware of this order because he knows that hallucinogenic drugs differ from other drugs of abuse in their capacity to:

   ◯ **A.** Create both stimulant and depressant effects

   ◯ **B.** Induce states of altered perception

   ◯ **C.** Produce severe respiratory depression

   ◯ **D.** Induce rapid physical dependence

213. A client with a history of abusing amphetamines abruptly stops her drug use. The nurse should give priority to assessing the client for:

   ◯ **A.** Depression and suicidal ideation

   ◯ **B.** Diaphoresis and tachypnea

   ◯ **C.** Muscle cramping and abdominal pain

   ◯ **D.** Tachycardia and euphoric mood

214. During the assessment of a laboring client, the nurse notes that the FHT are loudest in the upper left quadrant. The infant is most likely in which position?

- ○ **A.** Left mentum anterior
- ○ **B.** Left occipital anterior
- ○ **C.** Left sacral anterior
- ○ **D.** Left occipital transverse

215. The primary physiological alteration in the development of asthma is:

- ○ **A.** Bronchiolar inflammation and dyspnea
- ○ **B.** Hypersecretion of abnormally viscous mucus
- ○ **C.** Induction of histamine mucosal edema
- ○ **D.** Spasm of bronchiolar smooth muscle

216. A client with mania is busy investigating the unit and overseeing the activities of others. She is unable to finish her dinner. To help her maintain sufficient nourishment, the nurse should:

- ○ **A.** Serve high-calorie foods she can carry with her.
- ○ **B.** Encourage her appetite by sending out for her favorite foods.
- ○ **C.** Serve her small, attractively arranged portions.
- ○ **D.** Allow her in the unit kitchen for extra food whenever she pleases.

217. To maintain Bryant's traction, the nurse must make certain that the child's:

- ○ **A.** Hips are resting on the bed with the legs suspended at a right angle to the bed
- ○ **B.** Hips are slightly elevated above the bed with the legs suspended at a right angle to the bed
- ○ **C.** Hips are elevated above the level of the body on a pillow with the legs suspended parallel to the bed
- ○ **D.** Hips and legs are flat on the bed with the traction positioned at the foot of the bed

218. Which of the following signs is highly suggestive of impaired hearing in an infant?

- ○ **A.** The absence of the Moro reflex
- ○ **B.** The absence of babbling by age 7 months
- ○ **C.** A lack of eye contact when spoken to
- ○ **D.** A lack of hand gesture to indicate wants

219. After four days of extreme anxiety, a hospitalized toddler appears to settle in. He seems uncon-cerned when his parents come to visit. The nurse knows that:

    ○   **A.** He is experiencing detachment.

    ○   **B.** He has successfully adjusted to the hospital environment.

    ○   **C.** He has accepted hospitalization and seeing his parents too frequently will only renew his anxiety.

    ○   **D.** He has transferred his attachment to the nursing staff.

220. An order is written for a peak to be drawn on a client receiving Garamycin. The nurse is aware that he should contact the lab for them to draw the blood:

    ○   **A.** 15 minutes after the infusion

    ○   **B.** 30 minutes after the infusion

    ○   **C.** 1 hour after the infusion

    ○   **D.** 2 hours after the infusion

221. A client with an embolus is started on a continuous heparin infusion to run at 1,200 units per hour. The solution contains 12,500 units of heparin per 250 ml of normal saline. The IV set should be regulated to deliver how many milliliters per hour?

    ○   **A.** 12

    ○   **B.** 24

    ○   **C.** 36

    ○   **D.** 48

222. A client using a diaphragm should be instructed to:

    ○   **A.** Refrain from keeping the diaphragm in longer than eight hours.

    ○   **B.** Keep the diaphragm in a warm location.

    ○   **C.** Have the diaphragm resized if she gains five pounds.

    ○   **D.** Have the diaphragm resized if she has any surgery.

223. The nurse is providing postpartum teaching for a non-nursing mother. Which of the client's state-ments indicates the need for additional teaching?

    ○   **A.** "I'm wearing a support bra."

    ○   **B.** "I'm expressing milk from my breast."

    ○   **C.** "I'm drinking four glasses of fluid during a 24-hour period."

    ○   **D.** "While I'm in the shower, I'll keep the water from running over my breasts."

224. Damage to the VIII cranial nerve results in:

- ○ **A.** Air conduction loss
- ○ **B.** Sensorineural loss
- ○ **C.** Mixed hearing disorders
- ○ **D.** Tinnitus

225. A client is receiving vincristine. The client should be taught that the medication can:

- ○ **A.** Cause diarrhea
- ○ **B.** Change the color of her urine
- ○ **C.** Cause mental confusion
- ○ **D.** Cause changes in taste

226. Which of the following nursing interventions is essential when caring for a client who is receiving cyclophosphamide?

- ○ **A.** Monitoring vital signs q 1 hour
- ○ **B.** Carefully monitoring of urine output
- ○ **C.** Monitoring apical pulse
- ○ **D.** Assessing for signs of increased intracranial pressure

227. A client with AIDS has lesions from herpes simplex virus. He is receiving intravenous acyclovir. Which nursing intervention is most critical during the administration of acyclovir?

- ○ **A.** Limit the client's activity.
- ○ **B.** Encourage a high-carbohydrate diet.
- ○ **C.** Utilize an incentive spirometer to improve respiratory function.
- ○ **D.** Encourage fluids.

228. A danger following bone marrow transplantation is graft-host disease. The first sign of graft-host disease is:

- ○ **A.** Chest pain
- ○ **B.** Rash
- ○ **C.** ECG changes
- ○ **D.** Fever

229. A client is admitted for an MRI, a CT scan, and a myelogram. Which of the following medication orders should be questioned for the client who is to have a myelogram?

- ○ **A.** Ampicillin 250 mg PO q 6 hours
- ○ **B.** Motrin 400 mg PO q 4 hours PRN for headache
- ○ **C.** Seconal 50 mg HS PRN sleep
- ○ **D.** Darvon 65 mg PO q 4 hours for pain

230. A client admitted with a severe head injury following an MVA is placed on a ventilator and hyper-ventilation is maintained. The primary reason for maintaining hyperventilation is:

- ○ **A.** To increase oxygen to the brain
- ○ **B.** To dilate the cerebral blood volume
- ○ **C.** To increase the cerebral blood volume
- ○ **D.** To promote cerebral vasoconstriction and decrease cerebral blood flow

231. While monitoring the urine specific gravity of a client with a head injury, the nurse notes that the client's specific gravity is decreasing and is currently 1.004. The most likely explanation for this finding is:

- ○ **A.** The client is well hydrated.
- ○ **B.** The client is experiencing renal failure.
- ○ **C.** The client has adequate ADH secretion.
- ○ **D.** The client is experiencing diabetes insipidus.

232. The nurse should visit which of the following clients first?

- ○ **A.** The client with diabetes with a blood glucose of 95 mg/dl
- ○ **B.** The client with hypertension being maintained on Lisinopril
- ○ **C.** The client with chest pain and a history of angina
- ○ **D.** The client with Raynaud's disease

233. Following a stroke, a client is found to have receptive aphasia. This finding is consistent with damage to:

- ○ **A.** The frontal lobe
- ○ **B.** The parietal lobe
- ○ **C.** The temporal lobe
- ○ **D.** The occipital lobe

234. During the first 72 hours post CVA, the nurse should position the client:

    ○ **A.** Flat in bed with the head elevated on a small pillow

    ○ **B.** With the head of the bed elevated at 30° and the client's head in a midline neutral position

    ○ **C.** In semi-Fowler's and the knee gatch elevated

    ○ **D.** Flat in bed and lying on the side

235. A client has undergone a lumbar puncture for examination of the CSF. Which of the following findings should be considered abnormal?

    ○ **A.** Total protein 40 mg/100 ml

    ○ **B.** Glucose 60 mg/100 ml

    ○ **C.** Clear, colorless appearance

    ○ **D.** White blood cells 100/cu. mm

236. Which of the following interventions is appropriate when caring for a client who has lost function of cranial nerve V on the left side?

    ○ **A.** Helping the client select foods that are easy to swallow

    ○ **B.** Speaking to the client on his right side

    ○ **C.** Applying an eye patch to the left eye

    ○ **D.** Speaking to the client on his left side

237. Following a CT scan with contrast medium, the nurse should give attention to:

    ○ **A.** Maintaining bed rest for eight hours

    ○ **B.** Forcing fluids

    ○ **C.** Observing the puncture site for hemorrhage

    ○ **D.** Administering pain medication

238. A client whose father died from Huntington's chorea asks what the chances are that he will develop the disease. The nurse knows that the chances of the client developing the disease are:

    ○ **A.** 25%

    ○ **B.** 50%

    ○ **C.** 100%

    ○ **D.** 0%

239. Cataracts result in opacity of the crystalline lens. Which of the following best explains the functions of the lens?

- ○ **A.** The lens controls stimulation of the retina.
- ○ **B.** The lens orchestrates eye movement.
- ○ **C.** The lens focuses light rays on the retina.
- ○ **D.** The lens magnifies small objects.

240. A client scheduled for a fluorescein angiography is to have mydriatic eye drops instilled in both eyes one hour prior to the test. The nurse knows that the purpose of the medication is:

- ○ **A.** To anesthetize the cornea
- ○ **B.** To dilate the pupils
- ○ **C.** To constrict the pupils
- ○ **D.** To paralyze the muscles of accommodation

241. A client with a severe corneal ulcer has an order for Gentamycin gtt q 4 hours and Neomycin 1 gtt q 4 hours. Which of the following schedules should be used when administering the drops?

- ○ **A.** Allow five minutes between the two medications.
- ○ **B.** The medications can be used together.
- ○ **C.** The medications should be separated by a cycloplegic drug.
- ○ **D.** The medications should not be used in the same client.

242. While assessing a client with AIDS, the nurse notes a reddish-purple discoloration on the client's eyelid. This finding is most consistent with:

- ○ **A.** Cytomegalovirus retinitis
- ○ **B.** AIDS entropion
- ○ **C.** Retinitis pigmentosa
- ○ **D.** Kaposi's sarcoma

243. An elderly client has difficulty distinguishing colors. Which colors are often misinterpreted by elderly clients?

- ○ **A.** Orange
- ○ **B.** Violet
- ○ **C.** Red
- ○ **D.** White

244. The rationale for refrigerating urine specimens that cannot be analyzed immediately is:

- ○ **A.** Urine becomes more acidic and kills bacteria that might be present.

- ○ **B.** Urea breaks down into ammonia, causing urine to become more alkaline and promoting cellular breakdown.

- ○ **C.** Components in the urine become consolidated so that the urine cannot be analyzed.

- ○ **D.** Red cells appear in stagnant urine.

245. The client with enuresis is being taught regarding bladder retraining. The ability to remain continent depends on the:

- ○ **A.** Sympathetic nervous system

- ○ **B.** Parasympathetic nervous system

- ○ **C.** Central nervous system

- ○ **D.** Lower motor neurons

246. A client with a history of renal calculi passes a stone made up of calcium oxalate. Which of the following diet instructions should be given to the client?

- ○ **A.** Increase intake of meats, eggs, fish, plums, and cranberries.

- ○ **B.** Avoid citrus fruits and juices.

- ○ **C.** Avoid dark green, leafy vegetables.

- ○ **D.** Increase intake of dairy products.

247. Which of the following drugs would be least helpful for a client who is experiencing an acute attack of bronchial asthma?

- ○ **A.** Cromolyn sodium

- ○ **B.** Epinephrine

- ○ **C.** Metaproterenol

- ○ **D.** Theophylline

248. Which of the following interventions is most helpful in determining the need for oxygen therapy for a client with COPD?

- ○ **A.** Asking the client whether he needs O_2

- ○ **B.** Assessing the client's level of fatigue

- ○ **C.** Evaluating the hemoglobin level

- ○ **D.** Using a pulse oximeter on the client's ear lobe

249. The nurse is evaluating the security of the client's tracheostomy ties. Which of the following methods is used to assess for tie tightness?

    ◯ **A.** The nurse places one finger between the tie and the neck.

    ◯ **B.** The tracheostomy can be pulled slightly away from the neck.

    ◯ **C.** There are no tie marks present.

    ◯ **D.** The nurse uses a Velcro fastener instead of a tie.

250. Which of the following clients is at highest risk for developing sarcordosis?

    ◯ **A.** A 40-year-old Caucasian with a history of bronchitis atrial tachycardia

    ◯ **B.** A 30-year-old African American who is pregnant

    ◯ **C.** A 50-year-old Asian male with emphysema

    ◯ **D.** A 60-year-old Hispanic male with cancer

Practice Exam II

NCLEX-RN Exam Cram, Third Edition

1. At 26 weeks gestation, a client is admitted to the ER stating that she has been having a painless bloody vaginal discharge since last evening. The nurse should give priority to:

   ○ **A.** Reporting the findings to the physician

   ○ **B.** Evaluating the color of the discharge

   ○ **C.** Evaluating the client's vital signs

   ○ **D.** Applying an external fetal monitor

2. A four-year-old is scheduled for a routine tonsillectomy. Which of the following lab findings should be reported to the doctor?

   ○ **A.** A hemoglobin of 12 Gm

   ○ **B.** A platelet count of 200,000

   ○ **C.** A white cell count of 16,000

   ○ **D.** A urine specific gravity of 1.010

3. An elderly client with glaucoma is scheduled for a cholecystectomy. Which medication order should the nurse question?

   ○ **A.** Meperidine (Demerol)

   ○ **B.** Cimetadine (Tagamet)

   ○ **C.** Atropine (Atropine)

   ○ **D.** Promethazine (Phenergan)

4. Which of the following instructions would not be included in the discharge teaching for a client receiving chlorpromazine (Thorazine)?

   ○ **A.** Wear protective clothing when working outside.

   ○ **B.** Avoid eating aged cheese.

   ○ **C.** Carry hard candy to decrease dryness of the mouth.

   ○ **D.** Report a sore throat immediately.

5. The nurse knows that a client with right-sided hemiplegia understands teaching regarding ambulation with a cane if she states:

   ○ **A.** "I will hold the cane in my right hand."

   ○ **B.** "I will advance the cane and the right leg together."

   ○ **C.** "I will be able to walk only by using a walker."

   ○ **D.** "I will hold the cane in my left hand."

6. An elderly client who experiences nighttime confusion wanders from his room into the room of another client. The nurse can best help decrease the client's confusion by:

   ○ **A.** Assigning a nursing assistant to sit with him until he falls asleep

   ○ **B.** Allowing the client to room with another elderly client

   ○ **C.** Administering a bedtime sedative

   ○ **D.** Leaving a night light on during the evening and night shifts

7. A nursing assistant assigned to care for a client with a radium implant tells the nurse, "I don't want to be assigned to that radioactive patient." The best action for the nurse to take is to:

   ○ **A.** Tell her that the client's body helps shield the radiation and provide a lead-lined apron for use.

   ○ **B.** Point out that her behavior is uncaring.

   ○ **C.** Assign her to care for another client.

   ○ **D.** Ask the nursing assistant why she is afraid of the client.

8. A client with cancer of the stomach has a gastric resection. Which information should be included in the client's post-operative teaching?

   ○ **A.** He can eat any type of food he wants to eat.

   ○ **B.** Eating carbohydrates will give him extra energy.

   ○ **C.** He will be able to have only high-calorie liquids.

   ○ **D.** Increasing his fat intake will help promote healing.

9. A client with psychotic depression is receiving haloperidol (Haldol). Which of the following side effects is associated with haloperidol?

- ○ **A.** Akathesia
- ○ **B.** Cataracts
- ○ **C.** Diaphoresis
- ○ **D.** Polyuria

10. While assisting a doctor with a sterile dressing change, the nurse notices that the doctor has contaminated his left glove. Which action should the nurse take?

- ○ **A.** Hand the doctor another pair of gloves.
- ○ **B.** Tell the doctor that he has contaminated his gloves.
- ○ **C.** Say nothing but continue to assist with the dressing change.
- ○ **D.** Report the incident to the infection control nurse.

11. Which of the following is a common complaint of the client with end-stage renal failure?

- ○ **A.** Weight loss
- ○ **B.** Itching
- ○ **C.** Ringing in the ears
- ○ **D.** Bruising

12. The nurse caring for a client scheduled for an angiogram should prepare the client for the procedure by telling him to expect:

- ○ **A.** Dizziness as the dye is injected
- ○ **B.** Nausea and vomiting after the procedure is completed
- ○ **C.** A decreased heart rate for several hours after the procedure is completed
- ○ **D.** A warm sensation as the dye is injected

13. A client with Parkinson's disease complains of "choking" when he swallows. Which intervention will improve the client's ability to swallow?

- ○ **A.** Withholding liquids until after meals
- ○ **B.** Providing semi-liquid foods when possible
- ○ **C.** Providing a full liquid diet
- ○ **D.** Offering small, more frequent meals

14. Which of the following medication orders needs further clarification?

- ○ **A.** Darvocet -N (propoxyphene/acetaminophen) 100 mg q 4–6 hrs. PRN

- ○ **B.** Nembutal (pentobarbital) 100 mg at bedtime

- ○ **C.** Coumadin (sodium warfarin) 10 mg

- ○ **D.** Estrace (estradiol) 2 mg q day

15. The primary concern when providing care for an 18-month-old is:

- ○ **A.** The child can creep up stairs.

- ○ **B.** The child is not toilet trained.

- ○ **C.** The child drops objects handed to him.

- ○ **D.** The child cries when his mother leaves him with a stranger.

16. Which statement best explains the rationale for placing a client in Trendelenberg position during the insertion of a central line catheter?

- ○ **A.** It will make catheter insertion easier.

- ○ **B.** It will make the client more comfortable.

- ○ **C.** It will prevent ventricular tachycardia.

- ○ **D.** It will prevent the development of pulmonary emboli.

17. The doctor has ordered the removal of a Davol drain. Which of the following instructions should the nurse give to the client prior to removing the drain?

- ○ **A.** The client should be told to breathe normally.

- ○ **B.** The client should be told to take two or three deep breaths as the drain is being removed.

- ○ **C.** The client should be told to hold his breath as the drain is being removed.

- ○ **D.** The client should breathe slowly as the drain is being removed.

18. The best diet for the client with a thyroidectomy is one that is:

- ○ **A.** High in fiber

- ○ **B.** Low in sodium

- ○ **C.** High in iodine

- ○ **D.** Low in fiber

19. A client with chronic obstructive pulmonary disease is receiving O_2 at 2 L/min. per nasal cannula. He is anxious and short of breath, and his mental status is clouded. The nurse should:

○ **A.** Increase the O_2 to 3 L/min.

○ **B.** Monitor for signs of impending respiratory failure.

○ **C.** Maintain the O_2 at 2 L/min, but increase the humidity.

○ **D.** Change the oxygen delivery system from cannula to a mask.

20. Which of the following findings is associated with right-sided heart failure?

○ **A.** Shortness of breath

○ **B.** Nocturnal polyuria

○ **C.** Daytime oliguria

○ **D.** Crackles in the lungs

21. Which finding indicates a need for further assessment of the client scheduled for a magnetic resonance imaging?

○ **A.** The client is an insulin-dependent diabetic.

○ **B.** The client refuses a corner bed.

○ **C.** The client is allergic to shellfish.

○ **D.** The client has a history of asthma.

22. A client with a total knee replacement returns from surgery. Which finding requires immediate nursing intervention?

○ **A.** There is 30 mL of bloody drainage from the Davol drain.

○ **B.** The continuous passive motion machine is set on 90° flexion.

○ **C.** The client is unable to ambulate to the bathroom.

○ **D.** The client is complaining of muscle spasms.

23. A nurse assigned to the rural health clinic is to administer the Mantoux test to a group of factory workers. The nurse should administer the Mantoux test in the clients':

○ **A.** Thigh

○ **B.** Buttock

○ **C.** Forearm

○ **D.** Upper arm

24. A client with end-stage renal disease received a renal transplant two weeks ago. Which of the following is an early sign of rejection of the transplant?

○   **A.** Increased urinary output

○   **B.** Tenderness over the operative site

○   **C.** Decreased urinary output

○   **D.** Blood pressure of 150/90

25. The physician has ordered a lumbar puncture on a client suspected of having meningitis. Following the procedure, the nurse should:

○   **A.** Place the collection vials on ice.

○   **B.** Number the collection vials.

○   **C.** Rotate the collection vials to prevent settling.

○   **D.** Carry the second and third vials to the lab after discarding the first vial.

26. Which of the following postpartal clients is at greatest risk for hemorrhage?

○   **A.** A gravida 1 para 1 with an uncomplicated delivery of a seven-pound infant

○   **B.** A gravida 1 para 0 with a history of polycystic ovarian disease

○   **C.** A gravida 3 para 3 with a history of low birth weight infants

○   **D.** A gravida 4 para 3 with a Caesarean section

27. An eight-year-old admitted with an upper respiratory infection has an order for O_2 saturation via pulse oximeter. To ensure an accurate reading, the nurse should:

○   **A.** Place the probe on the child's abdomen.

○   **B.** Recalibrate the oximeter at the beginning of each shift.

○   **C.** Apply the probe and wait 15 minutes before obtaining a reading.

○   **D.** Place the probe on the child's finger or earlobe.

28. A client with polysubstance abuse has been admitted to the hospital for detoxification. Which of the following drugs represents the most serious life-threatening situation during the withdrawal period?

○   **A.** Methadone

○   **B.** Secobarbital

○   **C.** Heroin

○   **D.** Cocaine

29. A client with allergic rhinitis has an order for a long-acting nasal spray that contains oxymetzoline. The client should be instructed to use the spray as directed to prevent:

- ○ **A.** Bleeding tendencies
- ○ **B.** Increased nasal congestion
- ○ **C.** Nasal polyps
- ○ **D.** Tinnitus

30. An infant with Tetralogy of Fallot is discharged with a prescription for Lanoxin Elixir. The nurse should instruct the mother to:

- ○ **A.** Administer the medication using a nipple.
- ○ **B.** Administer the medication using the calibrated dropper in the bottle.
- ○ **C.** Administer the medication using a plastic baby spoon.
- ○ **D.** Administer the medication in a baby bottle with 1 ounce of water.

31. A client with schizophrenia is ready to begin participating in therapeutic activities. The nurse should suggest that the client:

- ○ **A.** Participate on the unit softball team
- ○ **B.** Attend a class on psychotropic medication
- ○ **C.** Participate in art activities with three other clients
- ○ **D.** Watch TV in the unit day room

32. A five-year-old with a suspected ventricular septal defect is scheduled for a cardiac catheterization. The child's mother asks the nurse, "Why does my little girl have to have that tube put into her heart?" The nurse should tell the mother that the cardiac catheterization will:

- ○ **A.** Identify how much her heart is enlarged
- ○ **B.** Show exactly where the defect is
- ○ **C.** Show whether the ventricles are enlarged
- ○ **D.** Determine the existence of a murmur

33. A client is seen in the clinic and determined to have a hydatidiform mole. Which diagnostic test can confirm the diagnosis of a hydatidiform mole?

- ○ **A.** An ultrasound
- ○ **B.** Alpha-fetoprotein
- ○ **C.** Human chorionic gonadotrophin
- ○ **D.** Lecithin sphingomyelin ratio

34. A client scheduled for electroconvulsive therapy tells the nurse, "I'm so afraid. What will happen to me during the treatment?" Which of the following statements is most therapeutic for the nurse to make?

- ○ **A.** "You will be given medicine to relax you during the treatment."
- ○ **B.** "The treatment will produce a controlled grand mal seizure."
- ○ **C.** "The treatment can produce nausea and headache."
- ○ **D.** "You can expect to be sleepy and confused for a time after the treatment."

35. A 14-year-old with leukemia tells the nurse, "All I really want to eat is frozen yogurt." The nurse should:

- ○ **A.** Explain the importance of eating a balanced diet.
- ○ **B.** Ask the dietician to talk with the client to find out which foods he prefers.
- ○ **C.** Ask the kitchen to send the yogurt.
- ○ **D.** Document the client's refusal to eat the diet as ordered.

36. The nurse reports that a client with a Mantoux test has an induration of 10 mm. The nurse knows that the induration indicates:

- ○ **A.** Infection with the tubercle bacillus
- ○ **B.** Exposure to the tubercle bacillus
- ○ **C.** Questionable exposure to the tubercle bacillus
- ○ **D.** No exposure to the tubercle bacillus

37. Which of the following cutaneous manifestations is associated with Lyme disease?

- ○ **A.** Annular rash
- ○ **B.** Papular crusts
- ○ **C.** Bullae
- ○ **D.** Plaques

38. A gravid client reports that a prior pregnancy ended in loss of the baby early in the pregnancy. Which of the following instructions should be given to the client?

- ○ **A.** She should refrain from sex during this pregnancy.
- ○ **B.** She should avoid stimulation of the breasts.
- ○ **C.** She should quit work until after the baby is born.
- ○ **D.** She should report any nausea and vomiting.

39. A client is admitted to the coronary care unit with an acute myocardial infarction. The pain associated with myocardial infarction results from:

   ○ **A.** Spasm of the coronary artery

   ○ **B.** Ischemia of the myocardium

   ○ **C.** Vasodilation of the coronary veins

   ○ **D.** Ischemia of the carotid artery

40. Following an arteriogram, the nurse should give priority to:

   ○ **A.** Allowing the client to rest

   ○ **B.** Administering O_2 via nasal mask

   ○ **C.** Checking the EKG monitor

   ○ **D.** Checking the pulses distal to the catheterization site

41. The most common complication following a myocardial infarction is:

   ○ **A.** Hyperkalemia

   ○ **B.** Cardiac dysrhythmia

   ○ **C.** Acute respiratory distress

   ○ **D.** Hypovolemic shock

42. Which of the following snacks would be suitable for a child with gluten-induced enteropathy?

   ○ **A.** A soft oatmeal cookie

   ○ **B.** Buttered popcorn

   ○ **C.** A peanut butter and jelly sandwich

   ○ **D.** Cheese pizza

43. Following a coronary artery bypass, a client develops a temperature of 102°. The nurse should notify the doctor because an elevation in temperature:

   ○ **A.** Increases the cardiac output

   ○ **B.** Decreases the cardiac output

   ○ **C.** Indicates a cardiac tamponade

   ○ **D.** Increases diaphoresis and the likelihood of hypothermia

44. A client with a family history of Huntington's disease asks the nurse for information on how the disease is transmitted. Which of the following statements indicates that she understands the nurse's teaching?

- ○ **A.** "The chances of my passing the disease to my child are 1 in 2."
- ○ **B.** "I have no chance of passing the disease to a male child, but a female child would carry the disease."
- ○ **C.** "I have no chance of passing the disease to a female child, but a male child will have the disease."
- ○ **D.** "The chances of my passing the disease to my child are 1 in 4."

45. A client is being discharged following insertion of a permanent set pacemaker. A client with a permanent set pacemaker should be taught:

- ○ **A.** To keep a loose dressing over the insertion site at all times
- ○ **B.** That the pacemaker will function continuously at a set rate
- ○ **C.** That increases in activity will require adjustments in the pacemaker setting
- ○ **D.** That he will have to modify his lifestyle to allow for afternoon rest periods

46. To prevent dislocation of a hip prosthesis following a total hip replacement, the nurse should:

- ○ **A.** Maintain the client's affected leg in an adducted position.
- ○ **B.** Maintain the client's affected hip in a flexed position.
- ○ **C.** Tell the client to remain in a supine position.
- ○ **D.** Place an abduction pillow between the client's legs.

47. To prevent symptoms of Raynaud's disease, the client should:

- ○ **A.** Avoid a high-sodium diet.
- ○ **B.** Take a brisk, 15-minute walk daily.
- ○ **C.** Avoid exposure to cold.
- ○ **D.** Increase her vitamin C intake.

48. A client with end-stage renal failure is to receive a kidney transplant from her sister. Prior to surgery, the client will be scheduled for:

   ○ **A.** An intravenous pyelogram

   ○ **B.** Hemodialysis

   ○ **C.** A voiding cystogram

   ○ **D.** A renal biopsy

49. A client is admitted with acute abdominal pain. Which of the following findings requires immediate attention?

   ○ **A.** BP 100/50, P 96, abdominal distention

   ○ **B.** Temperature 99°, flatulence, nausea

   ○ **C.** Urinary frequency and dysuria

   ○ **D.** Temperature 99.2°, amber-colored urine

50. The doctor has ordered furosemide (Lasix) 80 mg IV push over five minutes. The nurse should give priority to the:

   ○ **A.** Assessment of the client's output

   ○ **B.** Assessment of the client's BP

   ○ **C.** Assessment of the client's RR

   ○ **D.** Assessment of the client's neuro signs

51. A client complains of pain and burning from herpes zoster. Which of the following provides temporary relief?

   ○ **A.** Applying a topical corticosteroid

   ○ **B.** Blowing cool air over the affected area

   ○ **C.** Applying warm, moist compresses

   ○ **D.** Applying an antifungal ointment

52. The nurse obtains a unit of whole blood from the blood bank at 1300 but is unable to start the blood until 1335. The nurse should:

   ○ **A.** Keep the blood refrigerated on the unit.

   ○ **B.** Return the blood to the blood bank.

   ○ **C.** Administer the blood at 1335 and document the time it was hung.

   ○ **D.** Recognize that the blood can be kept on the unit for two hours without any special care.

53. Which of the following complications is associated with a below-the-knee amputation?

    ○ **A.** Hip contracture

    ○ **B.** Knee contracture

    ○ **C.** Abduction of the hip

    ○ **D.** Adduction of the hip

54. A client has returned to his room following an esophagoscopy. The nurse should give priority to assessing the client's:

    ○ **A.** Level of consciousness

    ○ **B.** Gag reflex

    ○ **C.** Urinary output

    ○ **D.** Movement of extremities

55. During the removal of a central venous catheter, the client becomes anxious, diaphoretic, and short of breath. The nurse should give priority to:

    ○ **A.** Turning the client to the left side

    ○ **B.** Turning the client to the right side

    ○ **C.** Raising the client's head

    ○ **D.** Placing the client flat

56. Which instruction should be included in the discharge teaching for a client with cataract surgery?

    ○ **A.** Over-the-counter eye drops can be used to treat redness and irritation.

    ○ **B.** The eye shield should be worn at night.

    ○ **C.** It will be necessary to wear special cataract glasses.

    ○ **D.** A prescription for medication to control postoperative pain will be needed.

57. Which of the following indicates that the client taking an anticoagulant needs further teaching?

    ○ **A.** The client states that he will report bruising.

    ○ **B.** The client states that he eats green, leafy vegetables at least three times weekly.

    ○ **C.** The client states that he will return to the doctor's office for scheduled lab work.

    ○ **D.** The client states that his insulin dose might have to be adjusted while he is taking an anticoagulant.

58. Which of the following indicates failure of a ventriculoperitoneal shunt?

   ❍ **A.** Projectile vomiting

   ❍ **B.** Abdominal distention

   ❍ **C.** Decreased urinary output

   ❍ **D.** Decreased blood pressure

59. During the discharge teaching of a client with Buerger's disease, the nurse should teach the client:

   ❍ **A.** Exercises for improving vascular return from the lower extremities

   ❍ **B.** The importance of wearing mittens or gloves

   ❍ **C.** Dietary choices for reducing triglycerides

   ❍ **D.** The role of weight-bearing exercises in preventing bone loss

60. Which of the following findings suggests a complication in a client with surgical removal of a pituitary tumor?

   ❍ **A.** Polyuria

   ❍ **B.** Anuria

   ❍ **C.** Oliguria

   ❍ **D.** Dysuria

61. A 19-year-old primigravida is admitted for observation due to a sudden increase in blood pressure. The doctor suspects a diagnosis of pregnancy-induced hypertension. Which of the following is considered a significant factor in the development of pregnancy-induced hypertension?

   ❍ **A.** Maternal age

   ❍ **B.** Nutritional status of mother

   ❍ **C.** Pre-pregnant weight

   ❍ **D.** History of hypertension

62. An eight-year-old is admitted with drooling, muffled phonation, and a temperature of 102.6°. The nurse should immediately notify the doctor because the child's symptoms are suggestive of:

   ❍ **A.** Strep throat

   ❍ **B.** Epiglottitis

   ❍ **C.** Laryngotracheo bronchitis

   ❍ **D.** Bronchiolitis

63. A client with severe hypertension is receiving captopril (Capoten). The nurse should instruct the client to report which of the following to the doctor?

   ○ **A.** Coughing

   ○ **B.** Drowsiness

   ○ **C.** Frequent urination

   ○ **D.** Hunger

64. The doctor has ordered an IV of magnesium sulfate for a gravida 1 para 0 with preeclampsia. Which of the following symptoms is an expected side effect of magnesium sulfate?

   ○ **A.** Oliguria

   ○ **B.** Hypersomnolence

   ○ **C.** Hyporeflexia

   ○ **D.** Bradypnea

65. Which of the following symptoms is commonly reported in children with attention deficit hyperactive disorder?

   ○ **A.** Facial twitching

   ○ **B.** Impulsivity

   ○ **C.** Poor appetite

   ○ **D.** Nonintentional tremor

66. Phototherapy is ordered for a newborn with physiologic jaundice. The nurse caring for the infant should:

   ○ **A.** Offer the baby sterile water between feedings of formula.

   ○ **B.** Apply an emollient to the baby's skin to prevent drying.

   ○ **C.** Wear a gown, gloves, and a mask while caring for the infant.

   ○ **D.** Place the baby on enteric isolation.

67. A veteran is admitted with a diagnosis of chronic post-traumatic stress disorder. After being placed in the treatment room, he begins to pace frantically and make references to "highway one." As the nurse approaches him, he retreats to the corner and sits on the floor with his arms and legs pulled tight to his body. The client's behavior suggests that he is experiencing a:

   ○ **A.** Hallucination

   ○ **B.** Phobic reaction

   ○ **C.** Delusion

   ○ **D.** Flashback

68. Which of the following behaviors is characteristic of the client with schizoid personality disorder?

   ○ **A.** Excessive emotional outbursts

   ○ **B.** Violation of the rights of others

   ○ **C.** Social detachment

   ○ **D.** Attention-seeking behaviors

69. The doctor has prescribed imipramine (Tofranil) for an elderly client with endogenous depression. The nurse should give priority to assessing the client's:

   ○ **A.** Fluid intake

   ○ **B.** Cardiac status

   ○ **C.** Respiratory effort

   ○ **D.** Urinary output

70. A teen hospitalized with anorexia nervosa is now permitted to leave her room and eat in the dining room. Which of the following nursing interventions should be included in the client's plan of care?

   ○ **A.** Weighing the client after she eats

   ○ **B.** Having a staff member remain with her for one hour after she eats

   ○ **C.** Placing high-protein foods in the center of the client's plate

   ○ **D.** Providing the client with child-sized utensils

71. A client receiving lithium carbonate (Eskalith) has a level of 4.5 mEq/L. The nurse should prepare the client for immediate:

   ○ **A.** Transfusion

   ○ **B.** Hemodialysis

   ○ **C.** Renal biopsy

   ○ **D.** Electrocardiogram

72. A 15-year-old is admitted following an MVA. Examination reveals that the client has a closed head injury, a linear fracture of the temporal bone, a fracture of the mandible, and multiple abrasions. On admission, he is very drowsy. Which of the following doctor's orders should the nurse question?

   ○ **A.** Elevate the head 30°.

   ○ **B.** Apply neomycin (Neosporin) ointment to abrasions.

   ○ **C.** Ampicillin (Polycillin) 500 mg IVPB q 6 hrs.

   ○ **D.** Meperidine (Demerol) 75 mg q 3–4 hrs. PRN for pain.

73. A client hospitalized with bipolar disorder, manic phase, begins to talk loudly, pace the floor, and shout commands to others in the day room as he quickly changes the TV channels. The nurse's first action should include:

   ○ **A.** Checking the client's medication order

   ○ **B.** Escorting the client from the day room

   ○ **C.** Placing the client in seclusion

   ○ **D.** Finding out whether the client's behavior is upsetting others in the day room

74. According to Erickson's stage of growth and development, the developmental task associated with middle childhood is:

   ○ **A.** Trust

   ○ **B.** Initiative

   ○ **C.** Independence

   ○ **D.** Industry

75. Procrastination, noncompliance, and intentional inefficiency are characteristics of:

   ○ **A.** Avoidant personality disorder

   ○ **B.** Antisocial personality disorder

   ○ **C.** Compulsive personality disorder

   ○ **D.** Passive-aggressive personality disorder

76. A five-year-old is admitted to the hospital with pneumonia. Her orders include chest physiotherapy, mist tent, and inhalation with acetylcysteine (Mucomyst). Which of the following measures should be included in her care?

   ○ **A.** Telling her to breathe in through her nose and breathe out through her mouth

   ○ **B.** Applying lotion to the exposed parts of her body

   ○ **C.** Checking her clothing and linen frequently for dampness

   ○ **D.** Obtaining a rectal temperature every 4 hours

77. The nurse should observe for side effects associated with the use of bronchodilators. A common side effect of bronchodilators is:

   ○ **A.** Tinnitus

   ○ **B.** Tachycardia

   ○ **C.** Ataxia

   ○ **D.** Hypotension

78. The nurse is reviewing the chart of a one-day-old infant. Which of the following data requires further action?

   ○ **A.** Heart rate of 128

   ○ **B.** Respiratory rate of 72

   ○ **C.** Hematocrit of 50%

   ○ **D.** Blood glucose of 60 mg/100 ml

79. A primigravida, 26 years old and 33 weeks gestation, is admitted to the hospital with painless vaginal bleeding. She reports that the bleeding, which started two hours ago, has lessened in amount. Which of the following measures should be included in the client's care?

   ○ **A.** Monitoring of cervical dilatation

   ○ **B.** Counting the number of pads used

   ○ **C.** Checking the pH of the vaginal fluid

   ○ **D.** Observing for Cullen's sign

80. The five-minute Apgar of a baby delivered by C-section is recorded as 9. The most likely reason for this score is:

   ○ **A.** The mottled appearance of the trunk

   ○ **B.** The presence of conjunctival hemorrhages

   ○ **C.** Cyanosis of the hands and feet

   ○ **D.** Respiratory rate of 20–28/min

81. A client with a history of repeated sinusitis and deviated septum has an order for a CAT scan. To prepare the client for the procedure, the nurse should:

   ○ **A.** Tell the client that she can have an analgesic for discomfort.

   ○ **B.** Tell the client that needles will be placed above and below her eyes during the procedure.

   ○ **C.** Tell the client that she will need to be still during the procedure.

   ○ **D.** Tell the client that she will have a radiopaque substance given by IV.

82. A five-month-old infant is admitted to the emergency room with a temperature of 103.6° and irritability. The mother states that the child has been listless for the past several hours and that he had a seizure on the way to the hospital. A lumbar puncture confirms a diagnosis of bacterial meningitis. The nurse should assess the infant for:

   ○ **A.** Periorbital edema

   ○ **B.** Tenseness of the anterior fontanel

   ○ **C.** Positive Babinski reflex

   ○ **D.** Negative scarf sign

83. A client with a bowel resection and anastamosis returns to his room with a nasogastric tube attached to intermittent suction. Which of the following observations indicates that the nasogastric suction is working properly?

   ○ **A.** The client's abdomen is soft.

   ○ **B.** The client is able to swallow.

   ○ **C.** The client has active bowel sounds.

   ○ **D.** The client's abdominal dressing is dry and intact.

84. The nurse is teaching the client with insulin-dependent diabetes the signs of hypoglycemia. Which of the following signs is associated with hypoglycemia?

   ○ **A.** Tremulousness

   ○ **B.** Slow pulse

   ○ **C.** Nausea

   ○ **D.** Flushed skin

85. An adolescent client has been hospitalized for two months for an eating disorder. She asks the nurse what to tell her classmates about her long absence. The nurse can best help the client by:

   ○ **A.** Having her practice changing the subject when asked personal questions

   ○ **B.** Helping her invent a believable explanation for her absence

   ○ **C.** Engaging her in role-playing activities that are likely to occur

   ○ **D.** Encouraging her to share her experiences with those who ask

86. Which of the following symptoms is associated with an exacerbation of multiple sclerosis?

   ○ **A.** Anorexia

   ○ **B.** Seizures

   ○ **C.** Diplopia

   ○ **D.** Insomnia

87. A client with AIDS is admitted with a diagnosis of *pneumocystis carinii* pneumonia. Shortly after his admission, he becomes confused and disoriented. He attempts to pull out his IV and refuses to wear an O$_2$ mask. Based on his mental status, the priority nursing diagnosis is:

   ○ **A.** Social isolation

   ○ **B.** Risk for injury

   ○ **C.** Ineffective coping

   ○ **D.** Anxiety

88. Which of the following observations of the newborn indicates the possibility of a birth injury related to forceps delivery?

   ○ **A.** Asymmetry of the mouth

   ○ **B.** Pectus excavatum

   ○ **C.** Caput succedaneum

   ○ **D.** Strabismus

89. The doctor has ordered ampicillin (Polycillin) 150 mg every 6 hours IV piggyback for an infant with meningitis. The suggested dose for infants is 25–50 mg/kg/day in equally divided doses. The infant weighs 7 kg. The nurse should:

   ❍ **A.** Give the medication as ordered.

   ❍ **B.** Give half the amount ordered.

   ❍ **C.** Give the ordered amount q 12 hrs.

   ❍ **D.** Check the order with the doctor.

90. A 31-year-old client is admitted to the psychiatric unit after cutting both wrists with a kitchen knife. The client has a diagnosis of borderline personality disorder. The most therapeutic approach by the nurse is one that is:

   ❍ **A.** Warm and nurturing

   ❍ **B.** Open and flexible

   ❍ **C.** Firm and consistent

   ❍ **D.** Nonintrusive and passive

91. Which of the following conditions is frequently related to the development of renal calculi?

   ❍ **A.** Gout

   ❍ **B.** Pancreatitis

   ❍ **C.** Fractured femur

   ❍ **D.** Disc disease

92. Which symptom is considered an adverse reaction to kanamycin (Kantrex)?

   ❍ **A.** Diminished hearing

   ❍ **B.** Hypotension

   ❍ **C.** Hepatomegaly

   ❍ **D.** Petechiae

93. Which of the following beverages is most appropriate for a client with renal failure?

   ❍ **A.** Prune juice

   ❍ **B.** Grape juice

   ❍ **C.** Apple juice

   ❍ **D.** Apricot juice

94. A client with AIDS is admitted for treatment of wasting syndrome. Which of the following dietary modifications can be used to compensate for the limited absorptive capability of the intestinal tract?

   ◯ **A.** Thoroughly cooking all foods

   ◯ **B.** Offering yogurt and buttermilk between meals

   ◯ **C.** Forcing fluids

   ◯ **D.** Providing small, frequent meals

95. The client has an IV in place when he returns for surgery. While examining the IV site, the nurse notices pallor, coolness, and edema. The nurse is aware that these are signs of:

   ◯ **A.** Infiltration

   ◯ **B.** Infection

   ◯ **C.** Thrombus formation

   ◯ **D.** Sclerosing of the vein

96. Which of the following toys is the most appropriate for a two-year-old with Tetralogy of Fallot?

   ◯ **A.** A toy horn

   ◯ **B.** A stethoscope

   ◯ **C.** A push-pull toy

   ◯ **D.** A shape sorter

97. While sitting in the cafeteria, a nurse overhears two students discussing a client admitted for chemical detoxification. The nurse should:

   ◯ **A.** Report the incident to the teacher.

   ◯ **B.** Report the incident to the nursing supervisor.

   ◯ **C.** Confront the students with their behavior.

   ◯ **D.** Ignore the students' behavior.

98. The treatment protocol for a client with acute lymphatic leukemia includes prednisone, methotrexate (MTX), and cimetadine (Tagamet). The purpose of the cimetadine is to:

   ◯ **A.** Decrease the secretion of pancreatic enzymes.

   ◯ **B.** Enhance the effectiveness of the methotrexate.

   ◯ **C.** Promote peristalsis.

   ◯ **D.** Prevent a common side effect of prednisone.

99. An elderly client is hospitalized for a transurethral prostatectomy. Which finding should be reported to the doctor immediately?

○ **A.** An hourly urinary output of 40–50 ml

○ **B.** Bright red urine with many clots

○ **C.** Dark red urine with few clots

○ **D.** Requests for pain med every four hours

100. A client has a repair of a hiatal hernia using a thoracic approach. During the immediate post-op period, the nurse should give priority to the nursing diagnosis of:

○ **A.** A change in appetite

○ **B.** Respiratory change

○ **C.** Anxiety

○ **D.** Activity intolerance

101. Which statement by the parent of a child with sickle cell anemia indicates an understanding of the disease:

○ **A.** "The pain he has is due to the presence of too many red blood cells."

○ **B.** "He will be able to go snow skiing with his friends as long as he stays warm."

○ **C.** "He will need extra fluids in the summer to prevent dehydration."

○ **D.** "There is very little chance that his brother will have sickle cell."

102. A toddler with otitis media has just completed antibiotic therapy. A recheck appointment should be made to:

○ **A.** Determine whether the ear infection has affected her hearing.

○ **B.** Make sure that she has taken all the antibiotic.

○ **C.** Document that the infection has completely cleared.

○ **D.** Obtain a new prescription in case the infection recurs.

103. The doctor has ordered nasogastric feedings for a client following a stroke. Prior to administering a tube feeding, the nurse should:

○ **A.** Discard any aspirant and begin the tube feeding.

○ **B.** Check for tube placement by checking the pH of the aspirant.

○ **C.** Attach the feeding tube to low suction 30 minutes before feeding.

○ **D.** Mix the feeding with 200 ml of water.

104. A nine-year-old is admitted with suspected rheumatic fever. Which finding is suggestive of Syndeham's chorea?

    ○ **A.** Irregular movements of the extremities and facial grimacing

    ○ **B.** Painless swellings over the extensor surfaces of the joints

    ○ **C.** Faint areas of red demarcation over the back and abdomen

    ○ **D.** Swelling, inflammation, and effusion of the joints

105. A child with croup is placed in a cool, high-humidity tent connected to room air. The primary purpose of the tent is to:

    ○ **A.** Prevent insensible water loss

    ○ **B.** Provide a moist environment with oxygen at 30%

    ○ **C.** Prevent dehydration and reduce fever

    ○ **D.** Liquefy secretions and relieve laryngeal spasm

106. A client complains of tingling and numbness in his right leg following application of a long leg cast. The client's discomfort is most likely the result of:

    ○ **A.** Reduced venous return

    ○ **B.** Bone healing

    ○ **C.** Arterial insufficiency

    ○ **D.** Nerve compression

107. The nurse is suctioning the tracheostomy of an adult client. The recommended pressure setting for performing tracheostomy suctioning on the adult is:

    ○ **A.** 40–60 mm Hg

    ○ **B.** 60–80 mm Hg

    ○ **C.** 80–120 mm Hg

    ○ **D.** 120–140 mm Hg

108. The physician has prescribed prednisone daily for a client with Addison's disease. The nurse knows that the medication is best administered at:

    ○ **A.** 0700

    ○ **B.** 1200

    ○ **C.** 1600

    ○ **D.** 2100

109. A client hospitalized with mania is racing wildly about the unit trying to organize the other clients into a game of ping pong. The nurse should:

   ◯ **A.** Send the client to the recreation room for art therapy.

   ◯ **B.** Take the client outside for a walk.

   ◯ **C.** Allow the client to continue because his activities are goal directed.

   ◯ **D.** Suggest that the clients do exercises to a video instead.

110. A client with a right lobectomy has a three-chamber closed chest drainage system. The nurse knows that the third chamber provides for:

   ◯ **A.** An air seal

   ◯ **B.** Drainage collection

   ◯ **C.** Suction control

   ◯ **D.** A water seal

111. A client is admitted with a diagnosis of myxedema. An initial assessment of the client would reveal the symptoms of:

   ◯ **A.** Slow pulse rate, weight loss, diarrhea, and cardiac failure

   ◯ **B.** Weight gain, lethargy, slowed speech, and a decreased respiratory rate

   ◯ **C.** Rapid pulse, constipation, and bulging eyes

   ◯ **D.** Decreased body temperature, weight loss, and an increased respiratory rate

112. Which of the following should be included in the discharge teaching of a client with a unilateral adrenalectomy?

   ◯ **A.** The client's need to pay close attention to skin care

   ◯ **B.** The client's need to restrict her dietary intake of sodium and protein

   ◯ **C.** The client's need to recognize signs of hypoglycemia

   ◯ **D.** The client's need for daily steroid medication

113. Prior to administering a tube feeding, the nurse obtains 50 ml of aspirant. The nurse should:

   ◯ **A.** Discard the aspirant and begin the tube feeding.

   ◯ **B.** Replace the aspirant and begin the tube feeding.

   ◯ **C.** Discard the aspirant and hold the tube feeding.

   ◯ **D.** Replace the aspirant and hold the tube feeding.

114. Which of the following meal choices is suitable for a six-month-old infant?

    ○ **A.** Egg white, formula, and orange juice

    ○ **B.** Apple juice, carrots, and whole milk

    ○ **C.** Rice cereal, apple juice, and formula

    ○ **D.** Melba toast, egg yolk, and whole milk

115. The physician has ordered a renal diet for a client with acute renal failure. The diet that is usually ordered for the client with acute renal failure is one that is:

    ○ **A.** Low in sodium and low in protein

    ○ **B.** Low in protein and high in potassium

    ○ **C.** High in protein and high in phosphorus

    ○ **D.** High in sodium and low in magnesium

116. A client with acute pancreatitis is started on solid food. Which of the following menu selections should be avoided?

    ○ **A.** Vanilla custard

    ○ **B.** Angel food cake

    ○ **C.** Sliced peaches

    ○ **D.** Applesauce

117. Which statement describes the contagious stage of varicella?

    ○ **A.** The contagious stage is one day prior to the onset of the rash until the appearance of vesicles.

    ○ **B.** The contagious stage lasts during the vesicular and crusting stages of the lesions.

    ○ **C.** The contagious stage is from the onset of the rash until the rash disappears.

    ○ **D.** The contagious stage is one day prior to the onset of the rash until all the lesions are crusted.

118. A client with insulin-dependent diabetes takes 20 units of NPH insulin at 7 a.m. The nurse should observe the client for signs of hypoglycemia at:

    ○ **A.** 8 a.m.

    ○ **B.** 10 a.m.

    ○ **C.** 3 p.m.

    ○ **D.** 5 a.m.

119. The nurse is reviewing the results of a sweat test taken from a child with cystic fibrosis. Which finding supports the client's diagnosis?

   ○ **A.** A sweat potassium concentration less than 40 mEq/L

   ○ **B.** A sweat chloride concentration greater than 60 mEq/L

   ○ **C.** A sweat potassium concentration greater than 40 mEq/L

   ○ **D.** A sweat chloride concentration less than 40 mEq/L

120. Following visitation, the nurse observes a client's wife sitting alone crying. When approached, the wife states, "I'm so worried about him." The best response by the nurse is:

   ○ **A.** "Are you worried about him being in the hospital?"

   ○ **B.** "Tell me what it is that worries you."

   ○ **C.** "Would you like to talk with the social worker assigned to your husband?"

   ○ **D.** "Would you like to talk with your husband's doctor?"

121. The nurse is planning care for a client with a detached retina. Which of the following nursing diagnoses should receive priority?

   ○ **A.** Alteration in comfort

   ○ **B.** Alteration in mobility

   ○ **C.** Alteration in skin integrity

   ○ **D.** Alteration in O_2 perfusion

122. When rendering aid to a client who appears to be choking, the nurse's first action should be to:

   ○ **A.** Administer a blow to the client's back.

   ○ **B.** Ask the client whether he can speak.

   ○ **C.** Administer a chest thrust.

   ○ **D.** Establish an airway.

123. While reviewing a chart of an elderly client, the nurse notes that the last recorded temperature for the preceding shift was 104°. There is no documented intervention. The nurse should:

   ○ **A.** Check the doctor's orders for an antipyretic.

   ○ **B.** Ask the client whether she has received any medication for her fever.

   ○ **C.** Call the nurse at home to validate whether the medication was given.

   ○ **D.** Retake the temperature.

124. Which of the following infractions can result in revocation of the nurse's license?

    ◯ **A.** Failure to render care during a natural disaster

    ◯ **B.** Suspected negligence

    ◯ **C.** Felony conviction

    ◯ **D.** Failure to pay license renewal fees

125. A client in labor has an order for Demerol 75 mg IM to be administered 10 minutes prior to delivery. The nurse should:

    ◯ **A.** Wait until the client is placed on the delivery table and administer the medication.

    ◯ **B.** Question the order.

    ◯ **C.** Give the medication IM during the delivery to prevent pain from the episiotomy.

    ◯ **D.** Give the medication as ordered.

126. The primary purpose for using a continuous passive movement (CPM) apparatus for a client with a total knee repair is to help:

    ◯ **A.** Prevent contractures

    ◯ **B.** Promote flexion of the artificial joint

    ◯ **C.** Decrease the pain associated with early ambulation

    ◯ **D.** Alleviate lactic acid production in the leg muscles

127. Prior to suctioning a tracheotomy, the nurse should:

    ◯ **A.** Suction the oropharynx.

    ◯ **B.** Administer oxygen.

    ◯ **C.** Change the inner cannula.

    ◯ **D.** Raise the head of the bed.

128. Which of the following statements describes Piaget's stage of concrete operations?

    ◯ **A.** Reflex activity proceeds to imitative behavior.

    ◯ **B.** The ability to see another's point of view increases.

    ◯ **C.** Thought processes become more logical and coherent.

    ◯ **D.** The ability to think abstractly leads to logical conclusions.

129. A client recently diagnosed with bipolar disorder expresses concern over taking lithium because "a lot of people have problems getting too much of it." The nurse should explain that lithium toxicity usually occurs when the client has an insufficient intake of:

   ○ **A.** Carbohydrates for energy

   ○ **B.** Protein for maintenance of cell integrity

   ○ **C.** Potassium for muscle contractility

   ○ **D.** Sodium and fluids for renal excretion

130. A client admitted to the psychiatric unit claims to be the "Son of God" and insists that he will not be confined by "mere mortals." The most likely explanation for the client's delusions is:

   ○ **A.** He is demonstrating a conversion reaction.

   ○ **B.** He has experienced a stressful event.

   ○ **C.** He has low self-esteem.

   ○ **D.** He is experiencing overwhelming anxiety.

131. Which of the following statements reflects Kohlberg's theory of the moral development of the preschool-age child?

   ○ **A.** Obeying adults is seen as correct behavior.

   ○ **B.** Showing respect for parents is seen as important.

   ○ **C.** Pleasing others is viewed as good behavior.

   ○ **D.** Behavior is determined by consequences.

132. An elderly client is suspected of having pernicious anemia. A diagnosis of pernicious anemia is made by:

   ○ **A.** Bone marrow aspiration

   ○ **B.** Quantitative assay

   ○ **C.** Weber test

   ○ **D.** Schilling test

133. As a nurse nears a client with paranoia, the client suddenly jumps up and screams, "Go away. I don't want you near me." Which statement is most appropriate for the nurse to make?

   ○ **A.** "I don't understand why you are angry with me."

   ○ **B.** "All right. I'll leave you alone."

   ○ **C.** "Can you tell me what has upset you?"

   ○ **D.** "I will leave because you asked me to, but I will be back in half an hour."

134. Which of the following instructions should be given to a client with emphysema who is discharged home on Theo-Dur (theophylline)?

   ○ **A.** Take the medication when you experience shortness of breath.

   ○ **B.** If you miss a dose, you can take twice the amount at the next scheduled time.

   ○ **C.** Be careful operating machinery because the medication causes drowsiness.

   ○ **D.** Take the medication with antacid or food to prevent gastric upset.

135. Which of the following actions should the nurse give priority to when providing care for a child hospitalized with child abuse?

   ○ **A.** Arrange playtime with age mates.

   ○ **B.** Maintain a consistent schedule of caregivers.

   ○ **C.** Allow unsupervised visitation with the parents.

   ○ **D.** Encourage the child to reveal the identity of his abuser.

136. The nurse is monitoring a client receiving a blood transfusion. Which symptom is associated with a transfusion reaction?

   ○ **A.** Dyspnea

   ○ **B.** Thirst

   ○ **C.** Nausea

   ○ **D.** Diarrhea

137. Routine admission lab studies are ordered for a client admitted with pneumonia. Which lab result indicates that the client is dehydrated?

   ○ **A.** Hematocrit 36%

   ○ **B.** Urine specific gravity 1.030

   ○ **C.** White cell count 12,200

   ○ **D.** Reticulocyte count 1%

138. The nurse is caring for an eight-year-old following a routine tonsillectomy. Which finding should be reported immediately?

   ○ **A.** Reluctance to swallow

   ○ **B.** Drooling of blood-tinged saliva

   ○ **C.** An axillary temperature of 99° F

   ○ **D.** Respiratory stridor

139. The physician has prescribed iron dextran (Imferon) for a client with severe anemia. The nurse should administer the medication:

  ○ **A.** By subcutaneous injection

  ○ **B.** Orally in orange juice

  ○ **C.** By Z-track injection

  ○ **D.** Orally in milk

140. The nurse is administering a soap suds enema when the client begins to complain of abdominal cramping and a desire to defecate. The nurse should:

  ○ **A.** Tell the client to hold her breath and bear down.

  ○ **B.** Quickly administer the remainder of the enema.

  ○ **C.** Tell the client to breathe more slowly.

  ○ **D.** Stop the enema and record the amount instilled.

141. The physician has ordered a paracentesis to relieve abdominal ascites in a client with advanced cirrhosis. Prior to the procedure, the nurse should give priority to:

  ○ **A.** Maintaining the client NPO for eight hours

  ○ **B.** Instructing the client to void

  ○ **C.** Shaving the client from the abdomen to the symphysis

  ○ **D.** Administering pain medication

142. The nurse is teaching a group of clients in the family planning clinic about barrier methods of birth control. Which statement is true regarding the use of a diaphragm?

  ○ **A.** Using a contraceptive gel allows safe removal of the diaphragm within two hours of intercourse.

  ○ **B.** The client should wash the diaphragm with soap and hot water and store it in its compact.

  ○ **C.** The client should have the diaphragm refitted if she gains or loses 10 pounds.

  ○ **D.** Barrier methods of birth control are contraindicated in clients with diabetes.

143. The physician has prescribed neomycin sulfate for a client scheduled for colorectal surgery. The nurse recognizes that neomycin sulfate prepares the bowel by:

  ❍ **A.** Decreasing bacteria

  ❍ **B.** Enhancing blood flow

  ❍ **C.** Promoting peristalsis

  ❍ **D.** Decreasing absorption

144. The nurse is assisting in the establishment of short-term goals for a client with diabetes mellitus. Which statement represents a short-term goal for a client with diabetes mellitus?

  ❍ **A.** The client will select a snack from the diabetic exchange.

  ❍ **B.** The client will differentiate symptoms of hyperglycemia and hypoglycemia.

  ❍ **C.** The client will administer insulin injections without assistance.

  ❍ **D.** The client will describe self-care to prevent complications of diabetes.

145. The nurse is preparing to administer meperidine (Demerol) 75 mg and promethazine (Phenergan) 25 mg by injection. The nurse should:

  ❍ **A.** Combine the medications in a 3-cc syringe with a 23-gauge, 1 1/2-inch needle.

  ❍ **B.** Administer the Demerol IM in the ventrogluteal and the Phenergan IM in the deltoid.

  ❍ **C.** Administer the Demerol IM in the vastus lateralis and the Phenergan SC in the deltoid.

  ❍ **D.** Combine the medications in a 3-cc syringe with a 25-gauge, 5/8-inch needle.

146. The doctor has prescribed acetaminophen (Tylenol) elixir with codeine for a client following a tonsillectomy. The nurse should tell the client to:

  ❍ **A.** Avoid taking the medication more often than prescribed.

  ❍ **B.** Warm the medication to make the taste more palatable.

  ❍ **C.** Avoid taking the medication before going to sleep.

  ❍ **D.** Store the medication in the refrigerator.

147. A client with a fractured hip is placed in Buck's traction. Buck's traction is an example of:

  ❍ **A.** Skeletal traction

  ❍ **B.** Skin traction

  ❍ **C.** Balanced suspended traction

  ❍ **D.** Manual traction

148. Which nursing intervention will help to correct the respiratory alkalosis associated with hyperventilation?

    ○ **A.** Having the client breathe slowly through her nose

    ○ **B.** Having the client breathe humidified air

    ○ **C.** Having the client breathe from her diaphragm

    ○ **D.** Having the client breathe into a bag

149. A sling is applied to a client's forearm for a sprained wrist. The nurse should apply the sling so that the wrist is:

    ○ **A.** Lower than the elbow

    ○ **B.** In alignment with the elbow

    ○ **C.** Higher than the elbow

    ○ **D.** Kept in a position of comfort

150. The physician has ordered the collection of a sputum specimen for a client suspected of having tuberculosis. Following collection of the specimen, the nurse should:

    ○ **A.** Perform postural drainage.

    ○ **B.** Provide mouth care.

    ○ **C.** Force fluids.

    ○ **D.** Provide oxygen via mask.

151. The physician has prescribed methylphenidate (Ritalin) for an eight-year-old client with attention deficit disorder. Which finding indicates that the medication is having the desired effect?

    ○ **A.** The client sleeps more soundly.

    ○ **B.** The client is more alert and active.

    ○ **C.** The client completes assigned tasks.

    ○ **D.** The client has more stable moods.

152. The nurse is assisting with the formulation of a nursing diagnosis for a client with full thickness burn injuries of the arms and chest. During the first 24 hours, the priority nursing diagnosis is:

    ○ **A.** Alteration in fluid volume deficit

    ○ **B.** Pain

    ○ **C.** Alteration in body image

    ○ **D.** Alteration in fluid volume excess

153. The nurse is admitting a client with a suspected duodenal ulcer. The client will most likely report that his abdominal discomfort lessens when he:

   ○ **A.** Avoids eating

   ○ **B.** Rests in a recumbent position

   ○ **C.** Eats a meal or snack

   ○ **D.** Sits upright after eating

154. The physician has ordered the insertion of a nasogastric tube for a client following a cerebral vascular accident. Which method is most useful in determining the proper tube placement?

   ○ **A.** Instilling 5 mL of air while listening over the epigastrium

   ○ **B.** Checking the acidity of the gastric aspirant

   ○ **C.** Placing the end of the tube in water and watching for bubbling

   ○ **D.** Measuring the tube from the tip of the nose to the top of the xiphoid

155. A client with Rocky Mountain spotted fever is receiving chloramphenicol (Chloromycetin). Which of the following lab tests should the nurse monitor?

   ○ **A.** Complete blood count

   ○ **B.** Serum calcium

   ○ **C.** Serum creatinine

   ○ **D.** Partial thromboplastin time

156. Abdominal ultrasound in a client with gallbladder disease reveals that the gallbladder is grossly enlarged with many stones. If gallstones obstruct the bile duct, the client's stools will become:

   ○ **A.** Black and tarry

   ○ **B.** Clay colored

   ○ **C.** Dark brown

   ○ **D.** Greenish yellow

157. When administering an intramuscular injection to a child with cystic fibrosis, the nurse should:

   ○ **A.** Cleanse the injection site with povidone iodine (Betadine).

   ○ **B.** Avoid placing pressure on the injection site.

   ○ **C.** Use an airlock with all injections.

   ○ **D.** Use the smallest needle possible.

158. Which laboratory result indicates that the condition of a client with cirrhosis is worsening?

○ **A.** Increased serum creatinine

○ **B.** Decreased blood urea nitrogen

○ **C.** Increased serum ammonia

○ **D.** Decreased total bilirubin

159. The nurse is assessing a newborn in the well baby nursery. Which finding should alert the nurse to the possibility of a cardiac anomaly?

○ **A.** Diminished femoral pulses

○ **B.** Harlequin's sign

○ **C.** Circumoral pallor

○ **D.** Acrocyanosis

160. A two-year-old is hospitalized with a diagnosis of Kawasaki's disease. A severe complication associated with Kawasaki's disease is

○ **A.** The development of Brushfield spots

○ **B.** The eruption of Hutchinson's teeth

○ **C.** The development of coxa plana

○ **D.** The creation of a giant aneurysm

161. Which action improves communication when the nurse is caring for the client with a hearing impairment?

○ **A.** Talk in a normal tone of voice but talk more slowly

○ **B.** Accentuate key words so that the client will understand

○ **C.** Talk louder to focus the client on needed information

○ **D.** Stand at the foot of the bed when talking with the client

162. When performing tracheostomy suction, the nurse should stop suctioning if the client's heart rate falls below:

○ **A.** 80 beats per minute

○ **B.** 70 beats per minute

○ **C.** 60 beats per minute

○ **D.** 50 beats per minute

163. The nurse is caring for a client with suspected retinal detachment of the right eye. Which subjective finding is most common in clients with retinal detachment?

   ○ **A.** Dull, throbbing pain

   ○ **B.** Veil-like loss of vision

   ○ **C.** Sudden blindness

   ○ **D.** Loss of color discrimination

164. The nurse is monitoring the intake and output of a client hospitalized with acute glomerulonephritis. Which finding suggests the presence of red blood cells in the client's urine?

   ○ **A.** The urine is smoky in appearance.

   ○ **B.** The urine is orange tinged.

   ○ **C.** The urine is cloudy in appearance.

   ○ **D.** The urine is dark yellow.

165. The physician has prescribed timolol (Timoptic) ophthalmic drops and gentamicin (Garamycin) ophthalmic ointment for a client with glaucoma and conjunctivitis. When administering eye drops and eye ointments to the same client, the nurse should:

   ○ **A.** Administer the drops, wait 5 minutes, and administer the ointment.

   ○ **B.** Administer the two medications together.

   ○ **C.** Administer the ointment, wait 30 minutes, and administer the drops.

   ○ **D.** Ask the physician to prescribe both medications as drops or ointments.

166. A client with cancer of the bladder has had a cystectomy with the formation of an ileal conduit. Which of the following describes an ileal conduit?

   ○ **A.** The urine drains into the small intestine.

   ○ **B.** The urine is eliminated with stool.

   ○ **C.** The urine is emptied from a reservoir using a catheter.

   ○ **D.** The urine is drained from an abdominal opening.

167. A client with a history of angina is scheduled for a cardiac catheterization. Before sending the client for the procedure, the nurse should:

   ○ **A.** Shave the client's groin and axilla.

   ○ **B.** Administer an antiemetic.

   ○ **C.** Insert an indwelling catheter.

   ○ **D.** Check the chart for a signed permit.

168. The nurse is instructing a home health client on how to obtain a 24-hour urine specimen. Which statement indicates that the client understands the nurse's teaching?

- ○ **A.** "I will need to strain all my urine before placing it in the collection bottle."

- ○ **B.** "I will need to keep the collection bottle in a cooler filled with ice."

- ○ **C.** "I will collect the urine specimen from a midstream voiding."

- ○ **D.** "I will need to clean the perineum and collect a sterile specimen."

169. The charge nurse is formulating a discharge teaching plan for a client with mild preeclampsia. The nurse should give priority to:

- ○ **A.** Teaching the client to report a nose bleed

- ○ **B.** Instructing the client to maintain strict bed rest

- ○ **C.** Telling the client to notify the doctor of pedal edema

- ○ **D.** Advising the client to avoid sodium sources in her diet

170. The nurse is caring for a client with end-stage renal disease. Which laboratory result is most indicative of advanced renal disease?

- ○ **A.** Elevated serum sodium

- ○ **B.** Decreased serum potassium

- ○ **C.** Elevated serum creatinine

- ○ **D.** Decreased serum calcium

171. The nurse is preparing to discharge a client who is taking an MAO inhibitor. The nurse should instruct the client to:

- ○ **A.** Wear protective clothing and sunglasses when outside.

- ○ **B.** Avoid cold preparations containing pseudoephedrine.

- ○ **C.** Drink at least eight glasses of water a day.

- ○ **D.** Increase his intake of high-quality protein.

172. The nursing staff of an inpatient psychiatric facility is composed of an RN, an LPN, and two nursing assistants. Which client should be assigned to the care of the RN?

- ○ **A.** A client with bipolar disorder with a morning lithium level of 1.3 mEq/L

- ○ **B.** A client with schizophrenia receiving chlorpromazine (Thorazine) with a WBC of 7,500

- ○ **C.** A client with major depression who is scheduled for ECT

- ○ **D.** A client with schizoaffective disorder who is receiving risperidone (Risperdal)

173. Which of the following meal selections is appropriate for a client with celiac disease?

- ○ **A.** Toast, jam, and apple juice
- ○ **B.** Peanut butter cookies and milk
- ○ **C.** Rice Krispies bar and milk
- ○ **D.** Cheese pizza and Kool-Aid

174. A client with hyperthyroidism is taking lithium carbonate (Lithobid) to inhibit thyroid hormone release. Which complaint by the client should alert the nurse to a problem with the client's medication?

- ○ **A.** The client complains of blurred vision.
- ○ **B.** The client complains of increased thirst and increased urination.
- ○ **C.** The client complains of increased weight gain over the past year.
- ○ **D.** The client complains of a sore throat and headache.

175. A client with an open reduction and internal fixation for a fractured hip is to begin ambulation. The hip was repaired using a compression plate and screws. The client will most likely begin ambulation with:

- ○ **A.** Full weight bearing on the affected leg
- ○ **B.** Nonweight bearing on the affected leg
- ○ **C.** Toe touch weight bearing on the affected leg
- ○ **D.** Weight bearing as tolerated on the affected leg

176. The physician has ordered intravenous fluid with potassium replacement for a pediatric client admitted with gastroenteritis and dehydration. Before adding potassium to the intravenous fluid, the nurse should:

- ○ **A.** Assess the urinary output.
- ○ **B.** Obtain arterial blood gases.
- ○ **C.** Perform a dextrostick.
- ○ **D.** Obtain a stool culture.

177. The nurse is formulating a plan of care for a client with community-acquired pneumonia. Which nursing diagnosis should receive priority?

- ○ **A.** Ineffective airway clearance
- ○ **B.** Activity intolerance
- ○ **C.** Altered nutrition
- ○ **D.** Risk for fluid volume deficit

178. A two-month-old infant has just received her first Tetramune injection. The nurse should tell the mother that the immunization:

    ○ **A.** Will need to be repeated when the child is four years of age

    ○ **B.** Is given to determine whether the child is susceptible to pertussis

    ○ **C.** Is one of a series of injections that protects against diphtheria, pertussis, tetanus, and *hemophilius influenza B*

    ○ **D.** Is a one-time injection that protects against the measles, the mumps, rubella, and vari-cella

179. A client with Addison's disease has been receiving glucocorticoid therapy. Which finding indicates a needed dosage adjustment?

    ○ **A.** Dryness of the skin and mucus membranes

    ○ **B.** Dizziness when rising to a standing position

    ○ **C.** A weight gain of six pounds in the past week

    ○ **D.** Difficulty in remaining asleep

180. A client with insulin-dependent diabetes receives an injection of 12 units of regular insulin at 7 a.m. The nurse should provide the client with a snack at:

    ○ **A.** 9 a.m.

    ○ **B.** 11 a.m.

    ○ **C.** 2 p.m.

    ○ **D.** 7 p.m.

181. A client admitted with pelvic inflammatory disease is suspected of having gonorrhea. The definitive diagnosis of gonorrhea is made by:

    ○ **A.** Cervical washing

    ○ **B.** Fluorescent stain of the discharge

    ○ **C.** Blood culture

    ○ **D.** Culture of vaginal discharge

182. The nurse is caring for an obstetrical client in early labor. After the rupture of membranes, the nurse should give priority to:

 ❍ **A.** Applying an internal monitor

 ❍ **B.** Assessing fetal heart tones

 ❍ **C.** Assisting with epidural anesthesia

 ❍ **D.** Inserting a Foley catheter

183. The physician has prescribed acyclovir (Zovirax) for a client with herpes simplex. Which statement is true regarding topical acyclovir?

 ❍ **A.** Topical acyclovir provides protection against reinfection with the herpes virus.

 ❍ **B.** Topical acyclovir provides immunity against herpes virus type 2.

 ❍ **C.** Topical acyclovir should be applied to herpetic lesions with a gloved hand.

 ❍ **D.** Topical acyclovir used on a daily basis will prevent future outbreaks of herpes.

184. The nurse is preparing a client with peritoneal dialysis for discharge. The nurse's discharge teaching should include:

 ❍ **A.** Instructing the client to notify the doctor if the dialysate return becomes cloudy

 ❍ **B.** Instructing the client to notify the doctor of back discomfort

 ❍ **C.** Instructing the client to notify the doctor if urinary output diminishes

 ❍ **D.** Instructing the client to notify the doctor of abdominal fullness

185. The nurse is ambulating a post-operative client when the client suddenly develops severe chest pain and dyspnea. The nurse's first action should be:

 ❍ **A.** To provide supplemental oxygen

 ❍ **B.** To obtain an electrocardiogram

 ❍ **C.** To ask the client to describe her pain

 ❍ **D.** To obtain a chest x-ray

186. A client with a transurethral prostatectomy is returned to his room with a Foley catheter in place. To decrease the possibility of a kink developing in the urethral penile sphincter, the nurse should:

 ❍ **A.** Tape the catheter to the client's abdomen.

 ❍ **B.** Tape the catheter to the client's upper thigh.

 ❍ **C.** Leave the untaped catheter between the client's legs.

 ❍ **D.** Place the catheter beneath the client's leg.

187. The nurse is providing dietary teaching for a group of prenatal patients. Which of the following dietary selections is the best source of calcium?

   ○ **A.** Yogurt (6 ounces)

   ○ **B.** Whole milk (8 ounces)

   ○ **C.** Cheddar cheese (1 ounce)

   ○ **D.** Ice cream (6 ounces)

188. The nurse is preparing a room for a client returning from a thyroidectomy. Which item should be placed at the bedside of a client with a thyroidectomy?

   ○ **A.** An ambu bag

   ○ **B.** A tracheostomy set

   ○ **C.** An oral airway

   ○ **D.** A padded tongue blade

189. The physician has prescribed colchicine for a client with an attack of gout. The nurse should teach the client about the symptoms of colchicine toxicity, which include:

   ○ **A.** Diarrhea

   ○ **B.** Headache

   ○ **C.** Fever

   ○ **D.** Itching

190. A newborn is born with a large meningomyelocele. To prevent trauma to the sac, the nurse should position the newborn:

   ○ **A.** Flat supine

   ○ **B.** Prone with his hips elevated

   ○ **C.** Prone with his head elevated

   ○ **D.** Side lying

191. Which of the following meal selections provides a low-cholesterol, low-saturated fat breakfast?

   ○ **A.** Rice cereal, skim milk, toast with margarine, and orange juice

   ○ **B.** French toast, margarine, syrup, ham, and coffee

   ○ **C.** Waffles, maple syrup, sausage, an orange, and tea

   ○ **D.** A bagel, cream cheese, a poached egg, and coffee

192. The physician has prescribed levothyroxine (Synthroid) for a client with myxedema. Which statement indicates that the client understands the nurse's teaching regarding the medication?

- ○ **A.** "I will take the medication each morning after breakfast."
- ○ **B.** "I will check my heart rate before taking the medication."
- ○ **C.** "I will report visual disturbances to my doctor."
- ○ **D.** "I will stop the medication if I develop gastric upset."

193. The nurse is obtaining the blood pressure of a client who is obese. To obtain a blood pressure reading, the nurse should use a cuff that is:

- ○ **A.** Two thirds the diameter of the client's upper arm
- ○ **B.** One half the diameter of the client's upper arm
- ○ **C.** One third the diameter of the client's upper arm
- ○ **D.** Three fourths the diameter of the client's upper arm

194. A client with cancer has been instructed to increase the amount of protein and calories in his diet. Which dietary selection is highest in protein and calories?

- ○ **A.** Toast with jelly, beef broth, and tea
- ○ **B.** Baked fish, a roll with butter, and steamed vegetables
- ○ **C.** Tomato soup, crackers, and ginger ale
- ○ **D.** Cheese with crackers, fruit yogurt, and tea

195. A client returns to the doctor's office 72 hours after receiving a tuberculin skin test. Which finding requires further evaluation?

- ○ **A.** Induration of 10 mm
- ○ **B.** Redness at the injection site
- ○ **C.** Bruised area at the injection site
- ○ **D.** Absence of skin change

196. The nurse is caring for a client with an ileal conduit. Which intervention best prevents excoriation and skin breakdown for a client with an ileal conduit?

- ○ **A.** Applying zinc oxide paste around the stoma
- ○ **B.** Spraying the skin with tincture of benzoin
- ○ **C.** Applying a well-sealed drainage bag
- ○ **D.** Covering the skin with an antiseptic dressing

197. The nurse is teaching a client with asthma to use purse-lipped breathing. The primary benefit of purse-lipped breathing is:

   ○ **A.** Increasing the amount of oxygen reaching the lungs

   ○ **B.** Mobilizing tenacious bronchial secretions

   ○ **C.** Promoting more rapid expiration of carbon dioxide

   ○ **D.** Preventing a collapse of the alveoli

198. The nurse is caring for a client with a radium implant for the treatment of cervical cancer. While caring for the client with a radioactive implant, the nurse should:

   ○ **A.** Provide emotional support by spending additional time with the client.

   ○ **B.** Stand at the foot of the bed when talking to the client.

   ○ **C.** Avoid handling items used by the client.

   ○ **D.** Wear a badge to monitor the amount of time spent in the client's room.

199. The physician has prescribed tamoxofen citrate (Nolvadex) for a client with a positive family history of breast cancer. An adverse effect of Nolvadex is:

   ○ **A.** Oliguria

   ○ **B.** Agranulocytosis

   ○ **C.** Increased skin oils

   ○ **D.** Headache

200. A six-year-old is admitted with a diagnosis of childhood autism. Which behavior is most typical of a child with autism?

   ○ **A.** Willingness to talk to strangers

   ○ **B.** Disinterest in inanimate objects

   ○ **C.** Engaging in ritualistic behavior

   ○ **D.** Dislike of music

201. The nurse is caring for a client hospitalized with bipolar disorder, manic phase. Which of the following snacks would be best for a client with mania?

   ○ **A.** Potato chips

   ○ **B.** Diet cola

   ○ **C.** An apple

   ○ **D.** A milkshake

202. A client scheduled for a femoral popliteal bypass is to be assigned to a semiprivate room. Which client would be the most suitable roommate for a client with a femoral popliteal bypass graft?

    ○ **A.** A client with a transphenoidal hypophysectomy

    ○ **B.** A client with respiratory sarcoidosis

    ○ **C.** A client with a diabetic ulcer

    ○ **D.** A client with a closed fracture of the femur

203. A client hospitalized with severe depression and suicidal ideation refuses to talk with the nurse. The nurse recognizes that the suicidal client has difficulty:

    ○ **A.** Expressing feelings of low self-worth

    ○ **B.** Discussing remorse and guilt for actions

    ○ **C.** Displaying dependence on others

    ○ **D.** Expressing anger toward others

204. The nurse is caring for a client with a fiberglass cast applied to a distal fracture of the right tibia. The client should be able to bear weight on the cast within:

    ○ **A.** 10 minutes

    ○ **B.** 30 minutes

    ○ **C.** 3 hours

    ○ **D.** 24 hours

205. A client is to be discharged following the removal of a cataract on her right eye. The nurse should tell the client to:

    ○ **A.** Wear the metal eye shield only during waking hours.

    ○ **B.** Report any eye pain to the doctor immediately.

    ○ **C.** Refrain from using a pillow under her head.

    ○ **D.** Avoid wearing dark glasses inside.

206. The physician has prescribed amitriptyline (Elavil) for a client with depression. The nurse should continue to monitor the client's affect because the maximal effects of tricyclic antidepressant medication does not occur for:

    ○ **A.** 48–72 hours

    ○ **B.** 5–7 days

    ○ **C.** 2–4 weeks

    ○ **D.** 3–6 months

207. A client receiving hydrochlorothiazide (HTZ) is instructed to increase her dietary intake of potassium. The best snack for a client requiring increased potassium is a(n):

- ○ **A.** Pear
- ○ **B.** Apple
- ○ **C.** Orange
- ○ **D.** Banana

208. The physician has ordered a low-magnesium diet for a client with end-stage renal failure. Which of the following diet selections should be removed from the client's meal tray?

- ○ **A.** Fruit compote
- ○ **B.** Spinach salad
- ○ **C.** Baked potato
- ○ **D.** Custard

209. A client with bipolar disorder receives lithium bid. Which observation is associated with lithium toxicity?

- ○ **A.** Hyporeflexia
- ○ **B.** Akathesia
- ○ **C.** Ataxia
- ○ **D.** Petechiae

210. Which of the following statements best describes the gross motor development of a two-year-old?

- ○ **A.** She skips without falling.
- ○ **B.** She walks up and down stairs.
- ○ **C.** She rides a tricycle.
- ○ **D.** She is able to broad jump.

211. The nurse is caring for a client following the removal of the thyroid. Immediately post-op, the nurse should:

- ○ **A.** Maintain the client in a semi-Fowler's position with her head and neck supported by pillows.
- ○ **B.** Encourage the client to turn her head from side to side to promote drainage of oral secretions.
- ○ **C.** Maintain the client in a supine position with sandbags placed on either side of her head and neck.
- ○ **D.** Encourage the client to cough and deep breath every two hours with her neck in a flexed position.

212. A toddler with Tetralogy of Fallot is hospitalized with a diagnosis of pneumonia. During the nursing assessment, the child develops a "tet" episode. The nurse should:

    ○ **A.** Provide the child his favorite toy.

    ○ **B.** Place the child in a supine position.

    ○ **C.** Pick the child up and comfort him.

    ○ **D.** Place the child in a lateral knee chest position.

213. A newly diagnosed diabetic is learning to administer her injections of NPH and regular insulin. Which statement indicates that the client understands the nurse's teaching regarding proper insulin administration?

    ○ **A.** "I will administer the NPH and regular insulin in two separate injections."

    ○ **B.** "I will withdraw the dose of regular insulin before withdrawing the NPH insulin."

    ○ **C.** "It does not matter which insulin is withdrawn first as long as the amount is correct."

    ○ **D.** "I will withdraw the dose of NPH insulin before withdrawing the regular insulin."

214. An elderly client with glaucoma has been prescribed timolol (Timoptic) eye drops. Timoptic should be used with caution in clients with a history of:

    ○ **A.** Diabetes

    ○ **B.** Gastric ulcers

    ○ **C.** Emphysema

    ○ **D.** Pancreatitis

215. A client hospitalized with chronic dyspepsia is diagnosed with gastric cancer. Which of the following is associated with an increased incidence of gastric cancer?

    ○ **A.** Dairy products

    ○ **B.** Carbonated beverages

    ○ **C.** Refined sugars

    ○ **D.** Luncheon meats

216. A two-year-old is hospitalized with suspected intussusception. Which finding is associated with intussusception?

    ○ **A.** Currant jelly stools

    ○ **B.** Projectile vomiting

    ○ **C.** Ribbon-like stools

    ○ **D.** Palpable mass over the flank

217. Three days after a cast is applied to a fracture of the right lower leg, the client begins to complain of pain beneath the cast. The nurse should give priority to:

- ○ **A.** Elevating the extremity
- ○ **B.** Administering pain medication
- ○ **C.** Explaining that cast pain is normal
- ○ **D.** Notifying the physician

218. The physician has prescribed an NSAID for a client with rheumatoid arthritis. During medication teaching, the nurse should tell the client that:

- ○ **A.** Taking the medication with milk will render it ineffective.
- ○ **B.** Fluids should be restricted to prevent renal excretion.
- ○ **C.** Taking the medication with food will lessen gastric upset.
- ○ **D.** Exposure to sunlight will cause bronze pigmentation.

219. A client is sent to the psychiatric unit for forensic evaluation after he is accused of arson. His tentative diagnosis is antisocial personality disorder. In reviewing the client's record, the nurse could expect to find:

- ○ **A.** A history of consistent employment
- ○ **B.** A below-average intelligence
- ○ **C.** A history of cruelty to animals
- ○ **D.** An expression of remorse for his actions

220. A 65-year-old female is planning for retirement. Which statement indicates that the client has achieved ego integrity?

- ○ **A.** "After retirement, I plan to join a senior's travel club."
- ○ **B.** "I need to consider selling my home and moving closer to my daughter."
- ○ **C.** "I've worked most all my life; I'm not sure how to spend my days now."
- ○ **D.** "Few of my relatives live past their seventies."

221. The nurse is making assignments for the nursing assistant. Which client should the nursing assistant be assigned to care for?

- ○ **A.** 70-year-old with Alzheimer's dementia
- ○ **B.** 65-year-old with total knee repair
- ○ **C.** 72-year-old with exploratory laparotomy
- ○ **D.** 80-year-old with diverticulitis

222. The nurse is providing dietary teaching for an elderly client living on a fixed income. Which food choices would provide the client with needed nutrients and be cost effective?

- ○ **A.** Potatoes, green beans, and bacon
- ○ **B.** Spinach, dried beans, and tomatoes
- ○ **C.** Ham, corn, and strawberries
- ○ **D.** Beef, cheese, and milk

223. Which of the following findings would be expected in an infant with biliary atresia?

- ○ **A.** Rapid weight gain and hepatomegaly
- ○ **B.** Dark stools and poor weight gain
- ○ **C.** Abdominal distention and poor weight gain
- ○ **D.** Abdominal distention and rapid weight gain

224. The nurse is caring for a client with Cushing's disease. The nurse should carefully assess the client for signs of:

- ○ **A.** Hypoglycemia
- ○ **B.** Infection
- ○ **C.** Hypovolemia
- ○ **D.** Hyperinsulinemia

225. A client is admitted with suspected pheochromocytoma. The physiological alteration associated with pheochromocytoma is:

- ○ **A.** An extreme elevation in blood pressure
- ○ **B.** Petechial rash across the chest and axilla
- ○ **C.** White flecks in the iris
- ○ **D.** Yellow creases at the nasolabial folds

226. A client with osteoporosis has been advised to increase the amount of calcium in her diet. Which food provides the most calcium?

- ○ **A.** An 8-ounce glass of milk
- ○ **B.** An ounce of cheddar cheese
- ○ **C.** A half cup of raw broccoli
- ○ **D.** A 4-ounce salmon croquette

227. The physician has ordered dressings with mafenide acetate (Sulfamylon) cream for a client with full thickness burns of his hands and arms. Before dressing changes, the nurse should give priority to:

   ○ **A.** Administering pain medication

   ○ **B.** Checking the adequacy of urinary output

   ○ **C.** Requesting a daily complete blood count

   ○ **D.** Obtaining a blood glucose by finger stick

228. A client with acquired immune deficiency syndrome is hospitalized with disseminated herpes zoster. Which medication is indicated for the client with disseminated herpes zoster?

   ○ **A.** Gentamicin (Garamycin)

   ○ **B.** Acyclovir (Zovirax)

   ○ **C.** Pentamidine (Pentam)

   ○ **D.** Immune globulin (Polygam)

229. A primigravida arrives at the labor unit stating that she is having contractions. Which statement describes the presence of true contractions?

   ○ **A.** True contractions begin in the lower abdomen.

   ○ **B.** True contractions have a consistent frequency.

   ○ **C.** True contractions lessen with physical activity.

   ○ **D.** True contractions wax and wane in intensity.

230. The nurse is caring for a client receiving aminophylline (Truphylline). Side effects associated with aminophylline include:

   ○ **A.** Irritability, rapid pulse, and palpitations

   ○ **B.** Slow pulse, increased appetite, and sweating

   ○ **C.** Nausea, vomiting, and increased blood pressure

   ○ **D.** Drowsiness, vomiting, and decreased blood sugar

231. The nurse is teaching a group of parents about gross motor development of the two-year-old. Which behavior is an example of the normal gross motor skills of the two-year-old?

   ○ **A.** She can pull a toy behind her.

   ○ **B.** She can copy a horizontal line.

   ○ **C.** She can build a tower of eight blocks.

   ○ **D.** She can broad jump.

232. A client with schizophrenia is experiencing auditory hallucinations and is admitted for evaluation and treatment. A suitable activity for a client with schizophrenia who is experiencing hallucinations is:

- ○ **A.** Watching a movie with other clients
- ○ **B.** Working on a large piece puzzle
- ○ **C.** Playing a game of solitaire
- ○ **D.** Walking and talking with the nurse

233. A patient with MRSA is being discharged from the hospital but will continue to receive wound care and intravenous antibiotics for the next week. The patient's nursing care needs will best be met in a(n):

- ○ **A.** Rehabilitation center
- ○ **B.** Skilled nursing center
- ○ **C.** Extended care facility
- ○ **D.** Assisted living home

234. A patient refuses to take his dose of oral medication. The nurse tells the patient that if he does not take the medication that she will administer it by injection. The nurse's comments can result in a charge of:

- ○ **A.** Battery
- ○ **B.** Malpractice
- ○ **C.** Assault
- ○ **D.** Negligence

235. A nursing student has been assigned to administer the client's morning medication. When administering the medication, the student nurse:

- ○ **A.** Has less accountability for administering medication than the registered nurse
- ○ **B.** Has the same accountability for administering medication as the registered nurse
- ○ **C.** Has no accountability for administering medication since she is a student nurse
- ○ **D.** Has more accountability than the licensed practical nurse but less accountability than the registered nurse

236. The nurse on a psychiatric unit fails to check the patient's lithium level and continues to administer the daily dose of lithium. The patient develops lithium toxicity that requires hemodialysis. The nurse's failure to check the patient's lithium level can result in charges of:

- ○ **A.** Battery
- ○ **B.** Assault
- ○ **C.** Intentional tort
- ○ **D.** Malpractice

237. A patient's employer telephones the unit and requests information regarding the patient's condition and expected length of hospitalization. The patient has not signed a consent form for information to be released to anyone other than his immediate family. If the nurse discusses the patient's information with anyone other than the immediate family, he is guilty of:

- ○ **A.** Breaking confidentiality
- ○ **B.** Slander
- ○ **C.** Malice
- ○ **D.** Libel

238. A pregnant diabetic client, 37 weeks gestation, is scheduled for an amniocentesis. The client asks the nurse the purpose of the test. The nurse should explain that the primary reason for performing an amniocentesis is:

- ○ **A.** To determine the effect of the diabetes on the fetus
- ○ **B.** To estimate the skeletal age of the fetus
- ○ **C.** To determine the maturity of the fetal lungs
- ○ **D.** To obtain information about aberrant fetal genes

239. The nurse is to administer digoxin elixir to a six-month-old with a congenital heart defect. The nurse obtains an apical pulse rate of 100. The nurse should:

- ○ **A.** Record the heart rate and call the physician.
- ○ **B.** Record the heart rate and administer the medication.
- ○ **C.** Administer the medication and recheck the heart rate in 15 minutes.
- ○ **D.** Hold the medication and recheck the heart rate in 30 minutes.

240. After receiving an annual influenza immunization, a client develops symptoms suggestive of Guillain-Barré syndrome. Which symptom is associated with Guillain-Barré syndrome?

- ○ **A.** Paresthesia and weakness of the lower extremities
- ○ **B.** Hyperactive deep tendon reflexes
- ○ **C.** Emotional lability
- ○ **D.** Flapping tremors of the hand and feet

241. The nurse is caring for a one-year-old with a history of prematurity. Which developmental finding requires further evaluation by the physician?

- ○ **A.** The child has been creeping forthree months.
- ○ **B.** The child can pull himself to a standing position.
- ○ **C.** The child uses a pincer grasp.
- ○ **D.** The child can sit with support.

242. A withdrawn, depressed client sits in the day room but refuses to participate in scheduled group activities. When implementing a plan of care, the nurse should:

- ○ **A.** Plan activity that will allow the client to interact with a staff member.
- ○ **B.** Tell the client that participation in group activities is expected.
- ○ **C.** Allow the client to select an activity that he can enjoy doing alone.
- ○ **D.** Ask the client to prepare a list of activities or hobbies he enjoys.

243. A mother of a three-year-old hospitalized with lead poisoning asks the nurse to explain the treatment for her daughter. The nurse's explanation is based on the knowledge that lead poisoning is treated with:

- ○ **A.** Gastric lavage
- ○ **B.** Chelating agents
- ○ **C.** Antiemetics
- ○ **D.** Activated charcoal

244. The nurse is implementing a plan of care for a client with myxedema. Based on the client's diagnosis, the nurse should:

- ○ **A.** Provide high-calorie snacks for the client.
- ○ **B.** Tell the client to elevate her feet when sitting.
- ○ **C.** Provide an additional blanket.
- ○ **D.** Perform urine checks for ketones.

245. An adolescent bodybuilder has been taking anabolic steroids to increase his weight and the size and definition of his muscles. Psychological effects of anabolic steroids include:

○ **A.** Confusion and self-doubt

○ **B.** Aggression and uncontrolled rage

○ **C.** Elation and excitability

○ **D.** Decreased inhibitions and humor

246. A female client with mania has become very expansive and insists on playing strip poker with a group of male clients. In anticipation of the game, the client begins to undress. The most therapeutic response by the nurse would be:

○ **A.** To observe the reaction of the other clients

○ **B.** To take the cards away from the group

○ **C.** To tell the client her behavior is inappropriate

○ **D.** To escort the client to her room

247. Following the death of a client, a nursing assistant begins to cry uncontrollably and is unable to provide care for the other assigned clients. The RN should:

○ **A.** Send the nursing assistant home for the remainder of the day.

○ **B.** Explain to the nursing assistant that she will have to learn to cope with loss.

○ **C.** Send the nursing assistant to the lounge and care for the clients herself.

○ **D.** Encourage the nursing assistant to express her feelings about dying.

248. An 18-month-old is scheduled for a cleft palate repair. The usual type of restraints for a child with a cleft palate repair is:

○ **A.** Elbow restraints

○ **B.** Full arm restraints

○ **C.** Wrist restraints

○ **D.** Mummy restraints

249. The nurse is caring for a client with bleeding from esophageal varices. The factor that most likely contributed to the development of esophageal varices is:

○ **A.** Exposure to hydrocarbons

○ **B.** Being morbidly obese

○ **C.** Heavy alcohol consumption

○ **D.** Adhering to a lacto-vegetarian diet

250. A client is being treated for cancer with linear acceleration radiation. The physician has marked the radiation site with a blue marking pen. The nurse should:

   ◯ **A.** Remove the unsightly markings with acetone or alcohol.

   ◯ **B.** Cover the radiation site with loose gauze dressing.

   ◯ **C.** Sprinkle baby powder over the radiated area.

   ◯ **D.** Refrain from using soap lotion on the marked area.

Answers to Practice Exam I

1. B	28. C	55. D	82. B
2. A	29. D	56. A	83. D
3. D	30. C	57. A	84. D
4. B	31. D	58. B	85. A
5. A	32. B	59. C	86. D
6. D	33. C	60. B	87. C
7. A	34. A	61. B	88. B
8. B	35. B	62. D	89. B
9. B	36. B	63. B	90. D
10. B	37. B	64. B	91. D
11. D	38. D	65. D	92. A
12. B	39. A	66. D	93. B
13. D	40. B	67. A	94. B
14. A	41. B	68. C	95. D
15. A	42. B	69. B	96. B
16. B	43. C	70. B	97. B
17. B	44. B	71. A	98. B
18. C	45. A	72. C	99. C
19. A	46. B	73. B	100. D
20. D	47. B	74. A	101. A
21. B	48. B	75. A	102. D
22. A	49. C	76. B	103. D
23. D	50. B	77. A	104. A
24. A	51. D	78. C	105. A
25. D	52. B	79. B	106. C
26. C	53. A	80. B	107. D
27. B	54. C	81. D	108. D

109. C	**138.** A	**167.** B	**196.** D	**225.** D
110. B	**139.** D	**168.** C	**197.** C	**226.** B
111. A	**140.** A	**169.** C	**198.** C	**227.** D
112. B	**141.** C	**170.** D	**199.** B	**228.** B
113. C	**142.** D	**171.** C	**200.** B	**229.** C
114. D	**143.** B	**172.** C	**201.** C	**230.** D
115. B	**144.** D	**173.** B	**202.** C	**231.** D
116. A	**145.** C	**174.** A	**203.** B	**232.** C
117. D	**146.** B	**175.** A	**204.** A	**233.** C
118. A	**147.** C	**176.** A	**205.** B	**234.** B
119. B	**148.** D	**177.** B	**206.** B	**235.** D
120. B	**149.** D	**178.** A	**207.** A	**236.** C
121. D	**150.** D	**179.** C	**208.** B	**237.** B
122. B	**151.** D	**180.** A	**209.** A	**238.** B
123. A	**152.** B	**181.** D	**210.** A	**239.** C
124. B	**153.** B	**182.** B	**211.** D	**240.** B
125. B	**154.** D	**183.** A	**212.** B	**241.** A
126. D	**155.** C	**184.** A	**213.** A	**242.** D
127. C	**156.** C	**185.** D	**214.** C	**243.** B
128. B	**157.** B	**186.** A	**215.** D	**244.** B
129. A	**158.** D	**187.** B	**216.** A	**245.** A
130. B	**159.** C	**188.** A	**217.** B	**246.** C
131. D	**160.** D	**189.** B	**218.** B	**247.** A
132. D	**161.** B	**190.** B	**219.** A	**248.** D
133. A	**162.** D	**191.** B	**220.** B	**249.** A
134. B	**163.** A	**192.** D	**221.** B	**250.** B
135. D	**164.** A	**193.** C	**222.** A	
136. A	**165.** B	**194.** A	**223.** B	
137. B	**166.** D	**195.** B	**224.** B	

Answer Rationales

1. Answer B is correct. Vanillymandelic acid is a test done to detect pheochromocytoma, an adrenal tumor that often leads to malignant hypertension. Collection of a 24-hour urine is required for a VMA level. Coffee, tea, bananas, cocoa products, vanilla products, aspirin, and medications containing aspirin should be eliminated for two days before the test, as well as the day of the test. In answers A, C, and D, these foods would not interfere with the test results.

2. Answer A is correct. Drainage of more that 100 mls per hour is considered excessive and should be reported immediately to the physician. The clients in answers B and D are stable. The client in answer C has an elevated temperature and should be seen after the client who is bleeding.

3. Answer D is correct. Reticulocytes are immature red blood cells. Effective treatment of pernicious anemia will result in an increase in the number of reticulocytes. A, B, and C are incorrect because neutrophils, basophils, and monocytes are white blood cells. These cells are not increased by the administration of B12 injections.

4. Answer B is correct. Phenelazine (Nardil) is an MAO inhibitor. Foods high in tyramine should be avoided to prevent hypertensive crisis. The foods in answers A, C, and D do not interfere with this medication.

5. Answer A is correct. Unilateral neglect is particularly evident in those with right cerebral hemisphere strokes. The client is unaware of the existence of his left or paralyzed side. The client is therefore often observed leaning to the left with his arm caught in the wheel of the wheelchair. When questioned, he believes he is sitting upright. Other behaviors associated with unilateral neglect include washing or dressing only one side of the body. Answer B is incorrect because the client is able to distinguish between two tactile stimuli. Answer C is incorrect because the client is able to complete range of vision without turning his head. Answer D is incorrect because the client is able to carry out cognitive and motor activity on the unaffected side at the same time.

6. Answer D is correct. Providing foods in sealed single-serving packages lessens the likelihood of introducing food-borne bacteria to a client with severe immunosuppression. A client with leukemia and neutropenia does not have to request disposable utensils, but the utensils should be washed in hot water. The client does not have to wear a mask when visitors are present, but contagious visitors should not visit. IV sites should be cleaned with an antiseptic solution.

7. Answer A is correct. Signing chart entries as a registered nurse before attaining legal status is an attempt to fraud or deceive the public. This action can result in prosecution by the board of nursing as well as civil courts. A *tort* is a wrongful act; *malpractice* is an action that results in harm to the client; and *negligence* is failing to care for a client and harm results.

8. Answer B is correct. The nursing assistant should be assigned to the most stable client. The infant with bronchiolitis and the two-year-old with periorbital cellulites will require skilled nursing observations and IV antibiotics. The one-year-old with a fractured tibia should be carefully assessed for possible child abuse.

9. Answer B is correct. Discrepancies in charting and record keeping for controlled substances should be reported first to the nursing supervisor. If necessary, after reporting to the nursing supervisor, the problem should be reported to others through the chain of command.

10. Answer B is correct. The client with a herniated lumbar disc can be more easily managed on the postpartum unit than the other clients. The client with a total knee replacement and the client with ulcerative colitis present a higher risk of infection. The client with severe depression requires one-on-one observation.

11. Answer D is correct. Oranges contain only trace amounts of sodium. All the other selections are high in sodium content.

12. Answer B is correct. Paroxysmal nocturnal dyspnea, orthopnea, and coughing are early signs of pulmonary edema. The client with a cerebral vascular accident with a tube feeding, the client with a mastectomy, and the client with Parkinson's disease are all stable.

13. Answer D is correct. Persons with Sjogren syndrome develop xerostomia (dry mouth), which can be alleviated by applications of saliva substitute. The other answers will not help the client with xerostomia.

14. Answer A is correct. The nursing assistant should be assigned to the most stable client. The client with a laparoscopic cholecystectomy is usually discharged the same day of surgery or the day after surgery. The clients in answers B, C, and D are not stable.

15. Answer A is correct. Relaxation decreases the grimacing and writhing that characterize athetoid cerebral palsy. Clients with athetoid cerebral palsy experience contraction of the muscles and muscle rigidity. The client does not have hypoactive deep tendon reflexes, and stretching reflexes are not increased with rest. Fine motor movements are also not improved by rest periods.

16. Answer B is correct. Pertussis, or whooping cough, is detected by culture of nasopharyngeal secretions. A specimen from the blood, stool, or urine is not needed.

17. Answer B is correct. A low-residue diet preoperatively decreases the amount of stool in the bowel. Postoperatively, a high-fiber diet will decrease the likelihood of constipation. The other diets are not ordered for the client with a hemorrhoidectomy.

18. Answer C is correct. Sitz baths will help decrease the amount of post-op swelling and discomfort in the perianal region. Medication given by suppository is not recommended; aspirin can increase bleeding; and ice is also not recommended.

19. Answer A is correct. The nurse can best assist the visually impaired client with ambulation by walking slightly in front and to the side of him. Allowing the client to hold onto the nurse's arm provides for the client to have some control. The other answers do not provide the most support for the client.

20. Answer D is correct. The presence of adventitious breath sounds (rales) can indicate the development of congestive heart failure. Pedal edema indicates right-sided congestive failure. A temperature of 99.2° should be monitored but does not need to be reported immediately. The blood pressure of 100/52 is slightly low but should be monitored.

21. Answer B is correct. Oral cyclosporine should be diluted in milk, chocolate milk, or orange juice and drank immediately because this helps with absorption and masks the taste. The glass should be rinsed and the residual drank to ensure that all the medication is taken. It should be stored at room temperature, and any medication remaining after two months should be discarded. It is taken for life. The client taking cyclosporins does not have to supplement with iron, store it in the refrigerator, or taper off the medication.

22. Answer A is correct. Protein breaks down into nitrogenous wastes that increase the workload of the kidneys. The other answers do not explain the reason for decreasing the amount of protein in the diet.

23. Answer D is correct. Second-degree partial thickness burns have formed blisters and are painful. The other answers describe more severe burns.

24. Answer A is correct. Imipramine and other tricyclic antidepressants can cause cardiac dysrhythmias and should not be used in those with known cardiac disease. The clients in answers B, C, and D can take Imipramine.

25. Answer D is correct. Urinary specific gravity indicates hydration status. Answers A and B do not indicate hydration. The fact that the client wets a diaper every four hours does not indicate the amount of each voiding or the hydration status.

26. Answer C is correct. The interaction of foods containing tyramine and MAO inhibitors produces a hypertensive crisis. An early indication of rising BP is headache. Answers A, B, and D do not indicate hypertension.

27. Answer B is correct. Traction is not being maintained when the foot plate is resting against the end of the bed. The use of the trapeze is allowed, the weights should be off the ground, and the ropes should be in the pulleys.

28. Answer C is correct. Restlessness, irritability, a slight increase in pulse rate, and rapid shallow respirations are indicative of pain. These symptoms are not indicative of fluid volume deficit, impending shock, or heart failure.

29. Answer D is correct. Meperidine, a narcotic, is a central nervous system depressant and should be used cautiously in a client with a head injury. The other orders are indicative for the treatment of this client.

30. Answer C is correct. A primary cause of bladder spasms is an obstructed catheter. Continuous irrigation will help prevent clot formation, but kinks in the catheter will prevent outflow. Offering oral fluids is of no help. If the catheter is obstructed, administration of an analgesic will offer little relief and mask symptoms. Massaging the symphysis can increase the pain.

31. Answer D is correct. A client with mandibular wires should keep a pair of wire cutters with her at all times. Saliva can be swallowed or spit out of the mouth, moving the lips will not interfere with the wiring, and cleaning the wires with saline is not necessary.

32. Answer B is correct. Following a cholecystectomy, a client will want to eat a diet low in fat because fat can continue to cause discomfort. He does not, however, have to eliminate it from his diet completely. A low-residue diet is not required, nor are low-protein or low-sodium diets.

33. Answer C is correct. Obesity is often associated with gallbladder disease. The other answers are not associated with it.

34. Answer A is correct. Osteomyelitis is an infection of the bone. The signs are fever, redness at the site, pain, and signs of cardiac adjustment such as tachycardia. Nausea and dehydration are not associated with it. Erythema or redness will be at the site and proximal to the site. Fatigue and lethargy are not directly associated with it.

35. Answer B is correct. A complication of renal disease is anemia due to a lack of erythropoetin. This leads to chronic hypoxia and heart enlargement. The others are not associated with renal disease.

36. Answer B is correct. The description in the stem is of a PVC. The others are incorrect assessments.

37. Answer B is correct. Clients taking Flagyl should not drink alcohol. If alcohol is consumed, the client will experience nausea and vomiting. Answer A is incorrect because the client can take the medication with juice. Answer C is incorrect because there is no need for eye exams. Answer D is incorrect because the medication is taken for 10 days.

38. Answer D is correct. The cardioversion should be synchronized to the QRS complex to prevent severe dysrhythmias. The others are incorrect timing.

39. Answer A is correct. *Kyphosis* is hump back or a forward curvature of the back. This frequently causes severe muscle spasms. Applying heat will help to relieve muscle spasms. Telling the client about relaxation exercises will not help. Administering a narcotic would help but will not be ordered routinely, and applying ice is not the best option.

40. Answer B is correct. Phenergan is an antiemetic. When given with Demerol, it helps to decrease the nausea, a side effect of that medication. It is not used to dry secretions, provide pain relief, or prevent infection.

41. Answer B is correct. The nurse, prior to taking the other actions, should validate with the client that he has been smoking. If this is the case, teaching is needed regarding the use of oxygen and the danger of fires. It will do no good to tell him that smoking is allowed only outside. Saying nothing is incorrect, and calling the head nurse is unnecessary at this time.

42. Answer B is correct. A stone in the ureter will block the outflow, so the output will decrease. If the stone is in the kidney, the output will increase. Answers A, C, and D are incorrect because there will not be an increased urinary output, unchanged output, or dark and foamy urine.

43. Answer C is correct. The client having a cystogram will be placed in the lithotomy position. Prone is on the abdomen, dorsal recumbent is on the back with the knees flexed, and left Sims' is side lying.

44. Answer B is correct. Glomerulonephritis is a disease of the glomeruli within the kidney. Postrenal disease is caused by diseases below the kidney; prerenal disease is caused by other diseases such as high blood pressure. Extrarenal is a distractor.

45. Answer A is correct. Zofran is an antiemetic given prior to chemotherapy or when other antiemetic drugs are not successful. It is not given for fever, pain, or anxiety.

46. Answer B is correct. Syphilis is a sexually transmitted infection most often treated with penicillin. Answer A is a cortisol preparation; answer C is an antiviral; answer D is a drug used for osteoporosis.

47. Answer B is correct. To prevent formation of thrombi in an infant with congenital heart disease, the nurse should provide for adequate hydration. A, C, and D are incorrect because they do not directly decrease the chances of a thrombi.

48. Answer B is correct. Thiazide diuretics are not potassium sparing; therefore, additional sources of potassium will be needed. There is no need to supplement calcium, magnesium, or folate.

49. Answer C is correct. The nurse should inquire about a screen to prevent the client from falling onto the gas heater. His cat provides a source of unconditional love. She cannot change the structure of his house or alter the fact that he lives alone.

50. Answer B is correct. Preschoolers have a keen sense of their bodies and fear the loss of body integrity. Answer A is incorrect because children during the preschool period are very aware of their environment. Answer C is untrue because children of this age are unable to conceptualize. Answer D is wrong because children do not resist any explanation. Simple explanations should be given to children undergoing surgery.

51. Answer D is correct. Overuse of antacids composed of calcium carbonate or sodium bicarbonate can cause metabolic alkalosis. Acetaminophen and aspirin can cause acidosis. Docusate is a laxative and, if overingested, can cause diarrhea and acidosis.

52. Answer B is correct. According to Orem's theory, the nurse should recognize when to intervene on behalf of the client and when to allow the client to act independently. Leaving the night light on will foster independence and provide for the client's safety. The other answers foster dependence.

53. Answer A is correct. The nurse should give priority to obtaining the client's vital signs every two hours. Withdrawal from alcohol contributes to delirium tremens or seizures with about 5%–15% of clients dying. Obtaining a complete drug history and lab work are important but can be done later. Answers B and D are incorrect because these options can be done after taking the vital signs. Starting an IV is unnecessary at this time, so answer C is wrong.

54. Answer C is correct. Furosemide is a loop diuretic that promotes fluid loss, thereby resulting in diminished rales in a client with congestive heart failure. Answer A is incorrect. Answer B is incorrect because the output would increase. Answer D is incorrect because the temperature has nothing to do with the use of Lasix.

55. Answer D is correct. Synergistic effects of alcohol and chlordiazepoxide contribute to oversedation and CNS depression. The other answers are unrelated to the use of Librium.

56. Answer A is correct. Only biopsy will allow for a definitive diagnosis. A pap smear is done for cervical cancer. A rectal exam will show enlargement but will not reveal whether the prostate is cancerous or benign. A phosphatase elevation will make the doctor suspect prostate cancer, but it is not definitive.

57. Answer A is correct. Improvement in the client's acidosis is reflected by decreases in CO_2 levels. Answer B is more subjective. Answer C pertains to metabolic acidosis, but a blood glucose within normal limits is unrelated. Answer D is also subjective.

58. Answer B is correct. Heparin levels are evaluated by checking the partial thromboplastin time as the test for coagulation. The diagnostic tests in Answers A, C, and D are used for oral anticoagulants.

59. Answer C is correct. Demonstration is a better indicator of understanding than repeating instructions. Asking questions or for additional materials might indicate a need for further teaching. Repeating the instructions is good but is not the best indicator.

60. Answer B is correct. Questioning the client allows for clarification of the client's feelings and fears regarding the procedure. Answer A is incorrect because it does not help the client to voice fears. In Answer C, the nurse is making inferences that can increase the client's fear. Answer D is a false reassurance.

61. Answer B is correct. Coumadin blocks the absorption of vitamin K. Green, leafy vegetables are good sources of vitamin K. If a client eats foods from this group more than two or three times per week, the dose of Coumadin will have to be adjusted to maintain a therapeutic level. The client does not have to take the medication on a empty stomach. Visual halos are not associated with Coumadin. As already stated, the client should decrease his intake of green, leafy foods.

62. Answer D is correct. The client with gallbladder disease needs a low-fat diet. Answer D provides a low-fat diet that is balanced in all the food groups. The other answers are higher in fats.

63. Answer B is correct. Looking at the operative site indicates that the client has accepted the change in body image. Verbalizing acceptance, asking for information, and remaining silent are not the best indicators of acceptance.

64. Answer B is correct. Aquamephyton is given to a newborn to promote clotting. Newborns are susceptible to bleeding because they lack the intestinal flora to produce vitamin K. This drug does not prevent hyperbilirubinemia, prevent hypoglycemia, or promote respiratory stability.

65. Answer D is correct. A client receiving cortisone retains sodium and water. He should therefore avoid a high-sodium diet. Answer D provides the most nutrition with the least amount of sodium. Answers A, B, and C are much higher in sodium.

66. Answer D is correct. Nothing by mouth (NPO) requires that the client refrain from eating, drinking, and using nicotine because nicotine stimulates gastric secretion. Answer A is incorrect because this answer has no bearing on the order to withhold cigarettes. Answer B is incorrect because the surgeon will tell the nurse the same thing. Answer C is incorrect because smoking might suppress the appetite but has no bearing on the order to withhold cigarettes prior to surgery.

67. Answer A is correct. If blood is administered through a single IV site, there should be an IV port close to the client so that emergency drugs can be administered in case of a reaction. If a reaction occurs, diphenhydramine (Benadryl) can be given. Acetaminophen (Tylenol) can be given prior to the transfusion. A tourniquet is unnecessary.

68. Answer C is correct. Measuring the extremity with a paper tape measure is the best way to assess the amount of edema in an extremity. Marking the area where the measurement was taken allows for future comparisons. Checking for extremity by pitting, or pushing in on the client's extremity, is more subjective. Weighing the client is also subjective. Observing the output tells fluid status but not in the extremity.

69. Answer B is correct. Play therapy that allows the child to bandage the doll's head best prepares the child for surgery. Touring the PICU would be too frightening for him, and he is too young to express his feelings verbally, so answers A and C are wrong. D is a good answer, but it is not the best way to prepare the child for a craniotomy.

70. Answer B is correct. A client with Parkinson's is at risk for falls. Answers A, C, and D are not directly associated with Parkinson's.

71. Answer A is correct. The nurse's first action should be to slow the rate of infusion. Tinnitus can signal beginning toxicity. If tinnitus persists after the IV is slowed, the nurse should call the doctor because a peak level should be drawn. Benadryl is not indicated.

72. Answer C is correct. The therapeutic level of heparin is 1 1/2–2 times the control. A therapeutic range for the activated partial thromboplastin time (APTT) is approximately 60–90 seconds. The antidote for heparin is protamine sulfate. (Note: The therapeutic range for the prothrombin time [PT] is approximately 1 1/2–2 times the control. The antidote for Coumadin is aquamephyton.) The other answers are incorrect calculations.

73. Answer B is correct. Cardiac complications of mechanical ventilation include hypotension. Positive pressures increase intrathoracic pressure and inhibit blood return to the heart, which leads to decreased cardiac output and hypotension. Hypocarpnia can occur with ventilation. Hypoperfusion and hyperthermia are not associated with mechanical ventilation.

74. Answer A is correct. The LPN with two years experience in labor and delivery is best suited to care for the new C-section client. Because the infant was large, there is the possibility of post-section complications, which would best be handled by a more experienced nurse. The other nurses have less experience.

75. Answer A is correct. Erratic fetal heart rates are best assessed by an internal fetal monitor. The word *erratic* does not imply that the fetal heart tones are low or that decelerations are present. Answer B is unnecessary at this time. Assisting the client with walking will make it more difficult to assess the fetal heart tones, so answer C is wrong. Answer D is wrong because there is no evidence of the need to move the client to the delivery room. The client is 8 cm dilated, so she is not ready for delivery.

76. Answer B is correct. A client with Cushing's disease has an elevated cortisol level. Elevations in cortisol suppress the inflammatory response and contribute to the development of infection. The other answers are of lesser priority.

77. Answer A is correct. A child with acute lymphocytic leukemia should be placed in reverse isolation until he is in remission. A child with hepatitis A should be placed on enteric isolation. A child with osteomyelitis or spasmodic laryngitis requires no special isolation.

78. Answer C is correct. A moribund client is one who is dying. The nurse should talk calmly with the client while continuing to assess the vital signs. Obtaining medication for agitation will suppress the respirations further. If the nurse stops taking the vital signs, she cannot evaluate the client's status.

79. Answer B is correct. Kefzol, a cephalosporin, should be avoided because cross sensitivities exist between the penicillins and cephalosporin. The other medications can be given.

80. Answer B is correct. Aminoglycosides, such as gentamycin, are both ototoxic and nephrotoxic. The other medications do not have these toxic effects.

81. Answer D is correct. The client's fears can be allayed by being told that pain is not associated with multiple sclerosis. Answer A is incorrect because a headache is not associated with exacerbations of multiple sclerosis. Answers B and C are not good answers because they do not address the fear of a worsening condition.

82. Answer B is correct. The client will need to improve the strength in her arms to assist with chair transfer. Because the injury is at the T-4 level, she will not be able to use her leg muscles, perform balancing exercises, or use her quadriceps muscles.

83. Answer D is correct. Walking with the nurse will provide the client with social contact, and physical activity will lessen the likelihood of hallucinations. Answer A is wrong because watching a movie with other clients will not help prevent hallucinations since interaction during the movie is minimal. Answers B and C are wrong because they are done alone and therefore do not provide the needed social contact.

84. Answer D is correct. Addison's disease results in volume depletion, which contributes to postural hypotension and dehydration. The other answers are associated with myxedema.

85. Answer A is correct. Hypersecretion of cortisol, a glucocorticoid, can result in emotional lability. Altered body image is not necessarily a symptom, and not enough data is given to support this assessment. Altered aldosterone levels are not directly associated with Cushing's. Altered coping is incorrect because there is no data to support this answer.

86. Answer D is correct. The woman who has delivered several term infants is more likely to experience extreme pain after delivery because the uterus is contracting with more difficulty in an attempt to decrease bleeding. The other women will have less pain.

87. Answer C is correct. Discussing the behavior with the client allows him the opportunity to discuss situations or feelings that might contribute to the new behavior. The other answers are incorrect because they will not address the problem.

88. Answer B is correct. The total to be infused (100 ml) divided by the total time in minutes (45) times the drip factor (10) equals 22 gtts per minute. The other answers are mathematically incorrect.

89. Answer B is correct. The nurse should check the tongs and traction each shift. A torque wrench should be kept at the bedside to tighten the device as needed. The other tools are not used for Crutchfield tongs.

90. Answer D is correct. Increases in FHR during movement is a normal finding and is considered reassuring. A fetal heart rate of 160–180 indicates tachycardia. A baseline variability of 20–30 BPM indicates a hyperactive pattern. Ominous implies bad.

91. Answer D is correct. Oxytocin induces uterine contractions. The desired effect is progressive dilation with contractions lasting fewer than 90 seconds. A, B, C are incorrect because these answers do not evaluate the effectiveness of IV oxytocin.

92. Answer A is correct. *Suppression* is conscious forgetting. *Repression*, or unconscious forgetting, is revealed through slips of the tongue, dreams, or hypnosis. *Denial* is simply denying the problem exists, and rationalization involves making excuses.

93. Answer B is correct. *Denial* is the failure to regard an event or feeling. The defense mechanisms associated with chemical dependency are denial and rationalization. In this situation, the client is using denial when he states, "I don't have a problem." *Displacement* is placing blame on others who are not a threat; *reaction formation* is reacting in the opposite manner than the feeling really held by the client. The defense mechanisms listed in answers A, C, and D are not reflected in the client's statement.

94. Answer B is correct. *Splitting* is the primary defense mechanism used by persons with borderline personality disorder. Clients who use splitting tend to see themselves and others as either all good or all bad. *Denial* is denying a problem; *projection* is projecting feelings onto others; and *rationalization* is trying to explain or make excuses for behavior.

95. Answer D is correct. *Reaction formation* is the expression of feelings opposite to your true feelings. *Transference* is transferring a like or dislike for someone because he reminds you of someone. *Rationalization* is explaining or making excuses for behavior, and *conversion reaction* is converting a psychological trauma into a physical ailment.

96. Answer B is correct. Laxatives are ordered prior to an IVP to evacuate the bowel and provide for better visualization of the kidney. Collection of a 24-hour urine is unnecessary; the client will be NPO after midnight; and radiopaque dye is given IV, not as tablets.

97. Answer B is correct. The three signs associated with renal cancer are dull flank pain, painless hematuria, and the presence of a costovertebral mass. Answers A, C, and D are symptoms of urinary tract infections.

98. Answer B is correct. The client receiving allopurinol should increase his fluid intake by 2–3 liters per day. Answers A and C are wrong because taking the medication 30 minutes before meals and taking the medication before going to bed are unnecessary. There is no risk of hypotension or dizziness, so answer D is incorrect.

99. Answer C is correct. Lipitor is given to decrease cholesterol levels. Lipitor is not given to decrease blood pressure, improve appetite, or to improve bone density, so the other answers are incorrect.

100. Answer D is correct. The nurse should monitor the color, temperature, and pulses in the procedural leg. Pressure should be maintained on the insertion site, and a 5-pound sandbag and ice packs (not warm wet packs) should be available in case of emergency. The procedural leg should be kept straight, not flexed, for six hours. Fluids should be encouraged—not withheld—to expedite excretion of the contrast dye.

101. Answer A is correct. Anasarca, severe generalized edema, is associated with a loss of albumin from the circulating blood volume. It is not associated with hypertension, hyperalbuminemia, or hyperthermia, so answers B, C, and D are wrong.

102. Answer D is correct. The most typical sign of a fractured hip is disalignment. Pain, paresthesia, and pulselessness are characteristics associated with all fractures, so answers A, B, and C are wrong.

103. Answer D is correct. Nausea, jitteriness, tachycardia, hypotension, and irritability are associated with aminophylline toxicity. Administering an antiemetic or a sedative will mask the symptoms of toxicity, making answers A and C wrong. The blood pressure might or might not be associated with the aminophylline, so answer B is incorrect.

104. Answer A is correct. The green-tinged fluid indicates meconium staining from fetal distress, as does the FHR of 110 BPM. Yellow malodorous discharge indicates infection, so answer B is wrong. Answer C is incorrect because there is no information to support this answer. Answer D is incorrect because polyhydramnios is an indication of a tracheoesophageal fistula.

105. Answer A is correct. Conversion reaction is the development of physical symptoms in response to emotional distress. Answers B, C, and D are not related to the situation given in the stem and are therefore incorrect.

106. Answer C is correct. The banana Popsicle provides a source of fluid, and the cold helps soothe the mucus membranes and provides for vasoconstriction. The fruit punch is red and the strawberry soda can be mistaken for blood, so answers A and B are wrong. Ice cream will thicken secretions, so answer D is wrong.

107. Answer D is correct. Nipride is administered in D5W and has a light brownish tint. A new bag should be prepared after 24 hours. Answer A is incorrect because the solution should be discarded if it is highly colored—that is, blue, green, or dark red. Answer B is wrong because the IV fluid has been chosen. Answer C is wrong because the stem says that the bag is already covered.

108. Answer D is correct. The client with opiate use has constricted pupils. However, opiate overdose results in dilated pupils due to cerebral anoxia. But because the stem doesn't mention overdose, answer A is incorrect. The client's speech will be slowed and her blood pressure will be decreased with opiate use, so answers B and C are incorrect.

109. Answer C is correct. Dilantin should not be administered any faster than 50 mg per minute. It should be given in normal saline to prevent crystallization in the tubing, so answers A and B are incorrect. This medication can be given IV push, so answer D is wrong.

110. Answer B is correct. Answer B is correct because the client's leg should be positioned with the hip slightly flexed. Use of a recliner allows for slight hip flexion and promotes comfort. The client should not be placed in a straight chair, and the hip should not be flexed more that 45°. Use of an abduction pillow prevents hip adduction. The hip should not be flexed 90°, so answer A is wrong. C is incorrect because supine is not the best position for this client. Answer D is incorrect because the right leg should not be adducted.

111. Answer A is correct. Autosomal recessive disorders arise when an affected gene is transmitted from each parent. Persons who carry the trait show no signs of the disorder. Answer B is incorrect because males are not affected by autosomal recessive disorders at twice the rate as females. Answers C and D are incorrect because they do not describe the inheritance pattern.

112. Answer B is correct. Infants should be making rudimentary sounds for speech by six weeks of age and certainly by three months. An infant who fails to coo or babble by three months should be evaluated for hearing loss. Answer A is too early to expect the infant to make sounds, so it is incorrect. Answers C and D are wrong because they are too late.

113. Answer C is correct. *Sublimation* is the channeling of unacceptable behaviors into behaviors that are socially acceptable. The other defense mechanisms have nothing to do with the situation, so answers A, B, and D are incorrect.

114. Answer D is correct. Turning objects upside down, moving objects from one location to another, and dropping items from the high chair all teach the child about spatial relationships. Turning the cup upside down is not a sign of misbehavior or a negative action, so answers A and C are incorrect. Answer B is incorrect because toddlers are not able to use thought processes to experience events and reactions.

115. Answer B is correct. Displacement is the transference of emotions onto another other than the intended target. Projection is projecting feelings onto others, making answer A wrong. Undoing is making up for loss, so answer C is wrong. Answer D is incorrect because compensation has nothing to do with abuse.

116. Answer A is correct. The names and addresses of the sexual contacts should be obtained. Chlamydia is treated with antibiotics such as tetracycline or ampicillin and is not treated with Flagyl, so answer B is incorrect. Instructing the client to avoid sexual relations is good, but it is best to tell her to use condoms, so answer C is wrong. Douching will do no good, making answer D wrong.

117. Answer D is correct. Ascorbic acid increases the absorption of iron. Taking the medication with a glass of milk will decrease the absorption of the medication, so answer A is wrong. Answer B is incorrect because, if the client takes the medication on an empty stomach, nausea can occur. Answer C is incorrect because it is an untrue statement.

118. Answer A is correct. An infant should be expected to double her birth weight by six months and triple her birth weight by 12 months of age. Baby girl A's weight gain might be due to overfeeding or the result of a metabolic disorder. Both instances would warrant follow-up. The other infants are within normal limits; therefore, answers B, C, and D are incorrect.

119. Answer B is correct. A pneumothorax results in tracheal deviation toward the unaffected side. Answers A and D are incorrect because there will be no breath sounds. Answer C is incorrect because the trachea will be deviated to the unaffected side, not the affected side.

120. Answer B is correct. The nurse should give priority to improving the client's oxygenation. Answers A, C, and D will come later and are therefore incorrect because the question asks for the priority action.

121. Answer D is correct. The client in acute pain experiences physiological arousal similar to the fight or flight response—for example, an increased (not decreased) heart rate, an increased BP, and dilated pupils. Answers A, B, and C are wrong because increased blood pressure, inability to concentrate, and dilated pupils are reactions to pain. The question asks which does not support an assessment of post-op pain, so answer D is correct.

122. Answer B is correct. The client receiving epidural anesthesia should be carefully monitored for respiratory depression that might result from plasma and central nervous system concentrations of the drug. Answer A is incorrect because seizure activity usually is not present with epidural anesthesia. The client will be lying down, so postural hypotension is not a risk, making answer C incorrect. Answer D is wrong because hematuria is not a risk.

123. Answer A is correct. Physiological responses to sensory alterations include increased urinary levels of catecholamines, 17-ketosteroids, and lutenizing hormones. Answers B, C, and D are incorrect because they are not related to catecholamines.

124. Answer B is correct. Refusal to look at the body or body part involved can indicate an alteration in body image, but this finding alone is not enough to make the nursing diagnosis. The most immediate diagnosis that can be made based on the available data is potential for infection. Answers A, C, and D are not immediate diagnoses, so they are incorrect.

125. Answer B is correct. *Proximodistal* development is defined as development from the axis of the body to the periphery. An infant can control the movement of his arms before he can control the movement of his fingers. Answer A refers to cephalocaudal, or head-to-tail, development; therefore, it is incorrect. Answer C refers to general-to-specific development; therefore, it is incorrect. Answer D refers to simple-to-complex development; therefore, it is incorrect.

126. Answer D is correct. Intracellular K+ quickly leaks from damaged cell membranes. Blood cells falling directly onto the ball or filter apparatus can break and release K+. Administering blood that is warmed to room temperature can grow bacteria but is not associated with potassium, so answer A is wrong. Answers B and C are wrong because administering blood that is 24 hours old is allowed and an 18-gauge needle is best.

127. Answer C is correct. Complications of the prolonged use of NG suction include dehydration, hypokalemia, hyponatremia, and metabolic alkalosis. The laboratory results in answers A, B, and D are within normal limits, so those answers are wrong.

128. Answer B is correct. Healing by a second intention results in extensive scar formation because the wound is left open and allowed to heal from the inside out. Answer A is incorrect because healing might not be accomplished in 10 days. Answer C is incorrect because third-degree healing does not take place from the inside out. Healing by first intention, not third intention, involves the use of staples or sutures, so answer D is incorrect.

129. Answer A is correct. Foods and fluids that promote urine alkalinity are discouraged. These include citrus fruits and juices, excessive milk and milk products, and carbonated beverages. Answers B, C, and D are incorrect because they indicate that the client understands.

130. Answer B is correct. The sixth cranial nerve is the abducens, which controls lateral movement of the eyes. The ability to chew is controlled by the fifth cranial nerve; the ability to swallow is controlled by the ninth cranial nerve; scalp sensation is controlled by the fifth cranial nerve.

131. Answer D is correct. Limiting salt intake will help prevent edema formation, which increases attacks of Meniere's syndrome. The other foods are allowed, so answers A, B, and C are incorrect.

132. Answer D is correct. Dark-skinned individuals often have a yellowish discoloration of the conjunctiva and sclera. Jaundice is better detected by observing the hard palate. A dark-skinned individual might have yellow sclera, and the palms and soles are not best, nor are the nail beds.

133. Answer A is correct. Evaluation of tissue turgor is best achieved by pinching the abdominal tissue or the tissue of the forehead while the client is in a supine position. Placing the client in other positions does not provide the most objective way of evaluating skin turgor, so answers B and D are incorrect. Pressing the skin is an incorrect method, making answer C wrong.

134. Answer B is correct. Side effects of Leukeran include ulcerations of the mouth and GI tract. Foods that are pureed or liquid are best tolerated. The other foods are more difficult to chew.

135. Answer D is correct. The client with myxedema should be placed on a low-sodium diet because cortisol causes sodium retention. The other foods are allowed.

136. Answer A is correct. Middle Easterners are typically Muslim, so they pray five times per day facing the southeast (if in the United States). Answers B and C are incorrect because most of these individuals do not need specially prepared foods and will take blood products. The medicine man is a healer in Hispanic and Native American communities, so answer D is incorrect.

137. Answer B is correct. A client receiving Adriamycin will have a decrease in neutrophils and other white blood cells, resulting in decreased immunity. Answer A is incorrect because it does not address the stem. Answer C is incorrect because providing a wig is presumptive. Answer D is incorrect because straining the urine is unnecessary.

138. Answer A is correct. Swimming is the best sport for a client with muscular dystrophy. The other sports put too much stress on the muscles and increase fatigue, so answers B, C, and D are wrong.

139. Answer D is correct. Liquid nitrogen leads to cell death and tissue destruction. Tissue freezing is followed by tenderness and hemorrhagic blister formation. Dry, crusty, and itchy skin occurs much later, so answer A is wrong. Oozing and painful skin occurs immediately after cryosurgery, so answer B is wrong. Dry and tender skin occurs much later, so answer C is wrong.

140. Answer A is correct. Viral cultures should be placed on ice. Answer B is wrong because bacterial cultures and fungal cultures, not viral cultures, are transported at room temperature. There is no need to double-bag it, so answer C is incorrect. Answer D is incorrect because there is special handling in that the nurse should wear gloves.

141. Answer C is correct. Clients with AIDS who develop herpes simplex lesions should be treated immediately with intravenous Acyclovir. The other medications are not used to treat herpes lesions, so answers A, B, and D are incorrect.

142. Answer D is correct. A *papule* is a small, elevated skin lesion less than 1.0 cm in diameter. Answer A is wrong because macules are larger. A *plaque* is a dry lesion, so answer B is wrong. Answer C is wrong because a *wheal* is a raised, well-circumscribed lesion that is firm to touch.

143. Answer B is correct. Infants do not crawl until 9 or 10 months of age. The injuries observed are not consistent with the history given by the mother. The statements in answers A, C, and D are possible, so they are incorrect.

144. Answer D is correct. Persistent vomiting leads to alkalosis. Answer A is incorrect because it is acidosis. Answer B is incorrect because it is alkalosis but is respiratory. Answer C is incorrect because it is acidosis.

145. Answer C is correct. Asking the client to swallow as the tube is advanced will facilitate insertion. Placing the tube in warm water will make it more difficult to insert, so answer A is wrong. The client should be placed with his head elevated, making answer B incorrect. If the client hyperextends his neck, it will open the epiglottis, so answer D is wrong.

146. Answer B is correct. Rinsing the mouth with normal saline will provide for oral hygiene and make the client more comfortable. The client should use a soft toothbrush or a gauge to clean his teeth, so answer A is wrong. Answer C is wrong because if hydrogen peroxide is used, it should be diluted. Use of lemon and glycerin swabs will cause drying, so answer D is wrong.

147. Answer C is correct. Clients with cystic fibrosis are unable to absorb fat-soluble vitamins. Water-soluble preparations of the fat-soluble vitamins are given daily. Answer A is wrong because a client with cystic fibrosis does not have metabolism that is increased. Answer B is incorrect because a child with cystic fibrosis can eat a well-balanced diet and still lack nutrients. A child with cystic fibrosis also does not have an increased excretion of water-soluble vitamins, making answer D incorrect.

148. Answer D is correct. The client should be positioned on the left side to limit the flow of saline out of the stomach and to help prevent aspiration. The positions in answers A, B, and C are not recommended and are therefore incorrect.

149. Answer D is correct. Long-term therapy for diabetes insipidus involves vasopressin. The client should be told to hold her breath while using the spray because inhalation can result in pulmonary problems. Vasopressin preparations include DDAVP, desmopressin, and lypressin. Answers A, B, and C are unnecessary steps and are therefore incorrect.

150. Answer D is correct. A client with a transphenoidal hypophysecectomy will have an incision in either the nose or mouth. These clients can use dental floss and mouth rinses but should not brush their teeth because they can cause trauma to the mouth or nose. Answer A is incorrect because there is no incision in the scalp. The client should not cough because this increases intracranial pressure, so answer B is wrong. He will be placed with his head elevated to facilitate breathing, so answer C is wrong.

151. Answer D is correct. *Pheochromocytoma* is a catecholamine-producing tumor of the adrenal gland. Pheochromocytoma tumors cause synthesis of epinephrine and norepinephrine. The results of this stimulation is tachycardia not bradycardia. Answers A, B, and C are expected results of this type of tumor.

152. Answer B is correct. A rapid corticotrophin stimulation test involves the administration of corticosyntropin .25 mg–1 mg IM or IV after obtaining a baseline level. Blood samples are taken 30 minutes and one hour after administration of the drug. If there is adrenocortical insufficiency, the cortisol response will decrease or be absent. Answers A, C, and D are incorrect because they are not associated with this exam.

153. Answer B is correct. The blood urea nitrogen is elevated due to metabolic acidosis. The white blood cell count will be normal, so answer A is incorrect. The potassium in answer C is within normal limits. If a client with Addison's disease is in metabolic acidosis, the potassium will be either increased or decreased depending on renal function. Therefore, answer C is wrong. The sodium in answer D is elevated. In Addison's, the sodium is decreased, so answer D is incorrect.

154. Answer D is correct. Fatty foods and xanthine-containing beverages such as tea, cola, and coffee affect the tone and contractility of the low esophageal sphincter. These substances lower esophageal pressure and allow gastric contents to flow back into the esophagus. The foods found in answers A, B, and C do not increase discomfort in clients with GERD, so those answers are wrong.

155. Answer C is correct. Semi-Fowler's position promotes drainage, which can relieve pain. Other relief measures include the use of analgesics, sitz baths, and heat applications to the lower abdomen. The positions in answers A, B, and D will not relieve pain and might increase it, so they are wrong.

156. Answer C is correct. Antimicrobial drugs such as sulfasalazine help prevent secondary infection, decrease the frequency of exacerbation, and block folic acid synthesis so that bacteria are more susceptible to destruction. The usual dosages is 3 gms daily in divided doses. Answer A is incorrect because exposure to sunlight is not specific to this drug. Answer B is incorrect because taking the medication with meals is not recommended; however, it should not be taken on an empty stomach because it can cause nausea. Answer D is incorrect because it is untrue.

157. Answer B is correct. Autonomic dysreflexia results from uninhibited sympathetic discharges. Symptoms include pounding headache, marked increase in the blood pressure, tachycardia, flushed skin, nasal congestion, and visual disturbances. Interventions include raising the head of the bed to high Fowler's position, checking the Foley catheter to ensure patency, administering antihypertensive medication, and notifying the doctor. After the client is stabilized, you should check for fecal impaction. Answers A, C, and D are not associated with the treatment of autonomic dysreflexia, so they are incorrect.

158. Answer D is correct. When the client with glomerulonephritis is improving, the sedimentation rate will decrease. Answer A is incorrect because a positive ASO titer indicates prior infection with a beta hemolytic streptococcal infection. Answer B is incorrect because an increased C reactive protein rate indicates inflammation. Changes in eosinophil counts are associated with allergic responses and infections with helminthes, so answer C is wrong.

159. Answer C is correct. Peanut butter, crackers, and cheese are high in protein and sodium. Orange juice is high in potassium. The client with acute renal failure should select a diet that is low in protein, sodium, and potassium. Therefore, answers A, B, and D are wrong.

160. Answer D is correct. The client with a transplant should eliminate foods that pose the threat of contamination. Answers A, B, and C are all processed foods, so they don't pose a threat of contamination and are therefore incorrect.

161. Answer B is correct. Swimming promotes controlled rhythmic breathing. Soccer and basketball are too strenuous, so answers A and C are incorrect. Construction of model cars uses glues with noxious vapors, which can aggravate respiratory conditions, making answer D incorrect.

162. Answer D is correct. Reed instruments such as the clarinet help promote purse-lipped breathing and prolong the expiratory phase of respiration. The instruments in answers A, B, and C do not assist with this, so they are wrong.

163. Answer A is correct. Bright red bleeding with many clots indicates arterial bleeding. The vital signs should be obtained and the doctor notified at once. Answer B is not associated with the symptoms, so it is incorrect. Answer C is incorrect because bright red bleeding after surgery is not normal. Answer D is wrong because applying traction will not help.

164. Answer A is correct. Potassium-sparing diuretics such as Aldactone, midomor, and dyrenium do not require additional sources of potassium in the diet, so answers B, C, and D are incorrect.

165. Answer B is correct. Answers A, C, and D are incorrect because citrus fruits, raisins, and melons all contain high levels of potassium.

166. Answer D is correct. Many people prefer to supplement their calcium intake with calcium-based antacids. If calcium supplements are used, they should be administered 30 minutes before meals to maximize absorption, so answer A is wrong. Calcium absorption is better if it is administered throughout the day rather than in a single dose, making answer B wrong. Calcium supplements do not cause stomach upset, so answer C is wrong.

167. Answer B is correct. The most common complication of hypocalcemia is overstimulation of the nerves and muscles. Tetany, which can progress to convulsions, indicates that the client's condition is worsening. Answer A is incorrect because a decreased level of consciousness is not associated with hypocalcemia. Tachycardia, not brachycardia, is associated with hypocalcemia, making answer C incorrect. Answer D is incorrect because respiratory depression is not directly related to hypocalcemia.

168. Answer C is correct. The resistance to the electrical current is greatest in the muscles surrounding the long bones; therefore, they are usually subjected to the greatest amount of damage due to heat. Answers A, B, and D are incorrect because skin, intrathoracic, and bones are not the most affected by electrical burns.

169. Answer C is correct. As glucose moves from the blood into the cell, potassium is moved from the extracellular to the intracellular fluid. A, B, and D are incorrect rationales because administering glucoses does not eliminate potassium, bind with potassium, or lower the blood glucose.

170. Answer D is correct. Severe shock leads to decreased pressure in the renal artery and constriction of the afferent arterioles of the nephrons. If the tubular basement membrane is destroyed, the renal tubular epithelium cannot regenerate and renal failure becomes chronic. Answers A and C are incorrect because during hypovolemic shock blood is sent to the heart and brain. The skin does not suffer the most damage, making answer B wrong.

171. Answer C is correct. The entire arm represents 9% of the total body surface, and the posterior trunk represents 18% of the total body surface. Answers A, B, and D are incorrect calculations.

172. Answer C is correct. According to the Parkland formula, three fourths of the calculated fluid volume should infuse within 16 hours of the burn injury. The remaining one fourth of the volume should infuse over the last eight hours. Answers A, B, and D are incorrect calculations.

173. Answer B is correct. Valium given IV is the drug of choice for status epilepitcus. Carbamazepine (Tegretol) is used to treat psychomotor seizures, so answer A is wrong. Clonazepam (Klonopin) is used to treat myoclonic seizures, so answer C is wrong. Valproic acid (Depakene) is used to treat absence seizures, making answer D incorrect.

174. Answer A is correct. Approximately 80% of the lithium dose is absorbed in the proximal tubule of the kidney. The amount of reabsorption depends on the concentration of sodium. A deficiency in sodium causes greater absorption, leading to toxicity. Lithium dosages are not related to potassium, chloride, or magnesium, so answers B, C, and D are wrong.

175. Answer A is correct. In the immediate post-burn period, enlargement of capillary pores allows plasma, electrolytes, and protein molecules to move into the interstitial space, which creates a deficit in the vascular fluid volume. The decrease in the vascular volume results in a drop in the mean arterial pressure. Although fluid is lost from the site, this is not the reason for the major loss, so answer B is incorrect. Answer C is incorrect because large amounts of epinephrine will not lead to shock. The release of epinephrine helps to prevent shock. Answer D is incorrect because even though epinephrine will lead to tachycardia, it does not lead to ineffective cardiac output and shock.

176. Answer A is correct. Nausea, vomiting, and diarrhea are all symptoms of colchicine toxicity. Answers B, C, and D are not signs of toxicity and are therefore incorrect.

177. Answer B is correct. Positioning the infant on the abdomen with the hips slightly elevated prevents trauma and pressure on the sac. The other positions do not relieve pressure on the site, so answers A, C, and D are incorrect.

178. Answer A is correct. Bacon, French toast, sausage, cream cheese, and eggs are all high in cholesterol, so answers B, C, and D are incorrect.

179. Answer C is correct. A ventriculoperitoneal shunt is used to remove excessive cerebrospinal fluid from the ventricles of the brain in clients with hydrocephalus. The presence of cerebrospinal fluid would be indicated by a positive glucose. A is incorrect because the doctor can be called after checking the fluid to assess for cerebrospinal fluid. If it is positive, the nurse should contact the doctor. Answers B and D are incorrect because it is not enough to mark the dressing or take no action because the client's condition will continue to deteriorate.

180. Answer A is correct. A hydrocele or fluid in the scrotal sac is indicated by the inability to reduce the swelling by trasillumination of the scrotum. Answers B, C, and D are wrong because they are not true statements.

181. Answer D is correct. Cheese and yogurt provide needed calories and protein while being acceptable sources for the client with cancer. Answers A and B are low in protein and are therefore wrong. Although fresh fruit and vegetables would provide needed vitamins, they are less likely to be tolerated, making answer C incorrect.

182. Answer B is correct. The child is experiencing symptoms of an allergic reaction, which can involve the respiratory system. Applying the tourniquet helps to slow the spread of the bee toxin, and the epinephrine helps to maintain cardiovascular stability. Answer A is wrong because 4 liters of oxygen is not enough to help relieve the pain and ischemia. Oxygen should be applied by mask. Answer C will be of little help, although Benadryl might be given after applying the tourniquet, so it is incorrect. Reassuring the client will not treat the allergic reaction, so answer D is incorrect.

183. Answer A is correct. Clients receiving Digoxin and Lasix are at risk for hypokalemia. They are not at risk for other electrolyte abnormalities, so answers B, C, and D are wrong.

184. Answer A is correct. *Lochia rubra* is the first bright red bleeding after delivery. Answer B is incorrect because lochia serosa contains serous fluid and lasts for approximately 7 days. Answer C is incorrect because lochia alba is clear and lasts approximately 4–6 weeks. There is no such thing as lochia canta, so answer D is wrong.

185. Answer D is correct. Diminished hepatic function and decreased liver enzymes contribute to slower metabolism and slower detoxification threshold, thereby increasing the risk of drug accumulation and toxic effect. Answers A, B, and C are incorrect because diminished hepatic function will not decrease the possibility of drug toxicity, prevent analgesics from being given, or reduce the blood level of certain drugs.

186. Answer A is correct. Barbiturates increase the liver's capability to metabolize drugs, including phenytoin (Dilantin). Large doses can be required to produce the desired effect. An increase in metabolism occurs, so answer B is incorrect. The dosage does need to be altered/increased, so answer C is wrong. The two drugs can be given together, making answer D wrong.

187. Answer B is correct. Skin preparations containing povidone-iodine should not used on those with known or suspected allergies to shellfish. Anesthetics and antibiotics do not contain iodine, so answers A and C are incorrect. There is no need to monitor the client's thyroid levels post-operatively, so answer D is incorrect.

188. Answer A is correct. Normal prothrombin time is 12–20 seconds. Prolonged prothrombin time increases the chance of post-op hemorrhage. The other laboratory results are within normal range, so answers B, C, and D are wrong.

189. Answer B is correct. Measures to prevent spinal headache include placing the client flat in bed for 6–12 hours as well as maintaining adequate hydration. Answer A is wrong because placing the client in a quiet room might help to treat a spinal headache, but it will not prevent the headache. Answer C is wrong because administering a PRN pain medication will also help to treat the headache but not prevent it. Raising the head of the bed is contraindicated, so answer D is wrong.

190. Answer B is correct. Initial treatment of autonomic dysreflexia includes elevating the head of the bed to 45° to create orthostatic hypotension. Taking the client's pulse and respirations should be done next, but not first, so answer A is incorrect. Placing the client flat, supine will increase the blood pressure, making answer C incorrect. Answer D is wrong because it requires a doctor's order.

191. Answer B is correct. Testicular exam should be performed monthly while the client is in the tub or shower. Answer A is incorrect because testicular exams need not be done bimonthly. Answer C is incorrect because testicular exams are not done using a small penlight. This method of examination is done to detect a hydrocele. Answer D is incorrect because testicular exams should be done monthly, not yearly.

192. Answer D is correct. Following diarrheal illnesses, the villi often become lactose intolerant; therefore, the client should be placed on a soy-based formula with gradual reintroduction of regular formula. Isomil is not less expensive than other formulas, so answer A is wrong. There is no evidence to support answer B, so it is incorrect. Answer C is incorrect because the fact that Isomil is an excellent rehydrated formula is not the reason to change the infant's diet.

193. Answer C is correct. *Petaling* the cast is covering the edges with cast batting to soften them and prevent the cast material from flaking inside the cast. Cutting down the cast down both sides is *bi-valving*, so answer A is wrong. Cutting a window in the cast is done to examine the incision, so answer B is incorrect. Answer D is wrong because it is a distractor.

194. Answer A is correct. Changing position, gently massaging the abdomen, and ambulating help the return of the irrigating solution. Answer B is incorrect because reducing the amount of irrigate is contraindicated since it changes the doctor's order. Answer C is incorrect because simply increasing oral intake will not help to evacuate the irrigant. Answer D is incorrect because placing a heating pad on the abdomen will not help to facilitate return of the irrigation fluid.

195. Answer B is correct. The nurse should give priority to assisting with the tube's progression by changing the client's position every two hours and by advancing the tube 3–4 inches as the physician directs. Answer A is wrong because the tube should not be irrigated routinely. Answer C is wrong because changing the tape is unnecessary. Answer D is incorrect because the tube is not connected to high continuous suction.

196. Answer D is correct. Ecchymosis around the umbilicus is known as *Cullen's sign* and is suggestive of retroperitoneal bleeding into the abdominal wall. Cullen's sign is not associated with neurological injury, ruptured spleen, or bowel perforation, so answers A, B, and C are incorrect.

197. Answer C is correct. Pancreatin supplies enzymes that assist in the digestion of fats. Drug management is determined to be effective when the stools become less fatty and less frequent. Answer A is a subjective answer, so it is incorrect. Answer B is incorrect because a weight loss of greater than 10 pounds can indicate that the client's condition is worsening, not improving. Answer D is incorrect because bruising is more subjective and might not indicate that the condition is improving.

198. Answer C is correct. Diabetes mellitus in the pregnant client places the infant at risk for changes in placental vasculature. Answer A is incorrect because, in and of itself, fetal movement is not adversely affected by diabetes. Answer B is incorrect because maternal insulin levels are not measured by a non-stress test. Answer D is wrong because fetal lung maturity is not measured by a non-stress test.

199. Answer B is correct. Renal agenesis is associated with oligohydramnios, or lower-than-normal amounts of amniotic fluid. Answers A, C, and D are incorrect because they are associated with polyhydramnios.

200. Answer B is correct. Aminophylline is a xanthine derivative that can cause central nervous system stimulation. Nervousness and tremulousness are common side effects. Answer A is wrong because central nervous system depression is not associated with xanthine use. Xanthines do not have an anticholinergic effect, so answer C is incorrect. Answer D is incorrect because cardiovascular depression is not associated with aminophylline.

201. Answer C is correct. Herpes zoster, also called *shingles*, is a viral infection that is treated with antiviral medications. It is not usually treated with the categories in answers A, B, and D, so they are incorrect.

202. Answer C is correct. Propranolol (Inderal) is a beta blocker that can produce bradycardia and bronchospasm. These facts would make this drug contraindicated in this client. The drugs in answers A, B, and D can be administered to this client, so those answers are wrong.

203. Answer B is correct. The client should be instructed to take her medication with meals to avoid gastric irritation. Answer A is incorrect because regular exercise is encouraged. Answer C is incorrect because applying hot compresses at night can lead to burns. Answer D is incorrect because weight-bearing exercises are encouraged, not avoided.

204. Answer A is correct. *Buck's traction* is a skin traction used to decrease muscle spasms. Buck's traction will not prevent the need for surgery, making answer B wrong. It also will not alleviate the pain associated with the fracture or prevent bleeding, so answers C and D are wrong.

205. Answer B is correct. Burns of the head and neck pose the immediate threat of airway compromise. The conditions in answers A, C, and D might be painful, but they do not present an immediate threat to life, so they are incorrect.

206. Answer B is correct. A PO_2 of 72% is very low. The normal is 95–105. Answer A is wrong because the BUN is normal. Answer C is wrong because the hemoglobin is low but does not have to be reported immediately. Answer D is wrong because the white blood cell count is normal.

207. Answer A is correct. Normal central venous pressure reading is approximately 5–10 cm of water. Answer B is incorrect because a carbon dioxide of 30 is low and does not indicate fluid overload. Answer C is incorrect because a hemoglobin of 18 is normal and does not indicate fluid overload. Answer D is wrong because the potassium is within normal limits.

208. Answer B is correct. The placenta produces insulinase, an insulin antagonist. As the pregnancy increases, so does the need for additional amounts of insulin. Answers A, C, and D are incorrect because they are untrue statements about insulin needs during pregnancy.

209. Answer A is correct. Lying on the left side takes the weight of the uterus off the vena cava and provides for greater perfusion to the kidneys. Answers B and D are incorrect because both Fowler's position and supine are on the client's back. Answer C is incorrect because Trendelenburg position is with the client's head down and legs elevated, which would make it more difficult to breath and increase the blood pressure.

210. Answer A is correct. Increasing dyspnea is associated with cardiac decompensation and congestive heart failure. The other symptoms are common to all pregnant clients, so answers B, C, and D are incorrect.

211. Answer D is correct. Opiates such as morphine should not be used because they cause spasms in the sphincter of Oddi. The other medications can be given to the client with pancreatitis, so answers A, B, and C are wrong.

212. Answer B is correct. Hallucinogens produce altered states of perception. Answer A is incorrect because hallucinogens do not produce both a stimulant and depressant effect. Answer C is incorrect because they do not produce severe respiratory depression. Answer D is incorrect because hallucinogens cause a psychological dependence, not a physical dependence.

213. Answer A is correct. Abrupt cessation of amphetamines produces depression and suicidal thinking. Clients withdrawing from amphetamines need to be watched closely for suicidal gestures. Barbituates cause B, so it's wrong. Answer C occurs when the client is withdrawing, so it's wrong. Answer D is incorrect because tachycardia and euphoria are not associated with withdrawal from amphetamines.

214. Answer C is correct. Fetal heart tones are best heard in the area between the scapula. If the fetus is in the left sacral anterior position, the fetal heart tones will be heard loudest in the upper left quadrant. Answers A, B, and D are incorrect positions if the heart tones are heard in the upper left quadrant.

215. Answer D is correct. Although all the choices are involved in the process of asthma, the primary physiological alteration involves spasms of the bronchiolar smooth muscle. Therefore, answers A, B, and C are wrong.

216. Answer A is correct. During periods of mania, the client might be unable to sit long enough to complete a meal. Providing high-calorie finger foods will allow the client to move about while maintaining adequate nutrition. Answers B, C, and D are not directed at the mania that the client is experiencing, so they are wrong.

217. Answer B is correct. To maintain Bryant's traction, the legs are suspended at a right angle to the bed with the hips slightly above the bed surface. Answers A, C, and D are incorrect because they do not describe the correct use of Bryant's traction.

218. Answer B is correct. Absence of babbling by age seven months suggests that the infant might not be able to hear. Answers A, C, and D are not related to impaired hearing and are therefore incorrect.

219. Answer A is correct. Toddlers are extremely sensitive to separation anxiety. Failure to respond to his parents indicates detachment. This is the third stage of separation anxiety. Answer B is incorrect because it does not indicate successful adjustment. Answer C is incorrect for the same reason. There is not enough data to support answer D, so it is incorrect.

220. Answer B is correct. A peak is the highest blood level. The peak should be drawn 30 minutes after the infusion. Answers A, C, and D are incorrect because they describe times inappropriate for drawing a peak level.

221. Answer B is correct. Each ml contains 50 units. To deliver 1,200 units per hour, the IV set must deliver 24 ml per hour. Answers A, C, and D are incorrectly calculated, so they are incorrect.

222. Answer A is correct. Due to the possibility of toxic shock syndrome, the client should remove the diaphragm in 6–8 hours. It should be kept in a cool place, not a warm one, so answer B is wrong. The diaphragm should be resized if the client gains 10 pounds or loses 10 pounds, not 5, so answer C is wrong. If the client has abdominal surgery, not any surgery, the diaphragm should be resized, so D is incorrect.

223. Answer B is correct. Expressing milk from the breast promotes milk production rather than facilitating drying of the milk. Answers A, C, and D indicate understanding, so they are incorrect.

224. Answer B is correct. Cranial nerve VIII damage results in sensorineural hearing loss. Answers A, C, and D are incorrect because the eighth cranial nerve does not control air conduction hearing loss, mixed hearing loss, or tinnitus.

225. Answer D is correct. Antineoplastic drugs such as Vincristine can cause changes in taste during or after administration. Vincristine does not cause the symptoms in answers A, B, or C, so they are incorrect.

226. Answer B is correct. Cyclophosphamide is toxic to the bladder and can case hemorrhagic cystitis. Monitoring vital signs every hour, monitoring the apical pulse, and assessing for intracranial pressure are not of particular concern with this medication because it does not have these side effects. Therefore, answers A, C, and D are incorrect.

227. Answer D is correct. Acyclovir is nephrotoxic, so the client must stay well hydrated. Answers A, B, and C are not necessary for the client taking acyclovir, making them incorrect.

228. Answer B is correct. A rash is usually the first sign of a graft-host disease. Chest pain and ECG changes are not directly associated with this, so answers A and C are incorrect. Answer D is incorrect because an extremely high fever might be a reaction, but a slight fever is expected.

229. Answer C is correct. Seconal is a barbiturate, and CNS depressants and stimulants, as well as phenothiazines, should not be given for 48 hours prior to a myelogram because they decrease the seizure threshold. Ampicillin is an antibiotic, Motrin is an NSAID, and Darvon is an analgesic, so they can all be given, making answers A, B, and D incorrect.

230. Answer D is correct. Hyperventilation to maintain a PCO_2 of 25–30 mm Hg causes vasoconstriction and leads to a decrease in cerebral blood volume. Answer A is wrong because the purpose of hyperventilation at this time is not to increase oxygen to the brain. Answers B and C are wrong because neither is its purpose to dilate the cerebral blood volume or to increase the blood volume.

231. Answer D is correct. The client with craniocerebral trauma is at risk for diabetes insipidus due to trauma to the pituitary gland. Answer A is incorrect because there is no data to support this answer. Answer B is incorrect because the client has had a head injury, not renal disease. Answer C is incorrect because the client with diabetes insipidus has inadequate antidiuretic hormone, not adequate.

232. Answer C is correct. The client in C needs further evaluation. Answer A is wrong because that client's blood glucose is within normal limits. Answer B is wrong because that client is maintained on his medication. Answer D is wrong because the client with Raynaud's disease is in no distress.

233. Answer C is correct. The temporal lobe contains the auditory center, where sounds are interpreted, and the association areas, where words are processed into coherent thought. The other answers are incorrect because they are not associated with receptive aphasia.

234. Answer B is correct. During the first 72 hours, the client is at greatest risk for cerebral edema and increased intracranial pressure. Elevating the head of the bed 30°–45° and maintaining the client's head midline in a neutral position facilitate venous drainage from the brain. The client should not be positioned flat because this can increase intracranial pressure. Because there is a history of clotting, the knee gatch should not be elevated.

235. Answer D is correct. The presence of white blood cells in the cerebrospinal fluid should be less than 5/cubic mm. An elevated white blood cell count indicates infection, tumors, or blood. Answers A, B, and C are incorrect because the levels are normal.

236. Answer C is correct. Loss of function of cranial nerve V results in loss of the blink reflex. The eye should be patched to prevent damage to the cornea. Answer A is incorrect because swallowing is not controlled by cranial nerve V. Answer B is incorrect because hearing is not involved with cranial nerve V. Answer D is incorrect for the same reason.

237. Answer B is correct. Contrast medium used in CT scans are excreted through the kidneys. Forcing fluids helps to remove the dye from the body. Answer A is incorrect because there is no need to maintain bed rest. There is no puncture site, so answer C is incorrect. Answer D is incorrect because there is no need to administer pain medication.

238. Answer B is correct. Huntington's chorea is inherited as an autosomal dominant disorder. The offspring of a parent with the disease has a 50% chance of developing the disease. Answers A, C, and D are incorrect calculations.

239. Answer C is correct. The lens bends light rays as they enter the pupil, causing them to fall on the retina. The lens does not control stimulation of the retina, making answer A wrong. Answer B is wrong because the lens does not orchestrate eye movement; this is done by the oculomotor nerve. Answer D is incorrect because the lens does not magnify small objects.

240. Answer B is correct. Mydriatics dilate the pupil. They do not anesthetize the cornea, so answer A is wrong. Mydriatics do not constrict the pupils, so answer C is wrong. Mydriatics do not paralyze the muscles of accommodation, so D is wrong.

241. Answer A is correct. If two medications are administered at the same time, administer the two drugsfive minutes apart starting with the eye drops. Answers B is incorrect because the medications should not be given together. C and D are incorrect because there is no need for a cycloplegic and the medication can be given to the same client.

242. Answer D is correct. Kaposi's sarcoma lesions are multifocal lesions with reddish purple discoloration or nodules that commonly appear on the lower fornix or eyelid. They are not associated with cytomegalovirus, AIDS entropion, or retinitis pigmentosa, so answers A, B, and C are incorrect.

243. Answer B is correct. Elderly clients often experience loss of color vision as they age. The colors that are often lost are blue, violet, and green. Answers A, C, and D are incorrect because these colors are more easily distinguished.

244. Answer B is correct. Urine that is allowed to stand at room temperature becomes more alkaline. Alkalinity of the urine promotes cellular breakdown. Abnormal urinary sediment can go undetected in stagnant urine. Answer A is untrue. Answer C is incorrect because, even if components of urine consolidate, the urine can still be analyzed. Answer D is incorrect because red cells would be present at the time the specimen is collected, they would not appear, so this is an untrue statement.

245. Answer A is correct. During bladder filling, the sympathetic nervous system fibers dominate and override detrusor muscle contractions. This prevents the involuntary emptying of the bladder. Bladder control is not directly dependent on the parasympathetic nervous system, the central nervous system, or the lower motor neurons; therefore, answers B, C, and D are wrong.

246. Answer C is correct. Dark green, leafy vegetables such as spinach contain oxalate. Answers A, B, and D are wrong because these foods are allowed with oxalate stones but are not allowed with uric acid stones.

247. Answer A is correct. Cromolyn sodium (Intal) is used before an attack and is of little use during an acute attack. Answers B, C, and D are used during an attack and are therefore incorrect.

248. Answer D is correct. The pulse oximeter uses waves of light and a sensor to measure oxygen saturation. Asking the client whether he needs oxygen is not adequate, so answer A is incorrect. Assessing the client's level of fatigue is also inadequate, so answer B is wrong. Evaluating the hemoglobin will not tell oxygen saturation, so answer C is wrong.

249. Answer A is correct. A properly secured tie allows space for only one finger to be placed between the tie and neck. Answers B and C are wrong because they are subjective. Although Velcro fasteners can be used, answer D does not assess whether the ties are correctly applied, so it is wrong.

250. Answer B is correct. Sarcordosis is most common in African-American females. The other clients are not at particular risk, so answers A, C, and D are incorrect.

Answers to Practice Exam II

1. D	28. B	55. A	82. B
2. C	29. B	56. B	83. A
3. C	30. B	57. B	84. A
4. B	31. C	58. A	85. C
5. D	32. B	59. A	86. C
6. D	33. A	60. A	87. B
7. A	34. A	61. A	88. A
8. B	35. C	62. B	89. D
9. A	36. B	63. A	90. C
10. A	37. A	64. B	91. A
11. B	38. B	65. B	92. A
12. D	39. B	66. A	93. D
13. B	40. D	67. D	94. D
14. C	41. B	68. C	95. A
15. A	42. B	69. B	96. D
16. A	43. A	70. B	97. C
17. B	44. A	71. B	98. D
18. A	45. B	72. D	99. B
19. B	46. D	73. B	100. B
20. B	47. C	74. D	101. C
21. B	48. B	75. D	102. C
22. B	49. A	76. C	103. B
23. C	50. B	77. B	104. A
24. C	51. B	78. B	105. D
25. B	52. B	79. B	106. D
26. D	53. B	80. C	107. C
27. D	54. B	81. C	108. A

109. B	**138.** D	**167.** D	**196.** C	**225.** A
110. C	**139.** C	**168.** B	**197.** D	**226.** A
111. B	**140.** C	**169.** A	**198.** D	**227.** A
112. D	**141.** B	**170.** C	**199.** B	**228.** B
113. B	**142.** C	**171.** B	**200.** C	**229.** B
114. C	**143.** A	**172.** A	**201.** D	**230.** A
115. A	**144.** A	**173.** C	**202.** D	**231.** A
116. A	**145.** A	**174.** B	**203.** D	**232.** D
117. D	**146.** A	**175.** C	**204.** B	**233.** B
118. C	**147.** B	**176.** A	**205.** B	**234.** C
119. B	**148.** D	**177.** A	**206.** D	**235.** B
120. B	**149.** C	**178.** C	**207.** D	**236.** D
121. B	**150.** B	**179.** C	**208.** B	**237.** A
122. B	**151.** C	**180.** A	**209.** C	**238.** C
123. D	**152.** A	**181.** D	**210.** B	**239.** B
124. C	**153.** C	**182.** B	**211.** A	**240.** A
125. B	**154.** B	**183.** C	**212.** D	**241.** D
126. B	**155.** A	**184.** A	**213.** B	**242.** A
127. B	**156.** B	**185.** A	**214.** C	**243.** B
128. C	**157.** D	**186.** B	**215.** D	**244.** C
129. D	**158.** C	**187.** A	**216.** A	**245.** B
130. C	**159.** A	**188.** B	**217.** D	**246.** D
131. D	**160.** D	**189.** A	**218.** C	**247.** D
132. D	**161.** A	**190.** B	**219.** C	**248.** A
133. D	**162.** D	**191.** A	**220.** A	**249.** C
134. D	**163.** B	**192.** B	**221.** A	**250.** D
135. B	**164.** A	**193.** A	**222.** B	
136. A	**165.** A	**194.** D	**223.** C	
137. B	**166.** D	**195.** A	**224.** B	

Answer Rationales

1. Answer D is correct. Painless vaginal bleeding is associated with placenta previa. The nurse should give priority to determining the status of the fetus. Answers B and C would be assessed before contacting the physician, as indicated in answer A.

2. Answer C is correct. Elevations in white cell count indicate the presence of infection that requires treatment prior to surgery. Answers A, B, and D are within normal limits and require no intervention.

3. Answer C is correct. Atropine is contraindicated in a client with glaucoma because it increases intraocular pressure. Answers A, B, and D are not contraindicated in a client with glaucoma.

4. Answer B is correct. Aged cheese, wine, and smoked or pickled meats should be avoided by a client taking an MAOI, not a phenothiazine such as Thorazine. Answers A, C, and D are included in the discharge teaching of a client receiving chlorpromazine (Thorazine).

5. Answer D is correct. The client will need to hold the cane in her left hand because of right-sided hemiplegia, which makes answer A incorrect. It will not be necessary for the client to advance the cane with her affected leg or to use a walker as stated in answers B and C.

6. Answer D is correct. Leaving a night light on during the evening and night shifts helps the client remain oriented to the environment and fosters independence. Answers A and B will not decrease the client's confusion. Answer C will increase the likelihood of confusion in an elderly client.

7. Answer A is correct. A radium implant provides a source of internal radiation. The nurse should explain that the client's body helps to shield those giving care from radiation but should also provide a lead-lined apron for use. Answers B, C, and D do not educate the nursing assistant regarding the client's treatment, so they are incorrect.

8. Answer B is correct. An increase in carbohydrates will provide energy and help decrease caloric expenditures following surgery. Answers A and C are incorrect statements. Answer D is incorrect because increased protein, not fat, is needed for healing.

9. Answer A is correct. Akathesia is an extrapyramidal side effect of many older antipsychotic medications such as haloperidol and chlorpromazine. Answers B, C, and D are not associated with the use of haloperidol.

10. Answer A is correct. The nurse should not allow the doctor to continue the dressing change without the use of sterile gloves. Answer B is incorrect because it implies that the doctor is negligent in his care. Answer C is incorrect because it places the client at risk for infection. Answer D is incorrect because infection could have been minimized or prevented by appropriate nursing care.

11. Answer B is correct. Pruritis, or itching, is caused by the presence of uric acid crystals on the skin, which is common in clients with end-stage renal failure. Answers A, C, and D are not associated with end-stage renal failure.

12. Answer D is correct. A client undergoing an angiogram will experience a warm sensation as the dye is injected. Answers A, B, and C are not associated with an angiogram.

13. Answer B is correct. Semi-liquids are more easily swallowed by a client with dysphagia than either liquids or solids; therefore, answer C is incorrect. Answers A and D are useful for a client with dumping syndrome following a gastrectomy, not a client with dysphagia.

14. Answer C is correct. There is no specified time or frequency for the ordered medication. Answers A, B, and D contain a specified time and frequency.

15. Answer A is correct. Falls constitute a major source of injury in toddlers. It will be important to provide safety measures such as stair guards. Answers B, C, and D are within the developmental norms for an 18-month-old; therefore, they are not a concern for the caregiver.

16. Answer A is correct. Placing the client in Trendelenburg position will engorge the vessels, make insertion of the catheter easier, and lessen the likelihood of air entering the central line. Answer B is incorrect because the client will not be more comfortable in Trendelenburg position. Answers C and D are not correct statements.

17. Answer B is correct. Taking deep breaths will decrease the discomfort experienced during removal of the drain. Answers A, C, and D are incorrect statements because they do not decrease the discomfort during removal of the drain.

18. Answer A is correct. Following a thyroidectomy, a client can develop symptoms of myxedema, which include constipation. The client should increase dietary fiber and fluid intake; therefore, answer D is incorrect. Answer B is incorrect because it is appropriate for a client with Cushing's disease. Answer C is incorrect because the client will not need to increase the intake of iodine.

19. Answer B is correct. Shortness of breath, anxiety, and cloudy mentation are associated with impending respiratory failure. Answer A might worsen the client's condition by robbing him of his CO_2 drive to breathe. Answer C is incorrect because increased humidity might increase the work of breathing. Answer D is incorrect because oxygen masks require oxygen settings greater than those tolerated by the client with COPD.

20. Answer B is correct. Increased voiding at night is a symptom of right-sided heart failure. Answers A, C, and D are incorrect because they are symptoms of left-sided heart failure.

21. Answer B is correct. An MRI requires the client to be confined in a small enclosure for a period of time. The client's refusal to accept a corner bed could indicate claustrophobia, so the client needs further assessment. An MRI is not contraindicated for clients with diabetes or asthma; therefore, answers A and D are incorrect. Answer C is incorrect because no contrast media is used.

22. Answer B is correct. The CPM machine should not be set at 90° flexion until the fifth postoperative day. Answers A, C, and D are expected findings and do not require immediate nursing intervention, so they are incorrect.

23. Answer C is correct. The proper site for the administration of the Mantoux test is the left forearm. Answers A, B, and D are incorrect because they are not proper locations for an intradermal injection.

24. Answer C is correct. Decreased urinary output is an early indication of renal transplant rejection. Answer A is an incorrect statement. Answer B is incorrect because tenderness over the operative site is expected. Answer D is incorrect because it is not a sign of transplant rejection.

25. Answer B is correct. The nurse should number the vials and take them to the lab for examination of protein, glucose, and cell count. Answer A is incorrect because the vials are not placed on ice. Answer C is incorrect because the vials should not be rotated. Answer D is an incorrect statement.

26. Answer D is correct. Multiparous clients have the greatest risk for postpartal hemorrhage; therefore, answers A, B, and C are incorrect statements.

27. Answer D is correct. The pulse oximeter should be placed on the child's finger or earlobe because blood flow to these areas is most accessible for measuring oxygen concentration. Answer A is incorrect because the probe cannot be secured to the abdomen. Answer B is incorrect because it should be recalibrated before application. Answer C is incorrect because a reading is obtained within seconds, not minutes.

28. Answer B is correct. A client withdrawing from barbiturates requires slow detoxification to prevent convulsions, delirium, tachycardia, and death. Answers A, C, and D are not associated with life-threatening symptoms during withdrawal; therefore, they are incorrect.

29. Answer B is correct. The overuse of nasal sprays containing oxymetazoline or phenylephrine can lead to rebound vasoconstriction and nasal congestion. Answer A is incorrect because it is a side effect of steroid nasal sprays. Answers C and D are incorrect because nasal polyps and tinnitus are not associated with the use of nasal sprays.

30. Answer B is correct. The medication should be administered using the calibrated dropper that comes with the medication. Answers A and C are incorrect because part of or all the medication could be lost during administration. Answer D is incorrect because part of or all the medication will be lost if the child does not finish the baby bottle.

31. Answer C is correct. The client should be encouraged to participate in quiet, nonchallenging activities with a few other clients. Answer A is incorrect because it will be overwhelming to the client. Answer B is incorrect at this time but will be appropriate as the client's condition continues to improve. Answer D is incorrect because solitary activities increase social isolation.

32. Answer B is correct. Cardiac catheterization will allow the doctor to determine the exact size and location of the defect. Answers A and C are incorrect because they are not symptoms of a ventricular septal defect. Cardiac catheterization does not determine the presence of murmurs; therefore, answer D is incorrect.

33. Answer A is correct. The presence of a hydatidiform mole is diagnosed using an ultrasound. Answer B is incorrect because it is the diagnostic test for neural tube defects. Answer C is incorrect because it is the diagnostic test to confirm pregnancy. Answer D is incorrect because it is the diagnostic test for fetal lung maturity.

34. Answer A is correct. The client will receive medication that relaxes his skeletal muscles and produces mild sedation. Answers B and D are incorrect because such statements increase the client's anxiety level. Nausea and headache are not associated with ECT, so answer C is incorrect.

35. Answer C is correct. A client receiving chemotherapy for leukemia usually develops ulceration of the oral mucosa. Cool soft foods such as ice cream and frozen yogurt are well tolerated. Answers A and B are incorrect because the child might not be able to eat a well-balanced diet of preferred foods because of the presence of mucosal ulceration. Answer D is incorrect because it does not take care of the client's nutritional needs; however, it is important to document the client's intake.

36. Answer B is correct. An induration of 10 mm or greater is considered to be a positive indication of exposure to the tubercle bacillus. Answers A, C, and D are incorrect statements.

37. Answer A is correct. Lyme disease produces a characteristic annular or circular rash sometimes described as a "bull's eye" rash. Answers B, C, and D are incorrect because they are not findings associated with Lyme disease.

38. Answer B is correct. Stimulation of the breasts and nipples can cause contractions that increase the likelihood of early termination of the pregnancy. Answer A is incorrect, although she should follow the doctor's recommendations regarding sexual intercourse early in the pregnancy. Answer C is incorrect because there is no indication that her work is detrimental to the pregnancy. Answer D is incorrect because nausea and vomiting are common in early pregnancy.

39. Answer B is correct. Ischemia of the myocardium produces crushing substernal pain that typically radiates to the left jaw and arm. Answers A, C, and D do not relate to the pain of myocardial infarction; therefore, they are incorrect.

40. Answer D is correct. The nurse should give priority to checking the pulses distal to the catheter insertion site as well as assessing the site for signs of bleeding. Answers A, B, and C are important but are not the main priority of care; therefore, they are incorrect.

41. Answer B is correct. The most common complication following a myocardial infarction is cardiac dysrhythmia, which is sometimes fatal. Answers A and C are incorrect because they are not common complications of myocardial infarction. Answer D is incorrect because the client would experience cardiogenic shock, not hypovolemic shock.

42. Answer B is correct. A client with gluten-induced enteropathy experiences symptoms after ingesting foods containing wheat, oats, barley, or rye. Corn or millet are thus substituted in the diet. Answers A, C, and D are incorrect because they contain foods that worsen the client's condition.

43. Answer A is correct. Elevations in temperature increase the client's oxygen requirements as well as the cardiac output; therefore, the doctor should be notified. Answer B is an incorrect statement because the cardiac output is increased, not decreased. Answer C is incorrect because an elevated temperature is not associated with cardiac tamponade. Answer D is incorrect because the client is kept on a cooling blanket to maintain hypothermia.

44. Answer A is correct. Huntington's disease is inherited as an autosomal dominant trait. There is a one in two, or 50%, chance that each child will be affected with the disease. Answer B is an incorrect statement. Answer C is incorrect because it refers to sex-linked disorders such as hemophilia. Answer D is incorrect because it refers to autosomal recessive disorders such as sickle cell anemia.

45. Answer B is correct. A permanent pacemaker will function at a continuous rate set by the physician. Answers A, C, and D are unnecessary; therefore, they are incorrect.

46. Answer D is correct. The client's leg should be maintained in an abducted position to prevent dislocation of the prosthesis. This is accomplished by the use of an abduction pillow. Answers A and B will increase the likelihood of dislocation of the prosthesis; therefore, they are incorrect. Answer C is unnecessary; therefore, it is incorrect.

47. Answer C is correct. Exposure to cold temperatures increases the peripheral vasospasms that characterize Raynaud's disease. Answers A and D are incorrect because they do prevent the symptoms of Raynaud's. Answer B will benefit the client with Buerger's but will not prevent the symptoms of Raynaud's.

48. Answer B is correct. Hemodialysis is scheduled before transplantation to rid the body of wastes and regulate the fluid and electrolyte balance. Answers A, C, and D are not performed on a client awaiting renal transplant; therefore, they are incorrect.

49. Answer A is correct. Decreased blood pressure, increased pulse rate, and abdominal distention are symptoms of altered bowel function and possible shock that require immediate intervention. Answer B is incorrect because it does not require immediate intervention. Answer C is incorrect because it suggests cystitis, which is treatable with antibiotics. Answer D is incorrect because there is no sign of illness that requires immediate intervention.

50. Answer B is correct. Administering furosemide (Lasix) too quickly by IV push method can lead to hypotension and shock. Answers A and C are incorrect because they do not apply to the administration of the medication. Answer D does not relate to the question; therefore, it is incorrect.

51. Answer B is correct. Blowing cool air over the affected site will help provide some relief from the pain and itching. Corticosteroids are contraindicated in the treatment of herpes; therefore, answer A is incorrect. Answer C is incorrect because warmth increases the itching and discomfort. Answer D is incorrect because herpes is caused by a virus, not a fungus.

52. Answer B is correct. Blood should not be kept on the unit longer than 30 minutes before administration. Answer A is incorrect because blood is not stored in the unit refrigerator. Answer C is incorrect because the blood has been kept on the unit and administered later than the allowable time. Answer D is an incorrect statement.

53. Answer B is correct. Knee contracture is a complication associated with below-the-knee amputation. Answer A is incorrect because it refers to a complication of above-the-knee amputation. Answers C and D are incorrect because they do not relate to the question.

54. Answer B is correct. The client's gag reflex is depressed prior to having an EGD. The nurse should give priority to checking for the return of the gag reflex before offering the client oral fluids. Answer A is incorrect because conscious sedation is used. Answers C and D are not affected by the procedure; therefore, they are incorrect.

55. Answer A is correct. The client has symptoms of an air embolus. Turning the client on the left side allows the air to be displaced to the right atrium, where it can be removed or absorbed. Answers B, C, and D are incorrect because they increase the likelihood of damage or death from the emboli.

56. Answer B is correct. The eye shield should be worn at night or when napping to prevent accidental trauma to the operative eye. Prescription eye drops, not over-the-counter eye drops, are ordered for the client; therefore, answer A is incorrect. The client might or might not require glasses following cataract surgery; therefore, answer C is incorrect. Answer D is incorrect because post-operative pain is not expected following cataract removal.

57. Answer B is correct. Green, leafy vegetables are rich in vitamin K, which decreases the effectiveness of the client's anticoagulant therapy. Answers A, C, and D are incorrect because they indicate that the client understands the nurse's teaching regarding his medication.

58. Answer A is correct. Projectile vomiting is a symptom of increased intracranial pressure that results from ventriculoperitoneal shunt failure. Answers B, C, and D are not symptoms associated with the failure of a ventriculoperitoneal shunt; therefore, they are incorrect.

59. Answer A is correct. The symptoms of Buerger's disease are improved by doing Buerger Allen exercises to improve vascular return from the lower extremities. Answer B is incorrect because it refers to Raynaud's disease. Answer C is not associated with Buerger's disease; therefore, it is incorrect. Answer D is incorrect because it refers to the prevention and treatment of osteoporosis.

60. Answer A is correct. Surgical manipulation of the pituitary can result in diabetes insipidus, which is characterized by polydipsia and polyuria. Answers B and C are symptoms of renal failure and are therefore incorrect. Answer D is a symptom of cystitis; therefore, it is incorrect.

61. Answer A is correct. The adolescent primigravida is particularly at risk for the development of pregnancy-induced hypertension. The nutritional status of the mother, prepregnant weight, and a history of hypertension are not significant factors in the development of PIH; therefore, answers B, C, and D are incorrect.

62. Answer B is correct. The child's symptoms are consistent with those of epiglottitis, an infection of the upper airway that can result in total airway obstruction. Symptoms of strep throat, laryngotracheobronchitis, and bronchiolitis are different from those presented by the client; therefore, answers A, C, and D are incorrect.

63. Answer A is correct. Persistent coughing is a sign of an allergic response to the medication. Answers B, C, and D are not associated with the use of captopril; therefore, they are incorrect.

64. Answer B is correct. Excessive sleeping is a common side effect of magnesium sulfate. Decreased urinary output, depressed reflexes, and slowed respirations are all signs of toxicity, not expected side effects; therefore, answers A, C, and D are incorrect.

65. Answer B is correct. The triad of symptoms commonly found in children with ADHD are inattentiveness, impulsivity, and excessive motor activity. Answers A, C, and D describe adverse effects from stimulant medications used to treat ADHD; therefore, they are incorrect.

66. Answer A is correct. Providing additional fluids will help the newborn eliminate excess bilirubin in the stool and urine. Answer B is incorrect because oils and lotions should not be used with phototherapy. Physiologic jaundice is not associated with infection; therefore, answers C and D are incorrect.

67. Answer D is correct. The client's symptoms are consistent with a flashback due to post-traumatic stress disorder. Answers A and C are incorrect because they are associated with psychotic disorders such as schizophrenia. Phobic reactions do not involve flashback episodes; therefore, answer B is incorrect.

68. Answer C is correct. Persons with schizoid personality disorder are generally described as withdrawn, reclusive, and loners. Answers A and D are incorrect because they describe the behaviors of a client with histrionic or borderline personality disorder. Answer B is incorrect because it describes the behaviors of a client with antisocial personality disorder.

69. Answer B is correct. An elderly client is likely to have changes in cardiac function. Because they are cardiotoxic, tricyclic antidepressants should be used with caution in clients with cardiac disease. Answers A, C, and D are important to assess but do not take priority over the client's cardiac status; therefore, they are incorrect.

70. Answer B is correct. Having a staff member remain with the client for one hour after meals will help prevent self-induced vomiting. Answer A is incorrect because the client will weigh more after meals, which can undermine treatment. Answer C is incorrect because the client will need a balanced diet and excess protein might not be well tolerated at first. Answer D is incorrect because it treats the client as a child rather than as an adult.

71. Answer B is correct. Lithium levels greater than 3.5 mEq/L are potentially fatal. At this level, the immediate use of dialysis is required to save the client's life. Answers A, C, and D do not relate to the client's care and are therefore incorrect.

72. Answer D is correct. Narcotics and sedatives are contraindicated in a client with a head injury. Answer A is incorrect because the client's head would be elevated. Answer B is incorrect because Neosporin or another topical antibiotic would be applied to the abrasions. Answer C is incorrect because the client would receive antibiotic therapy to prevent secondary infection.

73. Answer B is correct. Escorting the client from the day room allows him time to regain control of his behavior. Answers A and C are incorrect because these interventions would be done after the client has been removed from the day room. Answer D is incorrect because it has no bearing on appropriate care of the client.

74. Answer D is correct. According to Erikson's Psychosocial Developmental Theory, the developmental task of middle childhood is industry versus inferiority. Answer A is incorrect because it is the developmental task of infancy. Answer B is incorrect because it is the developmental task of the school-aged child. Answer C is incorrect because it is not one of Erikson's developmental stages.

75. Answer D is correct. Persons with passive-aggressive personality disorder display hostility through procrastination, noncompliance, and intentional inefficiency. Although psychiatrists no longer consider passive-aggressive personality disorder to be an official diagnosis, the condition is long term and problematic. Many clients can be helped through professional attention. Answer A is incorrect because its associated behaviors include shyness, aloofness, and social withdrawal. Answer B is incorrect because its associated behaviors include violation of the rights of others, lack of guilt or remorse, and failure to learn from mistakes. Answer C is incorrect because its associated behaviors including rigid perfectionism, lack of spontaneity, and over-seriousness.

76. Answer C is correct. The nurse should check the client's clothing and linen for wetness to prevent chilling. Answer A is incorrect because it is not necessary for her to exhale through her mouth. Answer B is incorrect because there is no indication that the client's skin needs lotion. Answer D is incorrect because a tympanic temperature would be obtained, not a rectal temperature.

77. Answer B is correct. A side effect of bronchodilators is tachycardia. Answers A and C are not associated with the use of bronchodilators; therefore, they are incorrect. Answer D is incorrect because hypotension is a sign of toxicity with some bronchodilators.

78. Answer B is correct. The respiratory rate of 72 is too rapid for a newborn. Answers A, C, and D are incorrect because they are within the normal range for the newborn.

79. Answer B is correct. The client's symptoms suggest placenta previa. Counting the number of pads and recording the amount of bleeding will best monitor the client's blood loss. Answer A is incorrect because a vaginal exam is contraindicated. Answer B is incorrect because the pH of the vaginal fluid will be influenced by the presence of bleeding. Answer D is incorrect because Cullen's sign indicates intra-abdominal bleeding.

80. Answer C is correct. Although cyanosis of the hands and feet is common in the newborn, it accounts for an Apgar score of less than 10. Answer A suggests cooling, which is not scored by the Apgar. Answer B is incorrect because conjunctival hemorrhages are not associated with the Apgar. Answer D is incorrect because it is within normal range as measured by the Apgar.

81. Answer C is correct. The client having a CAT scan of the sinuses will have to lie still in the prone position. Answer A is incorrect because there is no discomfort associated with a CAT scan. Answers B and D are inaccurate statements; therefore, they are incorrect.

82. Answer B is correct. Tenseness of the anterior fontanel indicates an increase in intracranial pressure. Answer A is incorrect because periorbital edema is not associated with meningitis. Answer C is incorrect because a positive Babinski reflex is normal in the infant. Answer D is incorrect because it relates to a preterm infant, not an infant with meningitis.

83. Answer A is correct. Nasogastric suction decompresses the stomach and leaves the abdomen soft and nondistended. Answer B is incorrect because it does not relate to the effectiveness of the NG suction. Answer C is incorrect because it relates to peristalsis, not the effectiveness of the NG suction. Answer D is incorrect because it relates to wound healing, not the effectiveness of the NG suction.

84. Answer A is correct. Tremulousness is an early sign of hypoglycemia. Answers B, C, and D are incorrect because they are symptoms of hyperglycemia.

85. Answer C is correct. Allowing the client to practice role-playing situations that she might later encounter will best prepare her for her return to school. Answers A, B, and D do not prepare the client as well as simulated role play; therefore, they are incorrect.

86. Answer C is correct. The most common sign associated with exacerbation of multiple sclerosis is double vision. Answers A, B, and D are not associated with a diagnosis or exacerbation of multiple sclerosis; therefore, they are incorrect.

87. Answer B is correct. The client's priority nursing diagnosis is based on his risk for self-injury. Answers A, C, and D focus on the client's psychosocial needs, which do not take priority over his physiological needs; therefore, they are incorrect.

88. Answer A is correct. Damage to the facial nerve and asymmetry of the mouth are associated with forceps delivery. Answer B is a chest deformity unrelated to forceps delivery; therefore, it is incorrect. Answer C is incorrect because it occurs as a result of prolonged labor and is unrelated to forceps delivery. Answer D is a normal finding in some newborns and is unrelated to forceps delivery; therefore, it is incorrect.

89. Answer D is correct. The recommended dose ranges from 175 mg to 350 mg per day. The order as written calls for 600 mg per day; therefore, the nurse should check the order with the doctor before giving the medication. Answer A is incorrect because the dosage exceeds the recommended amount. Answers B and C are incorrect because they involve changing the order, which requires a doctor's order.

90. Answer C is correct. The nurse should be firm and consistent when working with a client with borderline personality disorder. Answers A, B, and D are incorrect because they do not provide boundaries for the client.

91. Answer A is correct. Gout and renal calculi are the result of increased amounts of uric acid. Answer B is incorrect because it does not contribute to renal calculi. Answers C and D can result from decreased calcium levels. Renal calculi are the result of excess calcium; therefore, answers C and D are incorrect.

92. Answer A is correct. Diminished hearing and deafness are adverse reactions to amino-glycoside antibiotics. Answers B, C, and D are incorrect because they are not associated with the use of aminoglycosides.

93. Answer D is correct. A client with renal failure needs beverages that are low in potassium. A glass of apricot juice contains just 286 mg of potassium. Answers A, B, and C contain more potassium; therefore, they are incorrect. (Note: Prune juice contains 700 mg; grape juice contains 335 mg; and apple juice contains 296 mg.)

94. Answer D is correct. Providing small, frequent meals will compensate for limited absorptive capability and help reduce nausea. Answer A is incorrect because it does not compensate for limited absorption. Foods and beverages containing live cultures are discouraged for an immune-compromised client; therefore, answer B is incorrect. Answer C is incorrect because forcing fluids will not compensate for limited absorption and might increase nausea and vomiting.

95. Answer A is correct. Pallor, coolness, and edema at the IV site are signs of infiltration. Signs of infection, thrombus formation, and sclerosing of the vein include redness, warmth, and swelling; therefore, answers B, C, and D are incorrect.

96. Answer D is correct. A shape sorter is developmentally appropriate for a toddler and allows for quiet play. Answers A and C are incorrect because they require too much activity for a child with chronic hypoxia. Answer B is incorrect because it is too developmentally advanced for a toddler.

97. Answer C is correct. The students are violating confidentiality by discussing the client outside the area of care. The nurse should confront them with their behavior. Answers A and B are incorrect because their behavior should be confronted immediately rather than waiting for the teacher or nursing supervisor. Answer D is incorrect because it does not protect the client's right to confidential treatment.

98. Answer D is correct. A common side effect of prednisone is gastric ulcers, and cimetadine is given to help prevent the development of ulcers. Answers A, B, and C do not relate to the use of cimetadine; therefore, they are incorrect.

99. Answer B is correct. Bright red bleeding with many clots indicates arterial bleeding that requires surgical intervention. Answer A is within normal limits; therefore, it is incorrect. Answer C indicates venous bleeding, which can be managed by nursing intervention; therefore, it is incorrect. Answer D does not indicate excessive need for pain management that requires the doctor's attention; therefore, it is incorrect.

100. Answer B is correct. Repair of a hiatal hernia using a thoracic approach can cause the client to take shallow breaths, which can alter oxygen exchange. Answers A, C, and D do not relate specifically to the repair of a hiatal hernia, nor do they take priority over effective breathing; therefore, they are incorrect

101. Answer C is correct. The child will need additional fluids in summer to prevent dehydration that could lead to a sickle cell crisis. Answer A is not a true statement; therefore, it is incorrect. Answer B is incorrect because the activity will create a greater oxygen demand and precipitate sickle cell crisis. Answer D is not a true statement; therefore, it is incorrect.

102. Answer C is correct. The client should be assessed following completion of antibiotic therapy to determine whether the infection has cleared. Answer A would be done if there are repeated instances of otitis media; therefore, it is incorrect. Answer B is incorrect because the recheck appointment will not determine whether the child has completed all the medication. Symptoms of infection can resolve before the medication is finished. Answer D is incorrect because the purpose of the recheck is to determine whether the infection is gone, not to issue a prescription for treating future infections.

103. Answer B is correct. The nurse should confirm proper placement of the nasogastric tube prior to administering each feeding. Answer A is incorrect because it removes needed electrolytes with each feeding. Answer C is incorrect because suction is unnecessary. Answer D is incorrect because water is provided after the feeding.

104. Answer A is correct. A child with Syndeham's chorea will exhibit irregular movements of the extremities, facial grimacing, and labile moods. Answer B is incorrect because it describes subcutaneous nodules. Answer C is incorrect because it describes erythema marginatum. Answer D is incorrect because it describes polymigratory arthritis.

105. Answer D is correct. The primary reason for placing a child with croup under a mist tent is to liquefy secretions and relieve laryngeal spasms. Answer A is incorrect because it does not prevent insensible water loss. Answer B is incorrect because the oxygen concentration is too high. Answer C is incorrect because the mist tent does not prevent dehydration or reduce fever.

106. Answer D is correct. Numbness and tingling in an extremity immobilized by a cast are most likely the result of nerve compression. Answer A is incorrect because reduced venous return results in swelling of the extremity. Answer B is incorrect because numbness and tingling are not associated with bone healing. Answer C is incorrect because arterial insufficiency results in diminished or absent pulses in the extremity.

107. Answer C is correct. The recommended setting for performing tracheostomy suctioning for the adult is 80–120 mm Hg. Answers A and B are incorrect because the amounts of suction are too low. Answer D is incorrect because the amount of suction is excessive.

108. Answer A is correct. Steroid medication administered daily is given in the early morning to mimic the body's release of cortisol. Answers B, C, and D are incorrect because the times of administration are later in the day.

109. Answer B is correct. Taking the client outside for a walk away from the other clients will help provide a more calming activity and will show the client that the staff is interested in him. Answer A is incorrect because the client should be accompanied to the recreation room by a staff member. Answers C and D are incorrect because they will only increase his mania.

110. Answer C is correct. The third chamber is for suction control. Answer A is an incorrect statement. Answer B refers to the first chamber; therefore, it is incorrect. Answer D refers to the second chamber; therefore, it is incorrect.

111. Answer B is correct. Symptoms of myxedema include weight gain, lethargy, slowed speech, and decreased respirations. Answers A and D do not describe symptoms associated with myxedema; therefore, they are incorrect. Answer C describes symptoms associated with Graves's disease; therefore, it is incorrect.

112. Answer D is correct. Removal of the adrenal gland requires that the client receive daily steroid replacement. Answers A and C are incorrect because they apply to the client with diabetes mellitus. Answer B is incorrect because it applies to a client with renal or hepatic disease.

113. Answer B is correct. The nurse should replace the aspirant and begin the tube feeding. Answer A is incorrect because it removes electrolytes. Answer C is incorrect because it removes electrolytes and deprives the client of needed nourishment. Answer D is incorrect because there is no indication to hold the feeding.

114. Answer C is correct. Rice cereal, apple juice, and formula are suitable for a six-month-old infant's diet. Answers A, B, and D contain foods that have sources of protein that contribute to childhood allergies; therefore, they are incorrect.

115. Answer A is correct. A client with acute renal failure will be placed on a diet that restricts sodium, protein, potassium, and phosphorus. Answers B, C, and D would increase the amount of metabolic waste and electrolyte imbalance; therefore, they are incorrect.

116. Answer A is correct. A client with pancreatitis should have a low-fat, low-protein diet. Answers B, C, and D are suitable snacks for a client with pancreatitis; therefore, they are incorrect.

117. Answer D is correct. The contagious stage of varicella begins 24 hours prior to the onset of the rash and lasts until all the lesions are crusted. Answers A, B, and C are inaccurate regarding the time of contagion; therefore, they are incorrect.

118. Answer C is correct. A client taking NPH insulin should have a snack at midafternoon to prevent hypoglycemia. Answers A and B are incorrect because the times are too early for symptoms of hypoglycemia. Answer D is incorrect because the time is too late and the client would be in severe hypoglycemia.

119. Answer B is correct. A child with cystic fibrosis has sweat concentrations of chloride greater than 60 mEq/ L. Answers A and C are incorrect because they refer to potassium concentrations. Answer D is incorrect because the sweat concentration of chloride is too low.

120. Answer B is correct. The most therapeutic response is an open-ended one that allows the wife an opportunity to discuss her concerns about her husband's condition and care. Answers A, C, and D are incorrect because they are direct questions that do not encourage the wife to express her feelings.

121. Answer B is correct. A client with a detached retina will have limitations in mobility before and after surgery. Answer A is incorrect because a detached retina produces no pain or discomfort. Answers C and D do not apply to the client with a detached retina; therefore, they are incorrect.

122. Answer B is correct. If the client can speak, the airway is not obstructed. Answers A, C, and D are not the first actions the nurse should take; therefore, they are incorrect.

123. Answer D is correct. The nurse should retake the client's temperature to determine accuracy because no intervention was done. Answers A, B, and C depend on the client's present temperature reading; therefore, they are incorrect.

124. Answer C is correct. Torts (felonies) such as negligence, malpractice, and assault and battery, if proven, can result in revocation of the nurse's license. Answer A is incorrect because it is not punishable by law. Answer B is incorrect because wrongdoing is only suspected and has not been proven. Failure to pay the license renewal fees results in an inability to continue practice, not a revocation of the license; therefore, answer D is incorrect.

125. Answer B is correct. The nurse should question the order because administering a narcotic such as Demerol so close to the time of delivery can result in respiratory depression in the newborn. Answers A, C, and D are incorrect because they require administration of a narcotic immediately prior to or during delivery, which can cause respiratory depression in the newborn.

126. Answer B is correct. The primary purpose for the continuous passive motion machine is to promote flexion of the artificial joint. Answers A, C, and D do not describe the purpose of the CPM machine; therefore, they are incorrect.

127. Answer B is correct. Prior to suctioning, the client with a tracheostomy should be oxygenated at 100% via ambu or ventilator to prevent hypoxia. Answers A and C are done after suctioning the tracheostomy, not before; therefore, they are incorrect. Answer D is done last, so it is incorrect.

128. Answer C is correct. During concrete operations, the child's thought processes become more logical and coherent. Answer A is incorrect because it describes the sensorimotor stage of development. Answer B is incorrect because it describes the intuitive stage of development. Answer D is incorrect because it describes the formal operational stage of development.

129. Answer D is correct. Adequate amounts of sodium and fluids promote renal excretion and help to prevent lithium toxicity. Answers A, B, and C are not specific to a client taking lithium; therefore, they are incorrect.

130. Answer C is correct. Delusions of grandeur are associated with low self-esteem. Answer A is incorrect because conversion reaction is expressed as sensory or motor deficits. Answers B and D can cause an increase in the client's delusions but do not explain their purpose; therefore, they are incorrect.

131. Answer D is correct. According to Kohlberg, in the preconventional stage of development the behavior of a preschool child is determined by the consequences of his behavior. Answers A, B, and C describe other stages of moral development; therefore, they are incorrect.

132. Answer D is correct. The Schilling test is the diagnostic test for pernicious anemia. Answer A is incorrect because it is the diagnostic test for leukemia. Answer B does not apply to pernicious anemia; therefore, it is incorrect. Answer C refers to a hearing test for bone conduction; therefore, it is incorrect.

133. Answer D is correct. The client should be allowed some control; however, the nurse should contract with the client for a time to talk with him. Answer A is incorrect because the nurse is focused on her feelings rather than those of the client. Answer B is incorrect because it leaves the client to deal with his feelings alone. Answer C is a direct question that does not facilitate conversation; therefore, it is incorrect.

134. Answer D is correct. Theodur is a long-acting bronchodilator that can produce gastric upset if it is not taken with an antacid or food. Answer A is incorrect because the medication is taken on a regular schedule. Answer B is incorrect because it leads to over-medication. Answer C is incorrect because drowsiness is not a side effect of the medication.

135. Answer B is correct. Consistent caregivers give an abused child a sense of trust and security. Answer A is not a priority; therefore, it is incorrect. Answer C is incorrect because the nurse should observe the interaction between the parents and child. Answer D is incorrect because the child should not be pressured to talk about the abuse.

136. Answer A is correct. Shortness of breath, rash, and fever are symptoms of transfusion reaction. Answers B, C, and D are not associated with blood transfusion reaction.

137. Answer B is correct. Elevations in urine specific gravity indicate dehydration. Answers A, C, and D are within normal limits; therefore, they are incorrect.

138. Answer D is correct. Respiratory stridor is a clinical manifestation of partial airway obstruction. Answers A, B, and C are expected following a tonsillectomy; therefore, they are incorrect.

139. Answer C is correct. Imferon is administered deep IM using the Z-track method. Imferon is not administered by subcutaneous injection; therefore, answer A is incorrect. Answer B is incorrect because it refers to the administration of oral iron supplements. Answer D does not apply to the administration of Imferon; therefore, it is incorrect.

140. Answer C is correct. Telling the client to breathe more slowly will relax the abdominal muscles and make the procedure less uncomfortable. Answers A and B are incorrect because they interfere with the effectiveness of the procedure. Answer D is incorrect because the procedure may be stopped prematurely.

141. Answer B is correct. Having the client void prior to the paracentesis decreases the likelihood of the bladder being punctured. There is not need to hold the client NPO prior to the procedure; therefore, answer A is incorrect. Answer C is incorrect because the area does not need to be shaved. Answer D is incorrect because pain medication is not required prior to a paracentesis.

142. Answer C is correct. The client will need to have the diaphragm refitted if she gains or loses 10 pounds, has abdominal surgery, or has a baby. Answer A is incorrect because the diaphragm should remain in place for 6–8 hours. Answer B is incorrect because the diaphragm should not be washed with hot water. Answer D is not a true statement; therefore, it is incorrect.

143. Answer A is correct. Neomycin prepares the bowel for surgery by reducing the level of bacteria. Answers B, C, and D do not relate to the use of Neomycin; therefore, they are incorrect.

144. Answer A is correct. An appropriate short-term goal for a newly diagnosed diabetic is to be able to select a snack from the diabetic exchange. Answers B, C, and D are long-term goals; therefore, they are incorrect.

145. Answer A is correct. The two medications can be combined into one injection that will be given using a 23-gauge, 1 1/2-inch needle. There is no need to divide the medication into two injections given in two different locations; therefore, answers B and C are incorrect. Answer D is incorrect because the needle is not the right length.

146. Answer A is correct. The medication contains two ingredients, acetaminophen and codeine, which are harmful when taken in greater amounts than prescribed. Warming the medication will not make it more palatable; therefore, answer B is incorrect. Answer C is incorrect because the medication can be taken at bedtime. There is no need to store the medication in the refrigerator; therefore, answer D is incorrect.

147. Answer B is correct. Buck's traction is an example of skin traction used for a client with a fractured hip. Answers A, C, and D do not apply to Buck's traction; therefore, they are incorrect.

148. Answer D is correct. Having the client breathe into a bag or cupped hands will help to correct respiratory alkalosis due to hyperventilation. Answers A and C can slow the respirations but will not correct the respiratory alkalosis; therefore, they are incorrect. Answer B will soothe the client's mucus membranes but will not correct the respiratory alkalosis; therefore, it is incorrect.

149. Answer C is correct. The wrist should be kept higher than the elbow to minimize swelling. Answer A is incorrect because it will increase swelling and pain. Answer B will not minimize swelling; therefore, it is incorrect. Answer D is nonspecific and therefore incorrect.

150. Answer B is correct. The client should be allowed oral hygiene after the sputum collection. Answer A is not performed after the collection; therefore, it is incorrect. Answer C is incorrect because fluids are encouraged before the collection. Answer D is unnecessary for collection; therefore, it is incorrect.

151. Answer C is correct. Increased attention span is a desired effect of methylphenidate. Answer A is not associated with the medication; therefore, it is incorrect. Answer B is incorrect because the medication should not increase the child's activity level. Answer D is incorrect because the medication is not a mood stabilizer.

152. Answer A is correct. During the emergent phase of acute burn injury, the priority of care focuses on the client's fluid volume deficit or burn shock. Answers B, C, and D are not the top priority; therefore, they are incorrect.

153. Answer C is correct. Pain associated with duodenal ulcers is lessened if the client eats a meal or a snack. Answer A is incorrect because it makes the pain worse. Answer B refers to management of the client with dumping syndrome; therefore, it is incorrect. Answer D refers to the management of the client with gastroesophageal reflux; therefore, it is incorrect.

154. Answer B is correct. The best means for checking nasogastric tube placement is checking the acidity of the aspirant. Answers A and C are also checks for placement; however, they are not the best means, so they are incorrect. Answer D is a means of determining how far the tube should be inserted to reach the stomach; therefore, it is incorrect.

155. Answer A is correct. Agranulocytosis is an adverse reaction to chloramphenicol; therefore, the nurse should closely monitor the client's CBC. Answers B, C, and D are not associated with the use of the medication; therefore, they are incorrect.

156. Answer B is correct. Obstruction of the bile ducts results in clay-colored stools. Answer A is incorrect because it is associated with gastric bleeding. Answers C and D do not indicate biliary obstruction; therefore, they are incorrect.

157. Answer D is correct. The nurse should use the smallest needle possible when giving an injection to a child with cystic fibrosis to prevent bleeding. Answer A is incorrect because the site does not need cleaning with Betadine. Answer B is incorrect because pressure should be applied to the site after giving the injection. Answer C is unnecessary; therefore, it is incorrect.

158. Answer C is correct. Rising serum ammonia levels indicate that the client with cirrhosis is getting worse. Answer A indicates renal impairment; therefore, it is incorrect. Decreased blood urea nitrogen and decreased total bilirubin indicate improvement in the client's condition, so answers B and D are incorrect.

159. Answer A is correct. Diminished or absent femoral pulses are a sign of coarctation of the aorta. Answers B, C, and D are found in normal newborns and are not associated with cardiac anomaly; therefore, they are incorrect.

160. Answer D is correct. A severe complication associated with Kawasaki's disease is the development of a giant aneurysm. Answers A, B, and C are incorrect because they have no relationship to Kawasaki's disease.

161. Answer A is correct. When talking with the client who is hearing impaired, the nurse should sit beside the client and talk in a normal tone of voice more slowly. Talking louder and accentuating key words might actually distort sounds; therefore, answers B and C are incorrect. Answer D is incorrect because the nurse should sit near the client so that the client can benefit from lip reading.

162. Answer D is correct. A drop in heart rate during suctioning indicates vagal stimulation. If the client's heart rate drops below 50 beats per minute, suctioning should be discontinued. Answers A, B, and C are incorrect because the heart rates do not indicate vagal stimulation and bradycardia.

163. Answer B is correct. The presence of veil-like loss of vision is commonly reported by clients with retinal detachment. Answer A is incorrect because retinal detachment is pain free. Answer C is incorrect because retinal detachment does not result in sudden blindness. Loss of color discrimination is not a common symptom of retinal detachment; therefore, answer D is incorrect.

164. Answer A is correct. The urine of a client with acute glomerulonephritis (AGN) is dark or smoky in appearance due to the presence of RBCs and casts. Orange-tinged urine is not associated with AGN; therefore, answer B is incorrect. Answer C is incorrect because it indicates infection. Answer D indicates dehydration; therefore, it is incorrect.

165. Answer A is correct. Eye ointments should be applied five minutes after eye drops. Answer B is incorrect because the medications should not be used together. Answer C is incorrect because drops are applied before the ointment. Answer D is incorrect because a new order is not needed.

166. Answer D is correct. Urinary diversion with an ileal conduit allows the urine to drain from an opening on the surface of the abdomen. Answer A is incorrect because the urine does not drain into the small intestine. Answer B is incorrect because it describes a ureterosigmoidostomy. Answer C is incorrect because it describes an ileal reservoir or Kock pouch.

167. Answer D is correct. The nurse should check the chart for a signed permit before sending the client for a procedure such as cardiac catheterization. Answers A, B, and C are incorrect because they are unnecessary for a cardiac catheterization.

168. Answer B is correct. Collected specimens for a 24-hour urine for creatinine clearance are kept in a special container that is kept on ice. Answer A is unnecessary for a 24-hour urine collection; therefore, it is incorrect. Answers C and D refer to sterile or clean catch urine specimen collection not a 24-hour urine; therefore, they are incorrect.

169. Answer A is correct. A nosebleed in a client with mild preeclampsia indicates that the client's blood pressure might be elevated. Answer B is incorrect because the client will not need strict bed rest. Answer C is incorrect because pedal edema is common in a client with preeclampsia. Answer D is incorrect because the client does not need to avoid sodium, although she should limit or avoid high-sodium foods.

170. Answer C is correct. Elevations in serum creatinine indicate advanced renal disease. Answers A, B, and D are not specific to renal disease; therefore, they are incorrect.

171. Answer B is correct. Cold preparations containing pseudoephedrine should be avoided by a client taking an MAOI because the combination of medications can result in elevated blood pressure. Answer A is incorrect because it refers to a client taking an antipsychotic medication such as Thorazine. Answer C is not specific to a client taking an MAOI; therefore, it is incorrect. Answer D does not apply to the question; therefore, it is incorrect.

172. Answer A is correct. The client's morning lithium level is near the toxic level; therefore, the RN should care for the client. Answers B, C, and D can be cared for by an LPN or a nursing assistant.

173. Answer C is correct. Foods containing rice or millet are permitted for clients with celiac disease. Answers A, B, and D are not permitted because they contain flour made from wheat, which exacerbates the symptoms of celiac disease; therefore, they are incorrect.

174. Answer B is correct. Increased thirst and increased urination are signs of lithium toxicity. Answers A and D do not relate to the medication; therefore, they are incorrect. Answer C is an expected side effect of the medication; therefore, it is incorrect.

175. Answer C is correct. The client with ORIF of a fractured hip will begin ambulation with toe touch weight bearing on the affected leg. Answer A is incorrect because it places too much weight on the newly repaired hip. Answer B is incorrect because the client is allowed to bear minimal weight on the affected leg. Answer D is incorrect because it can place too much or too little pressure on the newly repaired hip.

176. Answer A is correct. During dehydration, the kidneys compensate for electrolyte imbalance by retaining potassium; therefore, the nurse should check for urinary output before adding potassium to the IV fluid. Answer B is incorrect because it measures respiratory compensation caused by dehydration. Answers C and D are incorrect because they do not relate to the administration of potassium replacement.

177. Answer A is correct. The primary nursing diagnosis for a client with any type of pneumonia is ineffective airway clearance. Activity intolerance, altered nutrition, and risk for fluid volume deficit are all applicable diagnoses, but they do not take priority over airway clearance; therefore, answers B, C, and D are incorrect.

178. Answer C is correct. The immunization protects the child against diphtheria, pertussis, tetanus, and *H. influenza B*. Answer A is incorrect because a second injection is given before four years of age. Answer B is not a true statement; therefore, it is incorrect. Answer D is incorrect because it is not a one-time injection, nor does it protect against measles, mumps, rubella, or varicella.

179. Answer C is correct. A weight gain of six pounds in a week in the client taking glucocorticoids indicates that the dosage should be modified. Answers A and B are not specific to the question; therefore, they are incorrect. Answer D is an expected side effect of the medication; therefore, it is incorrect.

180. Answer A is correct. Regular insulin peaks 2–3 hours after administration. If the insulin is given at 7 a.m., the snack should be given at 9 a.m. Answers B, C, and D are incorrect because the times are later than the peak.

181. Answer D is correct. The definitive diagnosis of gonorrhea is made by a culture of the vaginal discharge. Answer A is incorrect because cervical washings help diagnose cervical dysplasia, not gonorrhea. Answer B is incorrect because fluorescent stains help diagnose syphilis. Answer C is incorrect because blood cultures are not used to diagnose gonorrhea.

182. Answer B is correct. Assessing fetal heart tones reveals whether fetal distress occurred with rupture of the membranes. Answers A, C, and D are later interventions; therefore, they are incorrect.

183. Answer C is correct. The use of a gloved hand to apply the topical acyclovir will prevent transmission of the herpes virus to the caregiver. Answer A is incorrect because the medication does not protect against reinfection. Answer B is incorrect because the medication does not provide immunity. Answer D is incorrect because the medication will not prevent future outbreaks.

184. Answer A is correct. Cloudy dialysate return indicates infection and peritonitis, which require immediate antibiotic therapy. Answer C is incorrect because the client will not have urinary output. Answers B and D are incorrect because back discomfort and a sensation of abdominal fullness are commonly experienced by the client with peritoneal dialysis.

185. Answer A is correct. The client's symptoms suggest pulmonary emboli; therefore, the nurse's first action should be to apply supplemental oxygen. Obtaining a chest x-ray and electrocardiogram would be done after applying oxygen; therefore, answers B and D are incorrect. Answer C is incorrect because the information is not pertinent to the immediate care.

186. Answer B is correct. Taping the catheter to the client's upper thigh decreases the possibility of the catheter being kinked in the urethral penile sphincter. Answer A is incorrect because it does not decrease the possibility of the catheter being kinked in the urethral penile sphincter. Answer C is incorrect because it does not secure the catheter in place. Answer D is incorrect because it does not secure the catheter in place and it obstructs the flow of urine.

187. Answer A is correct. An average serving of yogurt contains approximately 400 mg of calcium. Answers B, C, and D contain lesser amounts of calcium; therefore, they are incorrect.

188. Answer B is correct. Obstruction of the upper airway by swelling is a post-operative complication of thyroidectomy; therefore, the nurse should keep a tracheostomy set at the client's bedside. Answers A, C, and D are ineffective in managing the client with an upper airway obstruction; therefore, they are incorrect.

189. Answer A is correct. Vomiting and diarrhea are adverse reactions or signs of colchicine toxicity. Headache, fever, and itching are side effects; therefore, answers B, C, and D are incorrect.

190. Answer B is correct. The newborn with a myelomeningocele should be positioned prone with the hips slightly elevated. This position helps to prevent pressure and trauma to the defect. Answer A is incorrect because it would place pressure on the defect, causing further nerve compromise. Answers C and D are incorrect because these positions would allow the weight of the defect to further stretch the nerve fibers, further compromising nerve tissue.

191. Answer A is correct. Rice cereal, skim milk, toast with margarine, and orange juice provide a well-balanced breakfast that is low in cholesterol and saturated fat. Answers B, C, and D contain animal products that are high in cholesterol and saturated fat; therefore, they are incorrect.

192. Answer B is correct. Levothyroxine increases metabolic rate and cardiac output. Adverse reactions include tachycardia and dysrhythmias; therefore, the client should be taught to check her heart rate before taking the medication. Answer A is incorrect because the client does not have to take the medication after breakfast. Answer C does not relate to the medication; therefore, it is incorrect. The medication should not be stopped because of gastric upset; therefore, answer D is incorrect.

193. Answer A is correct. The nurse should use a blood pressure cuff that is two thirds the diameter of the client's upper arm. Answers B and C will cause a false high reading; therefore, they are incorrect. Answer D will cause a false low reading; therefore, it is incorrect.

194. Answer D is correct. Cheese with crackers and yogurt is a good source of protein and calories. Answer A is incorrect because it is low in protein and calories. Answer B contains some protein but is low in calories; therefore, it is incorrect. Answer C does not contain protein and is low in calories; therefore, it is incorrect.

195. Answer A is correct. Indurations of 10 mm following a tuberculin skin test are generally considered positive and the client is evaluated for treatment with isonizid. Answer B is incorrect because the presence of redness following a tuberculin skin test is not considered significant. Answer C is incorrect because slight bruising can occur with administration of the test. Answer D is incorrect because it indicates a negative test.

196. Answer C is correct. The client's urine collection bag should form a good seal with the skin to prevent leakage and skin breakdown. Answer A is incorrect because it would prevent a good seal between the skin and bag. Tincture of benzoin would burn the delicate tissue; therefore, answer B is incorrect. Covering the skin with an antiseptic dressing would prevent a seal between the bag and skin; therefore, answer D is incorrect.

197. Answer D is correct. The use of purse-lipped breathing prevents a collapse of the alveoli by increasing the end expiratory pressure. Answers A, B, and C are incorrect because they have no relationship to the technique of purse-lipped breathing.

198. Answer D is correct. The nurse should wear a special badge when taking care of a client with a radioactive implant to measure the amount of time spent in the room. The nurse should limit the time of radiation exposure; therefore, answer A is incorrect. Standing at the foot of the bed of a client with a radioactive cervical implant increases the nurse's exposure to radiation; therefore, answer B is incorrect. The nurse does not have to avoid handling items used by the client; therefore, answer C is incorrect.

199. Answer B is correct. An adverse effect of tamoxifen (Nolvadex) is agranulocytosis. Answers A and C are not associated with the use of tamoxifen; therefore, they are incorrect. Answer D is a side effect, not an adverse effect; therefore, it is incorrect.

200. Answer C is correct. A child with autism engages in ritualistic behavior. Answer A is incorrect because the child does not talk to strangers. A child with autism prefers inanimate objects and likes music; therefore, answers B and D are incorrect.

201. Answer D is correct. The milkshake will provide needed calories and nutrients for a client with mania. Answers A and B are incorrect because they are high in sodium, which causes the client to excrete the lithium. Answer C has some nutrient value but not as much as the milkshake.

202. Answer D is correct. A client with a closed fracture poses little risk of infection for the post-operative client. Answers A, B, and C are incorrect because they pose a risk of infection to the post-operative client.

203. Answer D is correct. A suicidal client has difficulty expressing anger toward others. A depressed suicidal client frequently expresses feelings of low self-worth, feelings of remorse and guilt, and a dependence on others; therefore, answers A, B, and C are incorrect.

204. Answer B is correct. A cast made from fiberglass dries in 15 minutes and the client is able to bear weight within 30 minutes of application. Answer A is incorrect because the cast would not be dry enough to support weight bearing. Answer C is incorrect because the fiberglass cast can support weight bearing sooner than three hours. Answer D refers to a cast made of plaster of Paris; therefore, it is incorrect.

205. Answer B is correct. Pain following cataract surgery indicates a complication. Answer A is incorrect because the eye shield is worn while sleeping. Answer C is incorrect because the client should keep her head elevated 30°–45° post-operatively. Answer D is incorrect because sunglasses protect the client from the glare of lights or sunlight.

206. Answer D is correct. The maximal effects from tricyclic antidepressants might not be achieved for up to six months after the medication is started. Answers A and B are incorrect because the time for maximal effects is too brief. Answer C is incorrect because it refers to the time when initial symptomatic relief, rather than maximal effects, occurs.

207. Answer D is correct. Answers A, B, and C are incorrect because they contain lower amounts of potassium. (Note: The average sized banana contains 450 mg K+; the average sized pear contains 208 mg K+; the average sized apple contains 165 mg K+; and the orange contains 235 mg K+.)

208. Answer B is correct. The spinach salad contains 150 mg of magnesium. Answer A is incorrect because fruit is low in magnesium. A baked potato with the skin is high in potassium, not magnesium; therefore, answer C is incorrect. Answer D is high in calcium and protein, not magnesium; therefore, it is incorrect.

209. Answer C is correct. Ataxia can be seen in clients with lithium levels of 2.0–2.5 mEq/L. Hyerreflexia would be seen in the client rather than hyporeflexia; therefore, answer A is incorrect. Akathesia is an extrapyramidal side effect from antipsychotic medication; therefore, answer B is incorrect. Answer D is not specific to lithium use; therefore, it is incorrect.

210. Answer B is correct. A two year-old can walk up and down stairs, one foot at a time. Answers A and D are within the gross motor development of a five-year-old; therefore, they are incorrect. Answer C is within the gross motor development of a three-year-old, so it is incorrect.

211. Answer A is correct. Following a thyroidectomy, the client should be placed in semi-Fowler's position with the head and neck supported on pillows to decrease swelling that would place pressure on the airway. Answers B, C, and D are incorrect because they would increase the chances of post-operative complications that include bleeding, swelling, and airway obstruction.

212. Answer D is correct. Placing the child in a lateral knee position increases the blood flow back to the heart and lessens cerebral hypoxia. (The same effect is achieved when the child squats during a hypoxic attack.) Answers A and C provide comfort but do not increase blood flow back to the heart; therefore, they are incorrect. Answers B is incorrect because it does not increase blood flow back to the heart.

213. Answer B is correct. The dose of regular insulin is drawn into the syringe before the NPH insulin to prevent accidentally mixing rapid-acting insulin with time-released insulin. Answer A is incorrect because regular and NPH insulin can be given in one injection. Answers C and D contain inaccurate statements; therefore, they are incorrect.

214. Answer C is correct. Beta blockers such as timolol (Timoptic) can cause bronchospasm in a client with chronic obstructive pulmonary disease. Beta blockers such as timolol are prescribed for clients with diabetes, gastric ulcers, and pancreatitis; therefore, answers A, B, and D are incorrect.

215. Answer D is correct. Luncheon meats contain preservatives such as nitrites that have been linked to gastric cancer. Answers A, B, and C have not been found to increase the risk of gastric cancer; therefore, they are incorrect.

216. Answer A is correct. A child with intussusception has stools that contain blood and mucus, which are described as "currant jelly" stools. Answer B is a symptom of pyloric stenosis; therefore, it is incorrect. Answer C is a symptom of Hirschsprung's; therefore, it is incorrect. Answer D is a symptom of Wilms tumor; therefore, it is incorrect.

217. Answer D is correct. Pain three days after the application of a cast is a symptom of compartment syndrome, which requires immediate attention to bivalving or removing the cast. Answer A will reduce swelling but will do little to relieve the pain associated with compartment syndrome; therefore, it is incorrect. Answer B will not improve circulation to the extremity and will do little to lessen the pain of compartment syndrome; therefore, it is incorrect. Pain beneath the cast after three days is not normal, so answer C is incorrect.

218. Answer C is correct. Taking the medication with a meal or snack will lessen gastric upset caused by NSAIDs. Answers A and D are inaccurate statements; therefore, they are incorrect. Answer B is incorrect because fluids are needed to help renal excretion.

219. Answer C is correct. A history of cruelty to people and animals, truancy, setting fires, and a lack of guilt or remorse are associated with a diagnosis of conduct disorder in children, which becomes a diagnosis of antisocial personality disorder in adults. Answer A is incorrect because a client with antisocial personality disorder does not hold consistent employment. Answer B is incorrect because the client's IQ is usually higher than average. Answer D is incorrect because these clients lack guilt or remorse for wrongdoing.

220. Answer A is correct. Planning for travel with same-age peers is an example of ego integrity. Answers B, C, and D are examples of stagnation or ego despair; therefore, they are incorrect.

221. Answer A is correct. The nursing assistant should be assigned to care for a client with chronic health needs that mainly require assistance with the activities of daily living. Answers B, C, and D require skilled nursing care for acute health problems; therefore, they are incorrect.

222. Answer B is correct. Spinach provides vitamins and minerals; dried beans provide fiber, protein, and iron; and tomatoes provide vitamin C. Answer A is incorrect because it is not a well-balanced meal and bacon is high in fat and sodium. Answer C is incorrect because it is high in sodium and contains foods that are difficult for an elderly client to digest. Answer D is incorrect because beef is high in fat and cheese and milk can create problems for a client who is lactose intolerant.

223. Answer C is correct. An infant with biliary atresia has abdominal distention, poor weight gain, and clay-colored stools. Answers A, B, and D do not describe the symptoms associated with biliary atresia; therefore, they are incorrect.

224. Answer B is correct. Clients with Cushing's disease have an increase in cortisol levels that predispose them to infections. Answers A and C are incorrect because the client would have hyperglycemia and hypervolemia. Answer D is not associated with Cushing's disease; therefore, it is incorrect.

225. Answer A is correct. Pheochromocytoma is an adrenal tumor that causes an extreme elevation in blood pressure (malignant hypertension). Petechial rash across the chest and axilla is a symptom of pulmonary embolus; therefore, answer B is incorrect. White flecks in the iris, known as *Brushfield's spots*, are found in a child with Down syndrome; therefore, answer C is incorrect. Carotonemia, characterized by yellow creases at the nasolabial folds, can be found in the client who consumes an abundance of yellow vegetables; therefore, answer D is incorrect.

226. Answer A is correct. An 8-ounce glass of milk contains 290 mg of calcium. Answers B, C, and D contain lesser amounts; therefore, they are incorrect. (Note: An ounce of cheddar cheese contains 205 mg of calcium; half a cup of raw broccoli contains 175 mg of calcium; and a 4-ounce salmon croquette contains 165 mg of calcium.)

227. Answer A is correct. Sulfamylon produces a painful sensation when applied to the burn wound; therefore, the client should receive pain medication prior to dressing changes. Answers B, C, and D do not pertain to dressing changes with Sulfamylon; therefore, they are incorrect.

228. Answer B is correct. Acyclovir, an antiviral is used in the treatment of disseminated herpes zoster (shingles). Answers A, C, and D are not used in the treatment of viral infections therefore they are incorrect. Clients with acquired immune deficiency syndrome

229. Answer B is correct. True contractions are regular and consistent. True contractions do not have to begin in the lower abdomen; therefore, answer A is incorrect. Answer C is incorrect because true contractions do not lessen with activity. Answer D is incorrect because true contractions do not have a pattern of being strong and then weak—they are consistent.

230. Answer A is correct. Side effects of bronchodilators such as aminophylline include irritability, rapid pulse, and palpitations. Answer B is incorrect because bronchodilators cause the pulse to be rapid. Answer C is incorrect because a decreased blood pressure indicates toxicity rather than an expected side effect. Answer D is incorrect because bronchodilators such as aminophylline cause increased wakefulness, not drowsiness.

231. Answer A is correct. According to the Denver Developmental Screening Test, a child can pull a toy behind her by age 2 years. Answers B, C, and D are not accomplished until ages 4–5 years; therefore, they are incorrect.

232. Answer D is correct. The client is unable to actively hallucinate while talking with the nurse or other clients. Answers A, B, and C do not involve the client in an activity to minimize the hallucinations; therefore, they are incorrect.

233. Answer B is correct. Skilled nursing care centers are intermediate care facilities that offer care from a licensed nursing staff. Services provided include administration of intravenous medications, wound care, long-term ventilator management, and physical rehabilitation. Answers A, C, and D do not refer to agencies that provide the level of care needed by the patient with MRSA who is receiving IV antibiotics and wound care, therefore they are incorrect.

234. Answer C is correct. The nurse's comments are an example of assault. Assault refers to the intentional threat to bring about harmful or offensive contact. Battery refers to an intentional touching without consent therefore answer A is incorrect. Malpractice refers to negligence committed by a professional therefore answer B is incorrect. Negligence refers to conduct that falls below the standard of care therefore answer D is incorrect.

235. Answer B is correct. The student nurse has the same accountability for administering medication as the registered nurse. Answers A, C, and D are incorrect statements therefore they are wrong.

236. Answer D is correct. The nurse's failure to check the client's lithium level can result in a charge of malpractice since her nursing care fell below the acceptable standard of care. Answers A, B, and C do not apply to the situation therefore they are incorrect.

237. Answer A is correct. Sharing information about the patient's diagnosis, condition, or treatment results in the nurse's breaking the patient's confidentiality. Slander and libel refer to intentional torts that result in defamation of character therefore answers B and D are incorrect. Answer C is incorrect because malice refers to publishing false information with reckless disregard for the truth.

238. Answer C is correct. An amniocentesis at 37 weeks gestation will determine the maturity of the fetal lungs. Answer A is incorrect because it does not determine the effect of diabetes on the fetus. A sonogram determines the skeletal age of the fetus, not an amniocentesis; therefore, answer B is incorrect. Answer D involves an amniocentesis done in the first trimester; therefore, it is incorrect.

239. Answer B is correct. The infant's apical heart rate is within the accepted range for administering the medication. Answers A, C, and D are incorrect because the apical heart rate is suitable for giving the medication; therefore, there is no need to call the physician, recheck the heart rate, or withhold the medication.

240. Answer A is correct. Paresthesia and weakness of the lower extremities are symptoms of Guillain-Barré syndrome. Answer B is incorrect because the client would have hyporeactive reflexes. Answer C describes symptoms of a client with multiple sclerosis; therefore, it is incorrect. Answer D describes symptoms of hepatic coma; therefore, it is incorrect.

241. Answer D is correct. At one year of age, the infant should be able to sit without support. Answers A, B, and C are expected findings in the child at one year of age; therefore, they are incorrect.

242. Answer A is correct. A client who is depressed and withdrawn will work best in a one-to-one relationship with the nursing staff. Answer B is incorrect because it does not convey a sense of caring to the depressed client. Answer C is incorrect because the depressed client needs to be involved in activities with others. Answer D is incorrect because the depressed client frequently exhibits anhedonia, or lack of enjoyment in anything.

243. Answer B is correct. Chelating agents are used to treat clients with poisonings from heavy metals such as lead and iron. Answers A and D are used to remove noncorrosive poisons; therefore, they are incorrect. Answer C prevents vomiting; therefore, it is an incorrect response.

244. Answer C is correct. A client with myxedema can be made more comfortable by providing an extra blanket. Answer A is incorrect because the client needs low-calorie snacks. Answer B is incorrect because it does not specifically relate to a client with myxedema. Answer D is incorrect because it pertains to a client with diabetes mellitus.

245. Answer B is correct. Anabolic steroids can cause aggression and uncontrolled rage in the user. Answers A, C, and D do not describe the behavior of one who uses anabolic steroids; therefore, they are incorrect.

246. Answer D is correct. The client should be escorted to her room to protect her and to allow her an opportunity to regain control of her behavior. Answers A and B do not focus on the needs of the client; therefore, they are incorrect. Answer C should be done after the client is taken to her room; therefore, it is incorrect.

247. Answer D is correct. Talking with the nursing assistant regarding her feelings about death shows the most concern for her. Answer A is incorrect because it does not help the nursing assistant deal with her feelings. Answer B is incorrect because it is a non-empathetic response to the nursing assistant. Answer C is incorrect because it does not prepare the nursing assistant for future situations.

248. Answer A is correct. The least restrictive restraint for an infant with cleft lip and cleft palate repair is elbow restraints. Answers B, C, and D are more restrictive and unnecessary; therefore, they are incorrect.

249. Answer C is correct. *Esophageal varices* are varicosities of the esophagus that are the result of portal hypertension caused by chronic alcohol use. Answers A, B, and D are not causes of esophageal varices; therefore, they are incorrect.

250. Answer D is correct. The nurse should not use water, soap, or lotion on the area marked for radiation therapy. Answer A is incorrect because it would remove the marking. Answers B and C are unnecessary for a client receiving radiation; therefore, they are incorrect.

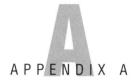

APPENDIX A

Things You Forgot

Throughout this book, we have tried to help you to simplify preparation for the NCLEX exam. This appendix includes information you have learned during nursing school but might have forgotten.

Therapeutic Drug Levels

Here are some of the therapeutic blood levels that are important for the nurse to be aware of when taking the NCLEX® exam:

- ▶ **Digoxin**: 0.5–2.0 ng/ml

- ▶ **Lithium**: 0.6–1.5 mEq/L

- ▶ **Dilantin**: 10–20 mcg/dl

- ▶ **Theophylline**: 10–20 mcg/dl

> **NOTE**
>
> Lab values vary by age and some books might have different reference values.

Vital Signs

Here are some of the normal ranges for vital signs:

- ▶ **Heart rate**: 80–100 beats per minute

- ▶ **Newborn heart rate**: 100–180 beats per minute

- ▶ **Respiratory rate**: 12–20 respirations per minute

- ▶ **Blood pressure**: systolic = 110–120 mm Hg; diastolic = 60–90 mm Hg

- ▶ **Newborn blood pressure**: systolic = 65 mm Hg; diastolic = 41 mm Hg

- ▶ **Temperature**: 98.6 +/-

Anticoagulant Therapy

These are the tests to be done for the client taking anticoagulants and their control levels. Remember that the therapeutic range is 1.5–2 times the control:

▸ **Coumadin (sodium warfarin) PT/Protime**: 12–20 seconds.

▸ **International normalizing ratio (INR)**: 2–3.

▸ **Antidote for sodium warfarin**: Vitamin K.

> **NOTE**
>
> Lab values vary by age and some books might have different reference values.

▸ **Heparin and heparin derivatives partial thromboplastin time (PTT)**: 30–60 seconds. If the client is taking Lovenox (enoxaparin), the nurse should check the platelet count because Lovenox can cause thrombocytopenia.

▸ **Antidote for heparin**: Protamine sulfate.

Intrapartal Normal Values

Here are some of the normal ranges to remember when caring for the client during the intrapartal period:

▸ **Fetal heart rate**: 120–160 beats per minute

▸ **Variability**: 6–10 beats per minute

▸ **Contractions**:

　▸ **Frequency of contractions**: Every 2–5 minutes

　▸ **Duration of contractions**: Less than 90 seconds

　▸ **Intensity of contractions**: Less than 100 mmHg

▸ **Amniotic fluid amount**: 500–1200 ml

Standard Precautions

Standard precautions are a set of guidelines for the nurse to take when caring for the client. These precautions protect the nurse from transmitting the disease to another client or to herself:

▶ Gloves should be worn when there is a chance of contact with blood and body fluids, when handling other potentially infected material, and when performing vascular access procedures.

▶ Gloves should be changed after each client contact and between contact procedures with the same client.

▶ Masks and protective eyewear should be worn when there is a likelihood of splashes or when body fluids might become airborne.

▶ Gloves and aprons should be worn during procedures in which there is the likelihood of splashes of blood or body fluids.

▶ Hand washing should be done immediately after contact with body fluids or other potentially infected material and as soon as gloves are removed.

▶ Needles and sharps should be disposed of in sharps containers. No recapping, bending, or breaking of needles should occur.

▶ Mouth-to-mouth resuscitation should be performed using a mouthpiece or other ventilation device.

> **CAUTION**
>
> Body fluids likely to transmit blood-borne disease include blood, semen, vaginal/cervical secretions, tissues, cerebral spinal fluid, amniotic fluid, synovial fluid, pleural fluid, peritoneal fluid, and breast milk. Body fluids not likely to transmit blood-borne disease unless blood is visible include feces, nasal secretions, sputum, vomitus, sweat, tears, urine, and saliva (the exception is during oral surgery or dentistry).

Airborne Precautions

Examples of infections caused by organisms suspended in the air for prolonged periods of time are tuberculosis, measles (rubella), and chickenpox. Place these clients in a private room. Healthcare workers should wear a HEPA mask or N-95 mask when dealing with such clients. These mask contain fine fibers and filter out particles, preventing them from passing through to the healthcare worker.

Droplet Precautions

Infections caused by organisms suspended in droplets that can travel 3 feet, but are not suspended in the air for long periods of time, are influenza, mumps, pertussis, rubella (German measles), diphtheria, pneumonia, scarlet fever, streptococcal pharyngitis, and meningitis. Place the client in a private room or in a room with a client who has the same illness. The clients should be no closer than 3 feet away from one another. Caregivers should wear a mask, and the door can remain open.

Contact Precautions

Infections caused by organisms spread by direct contact include RSV, scabies, colonization with MRSA, and VRE. Place the client in a private room or with a client with the same condition. Caregivers should wear gloves when entering the room and wear gowns to prevent contact with the client. Hands should be washed with an antimicrobial soap before leaving the client's room. Equipment used by the client should remain in the room and should be disinfected before being used by anyone else. The client should be transported only for essential procedures; during transport, precautions should be taken to prevent disease transmission.

Revised Life Support Guidelines (American Heart Association)

Frequently the American Heart Association releases guidelines for the care of the client experiencing dysrrhythmias. Refer to http://www.aafp.org/afp/2006050/practice.html for these guidelines.

Defense Mechanisms Often Used by Clients During Stressful Situations

Here is a quick reference to some of the defense mechanisms used by the client to help him cope with stressors:

▶ **Compensation**: The development of attributes that take the place of more desirable ones.

▶ **Conversion reaction**: The development of physical symptoms in response to emotional distress.

▶ **Denial**: The failure to regard an event or feeling.

▶ **Displacement**: The transference of emotions to another other than the intended.

▶ **Projection**: The transferring of unacceptable feelings to another person.

▶ **Rationalization**: The dismissal of one's responsibility by placing fault on another.

▶ **Reaction formation**: The expression of feelings opposite to one's true feelings.

▶ **Regression**: The returning to a previous state of development in which one felt secure.

▶ **Repression**: The unconscious forgetting of unpleasant memories.

▶ **Sublimation**: The channeling of unacceptable behaviors into behaviors that are socially acceptable.

▶ **Suppression**: The conscious forgetting of an undesirable memory.

Nutrition Notes

It is important for the nurse to be aware of different diets used in the disease processes we have discussed. Table A.1 provides a quick reference to help you remember the diets.

TABLE A.1   Dietary and Nutrition Notes to Remember

Diseases Being Treated	Foods to Include	Foods to Avoid
Bone marrow transplant clients	Cook or peel and wash all foods.	Avoid foods from salad bars, foods grown on or in the ground, and foods that are cultured.
Celiac/gluten-induced diarrhea	Milk, buttermilk, lean meats, eggs, cheese, fish, creamy peanut butter, cooked or canned juice, corn, bread stuffing from corn, cornstarch, rice, soybeans, potatoes, bouillon, and broth.	Malted milk, fat meats, luncheon meats, wheat, salmon, prunes, plums, rye, oats, barley, and soups thickened with gluten containing grains.
Congestive heart failure, hypertension	Meats low in cholesterol and fats, breads, starches, fruits, sweets, vegetables, dairy products.	Foods high in salts, canned products, frozen meats, cheeses, eggs, organ meats, fried foods, and alcohol.
Crohn's/ulcerative colitis	Meats, breads, starches, fruits, vegetables, dairy products.	Whole grains, legumes, nuts, vegetables with skins, prune juice, and gristly meats.

(continues)

TABLE A.1   *Continued*

Diseases Being Treated	Foods to Include	Foods to Avoid
Full liquid diets for clients who require a decrease in gastric motility	Milk, ice cream, soups, puddings, custards, plain yogurt, strained meats, strained fruits and vegetables, fruit and vegetable juices, cereal gruel, butter, margarine, and any component or combination of clear liquids.	All solid foods.
Lacto-vegetarian	Primary sources of protein, dairy products, peanut butter, legumes, soy analogs.	All meat products.
Peptic ulcer/hiatal hernia	Meats, breads, starches, fruits, vegetables, and dairy products.	Alcohol, coffee, chocolate, black or red pepper, chili powder, carminatives such as oil of peppermint and spearmint, garlic, onions, and cinnamon.
Radium implant clients	Same as for Crohn's and ulcerative colitis.	Same as for Crohn's and ulcerative colitis.
Renal transplant clients	Meats, dairy products, breads, starches, vegetables, and sweets.	Eggs, organ meats, fried or fatty food, foods containing salt, dried foods, salt substitutes, and fruits.

Immunization Schedule

It is important for the nurse to be aware of the recommended immunization schedule for various age groups. Figure A.1 provides a recommended schedule for infants and children through 6 years. Figure A.2 provides a recommended schedule for adolescent immunizations. Figure A.3 is a recommended schedule for adult immunizations.

For more detailed information, consult the CDC website at http://www.cdc.gov/vaccines/recs/schedules/default.htm.

Recommended Immunization Schedule for Persons Aged 0 Through 6 Years—United States · 2010

For those who fall behind or start late, see the catch-up schedule

Vaccine ▼ Age ▶	Birth	1 month	2 months	4 months	6 months	12 months	15 months	18 months	19-23 months	2-3 years	4-6 years
Hepatitis B[1]	HepB	HepB			HepB						
Rotavirus[2]			RV	RV	RV[2]						
Diptheria, Tetanus, Pertussis[3]			DTaP	DTaP	DTaP		DTaP				DTaP
Haemophilus influenzae type b[4]			Hib	Hib	Hib[4]	Hib					
Pneumococcal[5]			PCV	PCV	PCV	PCV					PPSV
Inactivated Poliovirus[6]			IPV	IPV		IPV					IPV
Influenza[7]						Influenza (Yearly)					
Measles, Mumps, Rubella[8]						MMR					MMR
Varicella[9]						Varicella					Varicella
Hepatitis A[10]						HepA (2 doses)				HepA Series	
Meningococcal[11]										MCV	

☐ Range of recommended ages for all children except certain high-risk groups   ☐ Range of recommended ages for certain high-risk groups

FIGURE A.1
Recommended Immunization Schedule for Persons Aged 0 through 6 Years.

Recommended Immunization Schedule for Persons Aged 7 Through 18 Years—United States · 2010

For those who fall behind or start late, see the catch-up schedule

Vaccine ▼ Age ▶	7-10 years	11-12 years	13-18 years
Tetanus, Diptheria, Pertussis[1]		Tdap	Tdap
Human Papillomavirus[2]		HPV (3 doses)	HPV series
Meningococcal[3]	MCV	MCV	MCV
Influenza[4]		Influenza (Yearly)	
Pneumococcal[5]		PPSV	
Hepatitis A[6]		HepA Series	
Hepatitis B[7]		HepB Series	
Inactivated Poliovirus[8]		IPV Series	
Measles, Mumps, Rubella[9]		MMR Series	
Varicella[10]		Varicella Series	

☐ Range of recommended ages for all children except certain high-risk groups   ☐ Range of recommended ages for catch-up Immunization   ☐ Range of recommended ages for certain high-risk groups

FIGURE A.2
Recommended Immunization Schedule for Persons Aged 7 through 18 Years.

Vaccine ▼ Age Group ▶	19-26 years	27-49 years	50-59 years	60-64 years	65 years
Tetanus, Diptheria, Pertussis (Td/Tdap)[1,*]	Substitute one-time dose for Td booster; then boost with Td every 10 years				Td booster every 10 years
Human Papillomavirus[2,*]	3 doses (females)				
Varicella[3,*]	2 doses				
Zoster[4]				1 dose	
Measles, Mumps, Rubella[5,*]	1 or 2 doses		1 dose		
Influenza[6,*]			1 dose annually		
Pneumococcal (polysaccharide)[7,8]		1 or 2 doses			1 dose
Hepatitis A[9,*]	2 doses				
Hepatitis B[10,*]	3 doses				
Meningococcal[11,*]	1 or more doses				

*Covered by the Vaccine Injury Compensation Program.

☐ For all persons in the category who meet the age requirements and who lack evidence of immunity (e.g., lack documentation of vaccination or have no evidence of prior infection)   ☐ Recommended if some other risk factor is present (e.g., based on Medical, occupational, lifestyle, or other indications)   ☐ No recommendation

FIGURE A.3
Recommended Immunization Schedule for Adults.

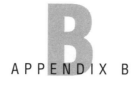

APPENDIX B

Need to Know More?

Pharmacology

http://www.druginfonet.com

http://www.fda.gov/search/databases.html

http://www.globalrph.com

http://www.mosbysdrugconsult.com

http://www.needymeds.com

http://www.nlm.nih.gov/medlineplus

http://www.nursespdr.com

Deglin, J., Vallerand, A. H. *Davis Drug Guide for Nurses*. Philadelphia: F.A. Davis, 2009.

Care of the Client with Respiratory Disorders

http://www.aaaai.org—The website for the American Academy of Allergy, Asthma, and Immunology

http://www.cdc.gov—The website for the Centers for Disease Control and Prevention

http://www.lungusa.org—The website for the American Lung Association

Ignatavicius, D., and Workman, S. *Medical Surgical Nursing: Critical Thinking for Collaborative Care*. 5th ed. Philadelphia: Elsevier, 2007.

Brunner, L., and Suddarth, D. *Textbook of Medical Surgical Nursing*. 12th ed. Philadelphia: Lippincott Williams & Wilkins, 2009.

LeMone, P., and Burke, K. in *Medical Surgical Nursing: Critical Thinking in Client Care*. 4th ed. Upper Saddle River, NJ: Pearson Prentice Hall, 2008.

Lewis, S., Heitkemper, M., Dirksen, S., Obrien, P,. and Bucher, L. *Medical Surgical Nursing: Assessment and Management of Clinical Problems*. 7th ed. Philadelphia: Elsevier, 2007.

Lehne, R. *Pharmacology for Nursing Care*. 7th ed. Philadelphia: Elsevier, 2009

Care of the Client with Genitourinary Disorders

http://www.kidney.org—The website for the National Kidney Foundation.

http://www.pkd.cure.org—The website for the Polycystic Kidney Disease Foundation.

Ignatavicius, D., and Workman, S. *Medical Surgical Nursing: Critical Thinking for Collaborative Care*. 5th ed. Philadelphia: Elsevier, 2007.

Brunner, L., and Suddarth, D. *Textbook of Medical Surgical Nursing*. 12th ed. Philadelphia: Lippincott Williams & Wilkins, 2009.

LeMone, P., and Burke, K. in *Medical Surgical Nursing: Critical Thinking in Client Care* 4th ed. Upper Saddle River, NJ: Pearson Prentice Hall, 2008.

Lewis, S., Heitkemper, M., Dirksen, S., Obrien, P., and Bucher, L. *Medical Surgical Nursing: Assessment and Management of Clinical Problems*. 7th ed. Philadelphia: Elsevier, 2007.

Lehne, R. *Pharmacology for Nursing Care*. 7th ed. Philadelphia: Elsevier, 2009.

Care of the Client with Hematological Disorders

http://www.americanhs.org—The website for the American Hemochromatosis Society

http://www.aplastic.org—The website for the Aplastic Anemia and MDS International Foundation

http://www.emedicine.com/med/topic3387.htm

http://www.hemophilia.org—The website for the National Hemophilia Foundation

http://www.marrow.org

http://www.nci.nih.gov—The website for the National Cancer Institute Information Center

http://www.ons.org—The website for the Oncology Nursing Society

http://www.sicklecelldisease.org—The website for the Sickle Cell Disease Association of America, Inc.

Brunner, L., and Suddarth, D. *Textbook of Medical Surgical Nursing*. 12th ed. Philadelphia: Lippincott Williams & Wilkins, 2009.

Lewis, S., Heitkemper, M., Dirksen, S., O'Brien, P., and Bucher, L. *Medical Surgical Nursing: Assessment and Management of Clinical Problems*. 7th ed. Philadelphia: Elsevier, 2007.

Fluid and Electrolytes and Acid/Base Balance

http://www.enursescribe.com

http://www.umed.utah.edu/ms2/renal

Ignatavicius, D., and Workman, S. *Medical Surgical Nursing: Critical Thinking for Collaborative Care*. 5th ed. Philadelphia: Elsevier, 2007.

Brunner, L., and Suddarth, D. *Textbook of Medical Surgical Nursing*. 12th ed. Philadelphia: Lippincott Williams & Wilkins, 2009.

Care of the Client with Burns

Ignatavicius, D., and Workman, S. *Medical Surgical Nursing: Critical Thinking for Collaborative Care*. 5th ed. Philadelphia: Elsevier, 2007.

Brunner, L., and Suddarth, D. *Textbook of Medical Surgical Nursing*. 12th ed. Philadelphia: Lippincott Williams & Wilkins, 2009.

LeMone, P., and Burke, K. in *Medical Surgical Nursing: Critical Thinking in Client Care*. 4th ed. Upper Saddle River, NJ: Pearson Prentice Hall, 2008.

Lewis, S., Heitkemper, M., Dirksen, S., Obrien, P., and Bucher, L. *Medical Surgical Nursing: Assessment and Management of Clinical Problems*. 7th ed. Philadelphia: Elsevier, 2007.

Lehne, R. *Pharmacology for Nursing Care*. 7th ed. Philadelphia: Elsevier, 2009.

Care of the Client with Sensory Disorders

http://www.afb.org—The website for the American Foundation for the Blind

http://www.loc.gov.nis—The website for the National Library Services for the Blind and Physically Handicapped

Ignatavicius, D., and Workman, S. *Medical Surgical Nursing: Critical Thinking for Collaborative Care*. 5th ed. Philadelphia: Elsevier, 2007.

Brunner, L., and Suddarth, D. *Textbook of Medical Surgical Nursing*. 12th ed. Philadelphia: Lippincott Williams & Wilkins, 2009.

LeMone, P., and Burke, K. in *Medical Surgical Nursing: Critical Thinking in Client Care*. 4th ed. Upper Saddle River, NJ: Pearson Prentice Hall, 2008.

Lewis, S., Heitkemper, M., Dirksen, S., Obrien, P., and Bucher, L. *Medical Surgical Nursing: Assessment and Management of Clinical Problems*. 7th ed. Philadelphia: Elsevier, 2007.

Lehne, R. *Pharmacology for Nursing Care*. 7th ed., Philadelphia: Elsevier, 2009.

Care of the Client with Neoplastic Disorders

http://www.abta.org—The website for the American Brain Tumor Association

http://www.cancer.gov—The website for the National Cancer Institute

http://www.komen.org—The website for the Susan G. Komen Breast Cancer Foundation

http://www.leukemia.org

http://www.leukemia-research.org

http://www.ons.org—The website for the Oncology Nursing Society

http://www.skincancer.org—The website for the Skin Cancer Foundation

Ignatavicius, D., and Workman, S. *Medical Surgical Nursing: Critical Thinking for Collaborative Care*. 5th ed. Philadelphia: Elsevier, 2007.

Brunner, L., and Suddarth, D. *Textbook of Medical Surgical Nursing*. 12th ed. Philadelphia: Lippincott Williams & Wilkins, 2009.

Care of the Client with Gastrointestinal Disorders

http://www.asge.org—The website for the American Society for Gastrointestinal Endoscopy

http://www.ccfa.org—The website for the Crohn's and Colitis Foundation

http://www.cdc.gov—The website for the Centers for Disease Control and Prevention

http://www.uoaa.org—The website for the United Ostomy Association

Brunner, L., and Suddarth, D. *Textbook of Medical Surgical Nursing*. 12th ed. Philadelphia: Lippincott Williams & Wilkins, 2009.

Ignatavicius, D., and Workman, S. *Medical Surgical Nursing: Critical Thinking for Collaborative Care*. 5th ed. Philadelphia: Elsevier, 2007.

Lewis,S., Heitkemper, M., Dirksen, S., O'Brien, P., and Bucher, L. *Medical Surgical Nursing: Assessment and Management of Clinical Problems*. 7th ed. Philadelphia: Elsevier, 2007.

Lemone, P., and Burke, K. *Medical-Surgical Nursing Critical Thinking in Client Care*. 4th ed. Upper Saddle River, NJ: Pearson Prentice Hall, 2008.

Care of the Client with Musculoskeletal and Connective Tissue Disorder

http://www.amputee-coalition.org—The website for the Amputee Coalition of America

http://www.niams.nih.gov—The website for the National Institute of Arthritis and Musculoskeletal and Skin Diseases

http://www.nof.org—The website for the National Osteoporosis Foundation

http://www.orthonurse.org—The website for the National Association of Orthopaedic Nurses

Ignatavicius, D., and Workman, S. *Medical Surgical Nursing: Critical Thinking for Collaborative Care.* 5th ed. Philadelphia: Elsevier, 2007.

Lewis, S., Heitkemper, M., Dirksen, S., O'Brien, P., and Bucher, L. *Medical Surgical Nursing: Assessment and Management of Clinical Problems.* 7th ed. Philadelphia: Elsevier, 2007.

Lemone, P., Burke, K. *Medical-Surgical Nursing Critical Thinking in Client Care.* 4th ed. Upper Saddle River, NJ: Pearson Prentice Hall, 2008.

Care of the Client with Endocrine Disorders

http://www.cdc.gov/diabetes—The website for the Centers for Disease Control and Prevention

http://www.diabetes.org—The website for the American Diabetes Association

http://www.diabetesnet.com—The website for the American Association of Diabetes Educators

http://www.eatright.org—The website for the American Dietetic Association

http://www.endo-society.org—The website for the National Endocrine Society

http://www.medhelp.org/nadf—The website for the National Adrenal Disease Foundation

http://www.niddk.nih.gov—The website for the National Diabetes Clearing House

http://www.pancreasfoundation.org—The website for the National Pancreas Foundation

http://www.thyroid.org—The website for the American Thyroid Association

Ignatavicius, D., and Workman, S. *Medical Surgical Nursing: Critical Thinking for Collaborative Care.* 5th ed. Philadelphia: Elsevier, 2007.

Brunner, L., and Suddarth, D. *Textbook of Medical Surgical Nursing.* 12th ed. Philadelphia: Lippincott Williams & Wilkins, 2009.

Care of the Client with Cardiac Disorders

http://www.americanheart.org—The website for the American Heart Association

http://www.nursebeat.com—The website for the *Nurse Beat: Cardiac Nursing Electronic Journal*

Ignatavicius, D., and Workman, S. *Medical Surgical Nursing: Critical Thinking for Collaborative Care.* 5th ed. Philadelphia: Elsevier, 2007.

Brunner, L., and Suddarth, D. *Textbook of Medical Surgical Nursing.* 12th ed. Philadelphia: Lippincott Williams & Wilkins, 2009.

Woods, A. "An ACE Up Your Sleeve and an ARB in Your Back Pocket," *Nursing Made Incredibly Easy*, Sept.–Oct. 2003, 36–42.

Care of the Client with Neurological Disorders

http://www.apdaparkinson.com—The website for the American Parkinson's Disease Association.

http://www.biausa.org—The website for the Brain Injury Association.

http://www.epilepsyfoundation.org—The website for the Epilepsy Foundation.

http://www.gbs-cidp.org—The website for the Guillain-Barré Syndrome Foundation.

http://www.nmss.org—The website for the National Multiple Sclerosis Society.

http://www.parkinson.org—The website for the National Parkinson's Foundation.

http://www.stroke.org—The website for the American Stroke Association.

Ignatavicius, D., and Workman, S. *Medical Surgical Nursing: Critical Thinking for Collaborative Care.* 5th ed. Philadelphia: Elsevier, 2007.

Lewis, S., Heitkemper, M., Dirksen, S., O'Brien, P., and Bucher, L. *Medical Surgical Nursing: Assessment and Management of Clinical Problems.* 7th ed. Philadelphia: Elsevier, 2007.

Lemone, P., and Burke, K. *Medical-Surgical Nursing Critical Thinking in Client Care.* 4th ed. Upper Saddle River, NJ: Pearson Prentice Hall, 2008.

Brunner, L., and Suddarth, D. *Textbook of Medical Surgical Nursing.* 12th ed. Philadelphia: Lippincott Williams & Wilkins, 2009.

Care of the Client with Psychiatric Disorders

http://www.nami.org—The website for the National Alliance on Mental Illness.

Kneisl, C., and Trigoboff, E. *Contemporary Psychiatric Mental Health Nursing*. 2nd ed. Upper Saddle River, NJ: Pearson Prentice Hall, 2009.

Townsend, M. *Essentials of Psychiatric Mental Health Nursing*. 4th ed. Philadelphia: F.A. Davis, 2008.

Lehne, R. *Pharmacology for Nursing Care*. 7th ed. Philadelphia: Elsevier, 2009.

Ball, J., and Bindler, R. *Pediatric Nursing: Caring for Children*. 4th ed. Upper Saddle River, NJ: Pearson Prentice Hall, 2008.

Maternal-Newborn Care

Lowdermilk, D. L., et al. (eds.). *Maternity and Women's Health Care*. 8th ed. St. Louis: C.V. Mosby, 2000.

McKinney, E., et al. (eds.). *Maternal-Child Nursing*. 2nd ed. St. Louis: W. B. Saunders, 2005.

Wong, D., et al. (eds.). *Maternal-Child Nursing Care*. 3rd ed. St. Louis: C.V. Mosby, 2002.

Care of the Pediatric Client

Hockenberry, M., and Wilson, D. , *Wong's Essentials of Pediatric Nursing* , 8th ed. St. Louis: Elsevier, 2009.

Ball, J., and Bindler, R. *Pediatric Nursing: Caring for Children*. 4th ed. Upper Saddle River, NJ: Pearson Prentice Hall, 2008.

www.aaai.org—American Academy of Allergy, Asthma, and Immunology

www.cdc.gov—Centers for Disease Control

www.lungusa.org—The American Lung Association

www.aafp.org—The American Academy of Family Practice

www.pathguy.com—Dr. Ed Friedlander, pathologist

www.cff.org—Cystic Fibrosis Foundation

www.candlelighters.org—Candlelighters Childhood Cancer Foundation

Cultural Practices Influencing Nursing Care

Brunner, L., and Suddarth, D. *Textbook of Medical Surgical Nursing*. 12th ed. Philadelphia: Lippincott Williams & Wilkins, 2009.

Ignatavicius, D., and Workman, S. *Medical Surgical Nursing: Critical Thinking for Collaborative Care*. 6th ed. Philadelphia: Elsevier, 2007.

Potter, P., and and Perry, A. *Fundamentals of Nursing*. 6th ed. St. Louis: C.V. Mosby, 2005.

Legal Issues in Nursing Practice

Tappen, R. *Nursing Leadership and Management: Concepts and Practice*. 5th ed. Philadelphia: F.A. Davis, 2004.

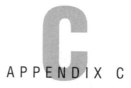
Calculations

Math calculation is an integral part of safe nursing care. This section is a review of the conversion tables and sample problems.

The Apothecary System of Measurement

Equivalents/Conversion Factors

- 1 minim = 1 drop

- 1 fluid dram = 60 minims

- 1 fluid ounce = 8 fluid drams

- 1 dram = 60 grains

- 30 ml = 2 tbs (tablespoons)

- 15 ml = 1 tbs

- 5 ml = 1 tsp (teaspoon)

The Household System of Measurement

Equivalents/Conversion Factors

- 1 teaspoon = 60 drops

- 2 tablespoon = 1 ounce

- 1 cup = 8 ounces

- 2 cups = 1 pint

- 2 pint = 1 quart

- 4 quarts = 1 gallon

- ▶ 1 pound = 16 ounces
- ▶ 1 teaspoon = 15–16 minims = 1 mL (milliliter)
- ▶ 2.2 pounds = 1 kilogram = 1000 gm (gram)

Metric Measurements

Equivalents/Conversion Factors

- ▶ 1 gr (grain) = 60–65 mg (milligram)
- ▶ 1 mg = 1000 mcg (microgram)
- ▶ 1 gm = 1000 mg = 15 gr
- ▶ 1 kg = 2.2 lbs

Test Your Math Skills

1. The doctor has ordered a nitroglycerin infusion to infuse at 15 mcg/minute. Available is 50 mg of nitroglycerin in 250 mL. A microdrop set is utilized to administer this medication. How many mL per hour will the nurse infuse? (In a microdrop set, the number of gtts per minute equals mL per hour.)

2. The doctor has ordered one unit of blood (500 mL) to be given over four hours. After verifying the order, calculate the rate in gtts/minute. (A 20 drop per mL blood set is available.)

3. The doctor has ordered 15 mg of Demerol (meperidine) for pain. Available is Demerol 25 mg per mL. How many mL will you administer?

4. The doctor has ordered 250 mg of Aldomet (methyldopa) for control of the client's primary hypertension. The pharmacy sent the medication labeled 1 tablet contains 125 mg. How many tablets will you administer?

5. The doctor has ordered 35 mg of Demerol (Meperidine) IM stat for pain. Available is 1 mL containing 50 mg. How many ml will you administer?

6. The doctor has ordered doxycycline (Vibramycin) 100 mg orally every 12 hours. The pharmacy sent the medication labeled 50 mg/5 mL. How many mL will you administer?

7. The doctor has ordered digoxin (Lanoxin) 0.25 mg orally qd (every day). The tablets are labeled 0.50 mg per tablet. How many tablets will you give?

8. The doctor has ordered a medication labeled gr 1/300 for atrial fibrillation. The cart contains a unidose container labeled 0.1 mg per tablet. How many tablets will you administer?

9. The doctor has ordered acetaminophen (Tylenol) gr 10 orally every four hours for headache. Available is 325 mg in one tablet. How many tablets will you administer?

10. The doctor has ordered glycopyrrolate (Robinul) 0.2 mg intramuscular. Available is 0.6 mg in one mL. How many mL will you administer?

11. The doctor has ordered phenytoin (Dilantin) 5 mg/kg of body weight to be given to the client with seizure disorder. Available is Dilantin 50 mg in 1 mL. How many mL will you administer to the client who weighs 110 pounds?

12. The doctor has ordered heparin 7500 units subcutaneously. Available is heparin 5000 units per mL. How many mL will you administer?

Answers

1. $$\frac{? \text{ ml}}{1 \text{ hour}} = \frac{250 \text{ ml}}{50 \text{ mg}} \times \frac{1 \text{ mg}}{1000 \text{ mcg}} \times \frac{15 \text{ mcg}}{1 \text{ minute}} \times \frac{60 \text{ minutes}}{1 \text{ hour}} = 4.5 \text{ or } 5 \text{ ml/hr}$$

(Note: In a microdrip set, $\dfrac{\text{ml}}{\text{hour}}$ is equal to gtts per minute.)

2. $$\frac{? \text{ gtt}}{1 \text{ minute}} = \frac{20 \text{ gtt}}{1 \text{ ml}} \times \frac{500 \text{ ml}}{4 \text{ hours}} \times \frac{1 \text{ hour}}{60 \text{ minutes}} = \frac{1000}{24} = 41.66 \text{ or } \frac{42 \text{ gtt}}{1 \text{ minute}}$$

3. $$? \text{ ml} = \frac{1 \text{ ml}}{25 \text{ mg}} \times \frac{15 \text{ mg}}{1} = 15 = .6 \text{ ml}$$

4. $$? \text{ tablet} = \frac{1 \text{ tablet}}{125 \text{ mg}} \times \frac{250 \text{ mg}}{1} = 250 \text{mg} = 2 \text{ tablets}$$

5. $$? \text{ ml} = \frac{1 \text{ ml}}{50 \text{ mg}} \times \frac{35 \text{ mg}}{1} = \frac{35}{50} = .7 \text{ ml}$$

6. $$? \text{ ml} = \frac{5 \text{ ml}}{50 \text{ mg}} \times \frac{100 \text{ mg}}{1} = \frac{500}{50} = 10 \text{ ml}$$

7. $$? \text{ tablet} = \frac{1 \text{ tablet}}{0.50 \text{ mg}} \times \frac{0.25 \text{ mg}}{1} = \frac{0.25}{0.50} = .5 \text{ tablet}$$

8. $$? \text{ tablets} = \frac{1/300 \text{ gr}}{1} \times \frac{1 \text{ tablet}}{0.1 \text{ mg}} = \frac{60 \text{ mg}}{1 \text{ gr}} = \frac{60/300}{1} = 2 \text{ tablets}$$

9. $$? \text{ tablets} = \frac{1 \text{ tablet}}{325 \text{ mg}} \times \frac{60 \text{ mg}}{1 \text{ gr}} = \frac{10 \text{ gr}}{1} = \frac{650}{325} = 2 \text{ tablets}$$

10. $$? \text{ ml} = \frac{1 \text{ ml}}{0.6 \text{ mg}} \times \frac{0.2 \text{ mg}}{1} = \frac{0.2}{0.6} = .3 \text{ ml}$$

11. $$? \text{ ml} = \frac{1 \text{ ml}}{50 \text{ mg}} \times \frac{5 \text{ mg}}{1 \text{ kg}} \times \frac{1 \text{ kg}}{2.2 \text{ lb}} \times \frac{110 \text{ lb}}{1} = \frac{550}{110} = 5 \text{ ml}$$

12. $$? \text{ ml} = \frac{1 \text{ ml}}{5000 \text{ units}} \times \frac{7500 \text{ units}}{1} = \frac{7500}{5000} = \frac{75}{50} = 1.5 \text{ ml}$$

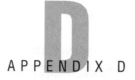

Most-Prescribed Medications in the United States

The NCLEX exam includes pharmacology as a subcategory under the area of physiological integrity. Because nurses are responsible for administering medications it is extremely important for the nurse to be aware of those drugs that are frequently prescribed. Table D.1 provides a listing of the most prescribed medications in the United States, including the generic and trade names of the medication, as well as primary uses and major concerns associated with the medication. Using this list will help you to prepare for these questions.

Information in this table was adapted from information found at the following sites/sources:

- http/apps.humana/marketing/documents.asp
- http://google.com
- *Davis's Drug Guide for Nurses*

TABLE D.1 Most-Prescribed Medications in the United States

Generic Name	Trade Name	Uses	Major Concerns
Acetaminophen	Tylenol	Analgesic	Watch for liver and kidney problems.
Albuterol	Proventil	Bronchodilator	This drug can cause tachycardia. The doctor needs to check blood levels for toxicity to this drug.
Alendronate	Fosamax	Osteoporosis	Remain upright for at least 30 minutes after taking to prevent gastroesophageal reflux disease (GERD). Take this drug with water.
Allopurinol	Zyloprim	Antigout	This client should drink at least eight glasses of water per day.
Alprazolam	Xanax	Antianxiety	This drug can be addictive.
Sertraline	Zoloft	Antidepressant	This drug can cause sedation.
Amiodipine	Norvasc	Antihypertensive	This drug can lead to hypotension.
Amitriptyline HCl	Elavil	Antidepressant	
Amoxicillin	Augmentin	Antibiotic	Watch for allergic reactions.
Atenolol	Tenormin	Antihypertensive	This drug can cause a drop in pulse rate, so check your pulse daily.
Azithromycin	Zithromax Z-Pak	Antibiotic	Watch for allergies.
Cephalexin	Keflex	Antibiotic	If you are allergic to cephalosporins, you might also be allergic to penicillin.
Cetirizine	Zyrtec	Antihistamine	
Clonazepam	Klonopin	Anticonvulsant	This drug should not be stopped abruptly.
Cyclobenzaprine HCl	Flexeril	Muscle relaxant	This drug can cause sedation.
Diazepam	Valium	Anticonvulsant/ antianxiety	Watch for allergies.
Doxazosin mesylate	Cardura	Antihypertensive	
Doxycycline hyclate	Vibramycin	Antibiotic	Women should not take this drug if pregnant.
Estrogen	Premarin	Hormone	This drug can increase the chances of blood clots.

TABLE D.1 Most-Prescribed Medications in the United States

Generic Name	Trade Name	Uses	Major Concerns
Fexofenadine	Allegra	Antihistamine	This drug can lead to dry mouth.
Furosemide	Lasix	Diuretic	This drug can lead to hypokalemia.
Glipizide	Glucotrol	Antidiabetic	Watch for hypoglycemia.
Hydrochlorothiazide	HCTZ	Diuretic	This drug can lead to hypokalemia.
Hydrocodone with acetaminophen	Lortab	Analgesic	Can be addictive.
Ibuprofen	Motrin	Analgesic/ anti-inflammatory	This drug can lead to hypertension and kidney disease.
Lansoprazole	Prevacid	Proton pump inhibitor/ antiulcer	Take the medication prior to meals.
Levothyroxin	Synthyroid	Hormone	Teach the client to check his pulse.
Levothyroxine	Levoxyl	Hormone	This drug can increase the chances of blood clotting.
Lisinopril	Zestril	Antihypertensive	This drug can lead to postural hypotension. Remain supine for at least 30 minutes when beginning the medication.
Lorazepam	Antivan	Anticonvulsant/ antianxiety	This drug can cause sedation.
Metformin	Glucophage	Antidiabetic	This drug should be stopped prior to a dye study such as a cardiac catheterization.
Metoprolol succinate	Toprol XL	Antihypertensive	The nurse needs to teach the client to check his pulse.
Metoprolol tartrate	Lopressor, Toprol	Antihypertensive	The client should be taught to check his pulse rate.
Montelukast	Singulair	Asthmatic medication	
Naproxen	Aleve	Analgesic	This drug can lead to hypertension and kidney disease.
Necon	Ortho-Novum 7/7/7	Oral contraceptive	This drug can increase the chances of blood clots.
Omeprazole	Prilosec	Proton pump inhibitor/ antiulcer	
Penicillin V potassium	Penicillin	Antibiotic	Watch for allergies.

(continues)

TABLE D.1 *Continued*

Generic Name	Trade Name	Uses	Major Concerns
Potassium chloride	K-Lyte	Supplement	The nurse should check renal function prior to giving the medication.
Prednisone	Deltasone	Anti-inflammatory	This drug can cause Cushing's syndrome. This drug can cause gastrointestinal problems.
Promethazine HCl	Phenergan	Antiemetic/antianxiety	
Rantidine HCl	Zantac	Histamine blocker/ antiulcer	Usually it is best to take this drug with meals.
Simvastatin	Zocor	Antilipidemic	This drug can cause liver problems and muscle soreness. Taking the drug at night will increase the drug's effectiveness. Do not take this drug with grapefruit juice.
Sulfamethoxazole	Septra, Bactrim	Antibiotic	This drug can cause gastrointestinal disturbance.
Trazodone HCl	Desyrel	Antidepressant	
Trinessa	Ortho TriClen	Oral contraceptive	This drug can increase chances of blood clotting.
Verapamil HCl	Calan	Antihypertensive/ antianginal	
Warfarin sodium	Coumadin	Anticoagulant	The nurse should teach the client to limit the intake of green leafy vegetables and watch for signs of bleeding.
Zolpidem	Ambien	Sleep aid	Allow at least eight hours of sleep time to prevent daytime drowsiness.

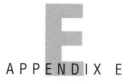

Alphabetical Listing of Nursing Boards in the United States and Protectorates

This appendix contains contact information for nursing boards found throughout the United States. The information found here is current as of this writing, but be aware that names, phone numbers, and websites do change. If the information found here is not completely current, most likely some of the information will be useful enough for you to still make contact with the organization. If all the information is incorrect, a helpful hint is to use an Internet search engine, such as Yahoo! or Google, and enter the name of the nursing board you are trying to contact. In addition, the following website keeps an up to date register of the different boards of nursing in the United States and its territories: https://www.ncsbn.org/515.htm. Most likely, you'll find some contact information. Also, if you don't have access to the Internet, contact your state government because they should be able to help you find the information you need.

Alabama Board of Nursing
770 Washington Avenue
RSA Plaza, Suite 250
Montgomery, AL 36104

Phone: 334-242-4060
Fax: 334-242-4360

Contact person: N. Genell Lee, MSN, JD, RN, Executive Officer
Website: http://www.abn.state.al.us/

Alaska Board of Nursing
550 West Seventh Avenue, Suite 1500
Anchorage, AK 99501-3567

Phone: 907-269-8161
Fax: 907-269-8196

Contact person: Nancy Sanders, PhD, RN, Executive Administrator
Website: http://www.dced.state.ak.us/occ/pnur.htm

American Samoa Health Services
Regulatory Board
LBJ Tropical Medical Center
Pago Pago, AS 96799

Phone: 684-633-1222
Fax: 684-633-1869

Contact person: Toaga Atuatasi Seumalo, MS, RN, Executive Secretary

Arizona State Board of Nursing
4747 North 7th Street, Suite 200
Phoenix, AZ 85014-3655

Phone: 602-771-7800
Fax: 602-771-7888

Contact person: Joey Ridenour, MN, RN, FANN, Executive Director
Website: http://www.azbn.gov/

Arkansas State Board of Nursing
University Tower Building
1123 S. University, Suite 800
Little Rock, AR 72204-1619

Phone: 501-686-2700
Fax: 501-686-2714

Contact person: Faith Fields, MSN, RN, Executive Director
Website: http://www.arsbn.org/

California Board of Registered Nursing
1625 North Market Boulevard, Suite N-217
Sacramento, CA 95834-1924

Phone: 916-322-3350
Fax: 916-574-8637

Contact person: Louise Bailey, MEd, RN, Interim Executive Officer
Website: http://www.rn.ca.gov/

California Board of Vocational Nurses and Psychiatric Technicians
2535 Capitol Oaks Drive, Suite 205
Sacramento, CA 95833

Phone: 916-263-7800
Fax: 916-263-7859

Contact person: Teresa Bello-Jones, JD, MSN, RN, Executive Officer
Website: http://www.bvnpt.ca.gov/

Colorado Board of Nursing
1560 Broadway, Suite 880
Denver, CO 80202

Phone: 303-894-2430
Fax: 303-894-2821

Contact person: Mark Merrill, Program Director
Website: http://www.dora.state.co.us/nursing/

Connecticut Board of Examiners for Nursing
Deptartment of Public Health
410 Capitol Avenue, MS# 13PHO
P.O. Box 340308
Hartford, CT 06134-0328

Phone: 860-509-7624
Fax: 860-509-7553

Contact person: Jennifer L. Filippone, Chief, Practitioner Licensing and Investigations
Section
Website: http://www.state.ct.us/dph/

Delaware Board of Nursing
861 Silver Lake Boulevard
Cannon Building, Suite 203
Dover, DE 19904

Phone: 302-744-4500
Fax: 302-739-2711

Contact person: David Mangler, MS, RN, Executive Director
Website: http://dpr.delaware.gov/boards/nursing/

District of Columbia Board of Nursing
Department of Health
Health Professional Licensing Administration
District of Columbia Board of Nursing
717 14th Street, NW
Suite 600
Washington, DC 20005

Phone: 877-672-2174
Fax: 202-727-8471

Contact person: Karen Scipio-Skinner, MSN, RNC, Executive Director
Website: http://hpla.doh.dc.gov/hpla/cwp/view,A,1195,Q,488526,hplaNav,I30661I,.asp

Florida Board of Nursing
Mailing address:
4052 Bald Cypress Way, BIN C02
Tallahassee, FL 32399-3252

Street address:
4042 Bald Cypress Way, Room 120
Tallahassee, FL 32399

Phone: 850-245-4125
Fax: 850-245-4172

Contact person: Joe Baker, Jr., Executive Director
Website: http://www.doh.state.fl.us/mqa/

Georgia Board of Nursing
237 Coliseum Drive
Macon, GA 31217-3858

Phone: 478-207-2440
Fax: 478-207-1354

Contact person: Sylvia Bond, RN, MSN, MBA, Executive Director
Website: http://www.sos.state.ga.us/plb/rn

Georgia State Board of Licensed Practical Nurses
237 Coliseum Drive
Macon, GA 31217-3858

Phone: 478-207-2440
Fax: 478-207-1354

Contact person: Sylvia Bond, RN, MSN, MBA, Executive Director
Website: http://www.sos.state.ga.us/plb/lpn

Guam Board of Nurse Examiners
#123 Chalan Kareta
Mangilao, Guam 96913-6304

Phone: 671-735-7407
Fax: 671-735-7413

Contact person: Margarita Bautista-Gay, RN, BSN, MN, Interim Executive Director
Website: http://www.dphss.guam.gov/

Hawaii Board of Nursing
King Kalakaua Building
335 Merchant Street, 3rd Floor
Honolulu, HI 96813

Phone: 808-586-3000
Fax: 808-586-2689

Contact person: Lee Ann Teshima, Executive Officer
Website: www.hawaii.gov/dcca/areas/pvl/boards/nursing

Idaho Board of Nursing
280 N. 8th Street, Suite 210
P.O. Box 83720
Boise, ID 83720

Phone: 208-334-3110
Fax: 208-334-3262

Contact person: Sandra Evans, MEd, RN, Executive Director
Website: http://ibn.idaho.gov/

Illinois Board of Nursing
James R. Thompson Center
100 West Randolph, Suite 9-300
Chicago, IL 60601

Phone: 312-814-2715
Fax: 312-814-3145

Contact person: Michele Bromberg, MSN, APN, BC, Nursing Act Coordinator
Website: http://www.idfpr.com/dpr/WHO/nurs.asp

Indiana State Board of Nursing
Professional Licensing Agency

402 W. Washington Street, Room W072
Indianapolis, IN 46204

Phone: 317-234-2043
Fax: 317-233-4236

Contact person: Sean Gorman, Board Director
Website: http://www.in.gov/pla/

Iowa Board of Nursing
RiverPoint Business Park
400 S.W. 8th Street, Suite B
Des Moines, IA 50309-4685

Phone: 515-281-3255
Fax: 515-281-4825

Contact person: Lorinda Inman, MSN, RN, Executive Director
Website: http://nursing.iowa.gov/

Kansas State Board of Nursing
Landon State Office Building
900 S.W. Jackson, Suite 1051
Topeka, KS 66612

Phone: 785-296-4929
Fax: 785-296-3929

Contact person: Mary Blubaugh, MSN, RN, Executive Administrator
Website: http://www.ksbn.org/

Kentucky Board of Nursing
312 Whittington Parkway, Suite 300
Louisville, KY 40222

Phone: 502-429-3300
Fax: 502-429-3311

Contact person: Charlotte F. Beason, EdD, RN, NEA, Executive Director
Website: http://www.kbn.ky.gov/

Louisiana State Board of Nursing
17373 Perkins Road
Baton Rouge, Louisiana 70810

Phone: 225-755-7500
Fax: 225-755-7585

Contact person: Barbara Morvant, MN, RN, Executive Director
Website: http://www.lsbn.state.la.us/

Louisiana State Board of Practical Nurse Examiners
3421 N. Causeway Boulevard, Suite 505
Metairie, LA 70002

Phone: 504-838-5791
Fax: 504-838-5279

Contact person: Claire Glaviano, BSN, MN, RN, Executive Director
Website: http://www.lsbpne.com/

Maine State Board of Nursing
158 State House Station
Augusta, ME 04333

Street address (for FedEx & UPS):
161 Capitol Street
Augusta, ME 04333

Phone: 207-287-1133
Fax: 207-287-1149

Contact person: Myra Broadway, JD, MS, RN, Executive Director
Website: http://www.maine.gov/boardofnursing/

Maryland Board of Nursing
4140 Patterson Avenue
Baltimore, MD 21215

Phone: 410-585-1900
Fax: 410-358-3530

Contact person: Patricia Ann Noble, MSN, RN Executive Director
Website: http://www.mbon.org/

Massachusetts Board of Registration in Nursing
Commonwealth of Massachusetts
239 Causeway Street, Second Floor
Boston, MA 02114

Phone: 617-973-0900
Fax: 617-973-0984

Contact person: Rula Faris Harb, MS, RN, Acting Executive Director
Website: http://www.mass.gov/dpl/boards/rn/

Michigan/DCH/Bureau of Health Professions
Ottawa Towers North
611 W. Ottawa, 1st Floor
Lansing, MI 48933

Phone: 517-335-0918
Fax: 517-373-2179

Contact person: Amy Shell, Executive Officer
Website: http://www.michigan.gov/healthlicense

Minnesota Board of Nursing
2829 University Avenue SE
Suite 200
Minneapolis, MN 55414

Phone: 612-617-2270
Fax: 612-617-2190

Contact person: Shirley Brekken, MS, RN, Executive Director
Website: http://www.nursingboard.state.mn.us/

Mississippi Board of Nursing
1080 River Oaks Drive
Flowood, MS 39232

Phone: 601-664-9303
Fax: 601-664-9304

Contact person: Melinda E. Rush, DSN, FNP, Executive Director
Website: http://www.msbn.state.ms.us/

Missouri State Board of Nursing
3605 Missouri Boulevard
P.O. Box 656
Jefferson City, MO 65102-0656

Phone: 573-751-0681
Fax: 573-751-0075

Contact person: Lori Scheidt, BS, Executive Director
Website: http://pr.mo.gov/nursing.asp

Montana State Board of Nursing
301 South Park
P.O. Box 200513
Helena, MT 59620-0513

Phone: 406-841-2345
Fax: 406-841-2305

Contact person: Vacant
Website: http://www.nurse.mt.gov

Nebraska Board of Nursing
301 Centennial Mall South
Lincoln, NE 68509-4986

Phone: 402-471-4376
Fax: 402-471-1066

Contact person: Diana Baker, MSN, RN, Executive Director
Website: http://www.hhs.state.ne.us/crl/nursing/nursingindex.htm

Nevada State Board of Nursing
5011 Meadowood Mall, Suite 300
Reno, NV 89502

Phone: 775-687-7700
Fax: 775-687-7707

Contact person: Debra Scott, MS, RN, FRE, Executive Director
Website: http://www.nursingboard.state.nv.us/

New Hampshire Board of Nursing
21 South Fruit Street, Suite 16
Concord, NH 03301-2341

Phone: 603-271-2323
Fax: 603-271-6605

Contact person: Margaret Walker, MBA, BSN, RN, Executive Director
Website: http://www.state.nh.us/nursing/

New Jersey Board of Nursing
P.O. Box 45010
124 Halsey Street, 6th Floor
Newark, NJ 07101

Phone: 973-504-6430
Fax: 973-648-3481

Contact person: George Hebert, Executive Director
Website: http://www.state.nj.us/lps/ca/medical/nursing.htm

New Mexico Board of Nursing
6301 Indian School Road, NE
Suite 710
Albuquerque, NM 87110

Phone: 505-841-8340
Fax: 505-841-8347

Contact person: Deborah Walker, MSN, RN, Executive Director
Website: http://www.bon.state.nm.us/

New York State Board of Nursing
Education Building
89 Washington Avenue
2nd Floor West Wing
Albany, NY 12234

Phone: 518-474-3817, extension 120
Fax: 518-474-3706

Contact person: Barbara Zittel, PhD, RN, Executive Secretary
Website: http://www.nysed.gov/prof/nurse.htm

North Carolina Board of Nursing
4516 Lake Boone Trail
Raleigh, NC 27607

Phone: 919-782-3211
Fax: 919-781-9461

Contact person: Julia L. George, RN, MSN, FRE, Executive Director
Website: http://www.ncbon.com/

North Dakota Board of Nursing
919 South 7th Street, Suite 504
Bismarck, ND 58504

Phone: 701-328-9777
Fax: 701-328-9785

Contact person: Constance Kalanek, PhD, RN, Executive Director
Website: http://www.ndbon.org/

Northern Mariana Islands
Commonwealth Board of Nurse Examiners
P.O. Box 501458
Saipan, MP 96950

Phone: 670-234-8950, ext. 3587
Fax: 670-664-4813

Contact person: Sinforosa D. Guerrero, Executive Officer Designee

Ohio Board of Nursing
17 South High Street, Suite 400
Columbus, OH 43215-3413

Phone: 614-466-3947
Fax: 614-466-0388

Contact person: Betsy J. Houchen, RN, MS, JD, Executive Director
Website: http://www.nursing.ohio.gov/

Oklahoma Board of Nursing
2915 N. Classen Boulevard, Suite 524
Oklahoma City, OK 73106

Phone: 405-962-1800
Fax: 405-962-1821

Contact person: Kimberly Glazier, MEd, RN, Executive Director
Website: http://www.ok.gov/nursing/

Oregon State Board of Nursing
17938 S.W. Upper Boones Ferry Road
Portland, OR 97224

Phone: 971-673-0865
Fax: 971-673-0684

Contact person: Holly Mercer, JD, RN, Executive Director
Website: http://www.osbn.state.or.us/

Pennsylvania State Board of Nursing
P.O. Box 2649
Harrisburg, PA 17105-2649

Phone: 717-783-7142
Fax: 717-783-0822

Contact person: Laurette D. Keiser, RN, MSN, Executive Secretary/Section Chief
Website: http://www.dos.state.pa.us/bpoa

Commonwealth of Puerto Rico Board of Nurse Examiners
800 Roberto H. Todd Avenue
Room 202, Stop 18
Santurce, PR 00908

Phone: 787-725-7506
Fax: 787-725-7903

Contact person: Roberto Figueroa, RN, MSN, Executive Director of the Office of
Regulations and Certifications of Health Care Professions

Rhode Island Board of Nurse Registration and Nursing Education
105 Cannon Building
Three Capitol Hill
Providence, RI 02908

Phone: 401-222-5700
Fax: 401-222-3352

Contact person: Pamela McCue, MS, RN, Executive Officer
Website: http://www.health.ri.gov/

South Carolina State Board of Nursing
Mailing Address:
P.O. Box 12367
Columbia, SC 29211

Physical Address:
Synergy Business Park, Kingstree Building
110 Centerview Drive, Suite 202
Columbia, SC 29210

Phone: 803-896-4550
Fax: 803-896-4525

Contact person: Joan K. Bainer, MN, RN, NE, BC, Administrator
Website: http://www.llr.state.sc.us/pol/nursing

South Dakota Board of Nursing
4305 South Louise Avenue, Suite 201
Sioux Falls, SD 57106-3115

Phone: 605-362-2760
Fax: 605-362-2768

Contact person: Gloria Damgaard, RN, MS, Executive Secretary
Website: http://www.state.sd.us/doh/nursing/

Tennessee State Board of Nursing
227 French Landing, Suite 300
Heritage Place MetroCenter
Nashville, TN 37243

Phone: 615-532-5166
Fax: 615-741-7899

Contact person: Elizabeth Lund, MSN, RN, Executive Director
Website: http://health.state.tn.us/Boards/Nursing/index.htm

Texas Board of Nurse Examiners
333 Guadalupe, Suite 3-460
Austin, TX 78701

Phone: 512-305-7400
Fax: 512-305-7401

Contact person: Katherine Thomas, MN, RN, Executive Director
Website: http://www.bon.state.tx.us/

Utah State Board of Nursing
Heber M. Wells Building, 4th Floor
160 East 300 South
Salt Lake City, UT 84111

Phone: 801-530-6628
Fax: 801-530-6511

Contact person: Laura Poe, MS, RN, Executive Administrator
Website: http://www.dopl.utah.gov/licensing/nursing.html

Vermont State Board of Nursing
Office of Professional Regulation
National Life Building North F1.2
Montpelier, Vermont 05620-3402
Phone: 802-828-2396
Fax: 802-828-2484

Contact person: Mary L. Botter, PhD, RN, Executive Director
Website: http://www.vtprofessionals.org/opr1/nurses/

Virgin Islands Board of Nurse Licensure
Veterans Drive Station
St. Thomas, VI 00803

Phone: 340-776-7397
Fax: 340-777-4003

Contact person: Winifred Garfield, CRNA, RN, Executive Secretary

Virginia Board of Nursing
Mailing Address:
P.O. Box 304247, Veterans Drive Station
St. Thomas, Virgin Islands 00803

Physical Address (For FedEx and UPS):
Virgin Island Board of Nurse Licensure
#3 Kongens Gade (Government Hill)
St. Thomas, Virgin Islands 00802
Phone: 340-776-7131
Fax: 340-777-4003

Contact person: Diane Ruan-Viville, MA, BSN, RN, Executive Director
Website: http://www.vibnl.org/

Washington State Nursing Care Quality Assurance Commission
Department of Health
HPQA #6
310 Israel Road SE
Tumwater, WA 98501-7864

Phone: 360-236-4700
Fax: 360-236-4738

Contact person: Paula Meyer, MSN, RN, Executive Director
Website: http://www.doh.wa.gov/hsqa/professions/nursing/default.htm

West Virginia Board of Examiners for Registered Professional Nurses
101 Dee Drive
Charleston, WV 25311

Phone: 304-558-3596
Fax: 304-558-3666

Contact person: Laura Rhodes, MSN, RN, Executive Director
Website: http://www.wvrnboard.com/

West Virginia State Board of Examiners for Licensed Practical Nurses
101 Dee Drive
Charleston, WV 25311

Phone: 304-558-3572
Fax: 304-558-4367

Contact person: Lanette Anderson, RN, BSN, JD, Executive Director
Website: http://www.lpnboard.state.wv.us/

Wisconsin Department of Regulation and Licensing
Mailing Address:
P.O. Box 8935
Madison, WI 53708-8935

Physical Address:
1400 E. Washington Avenue
Madison, WI 53703

Phone: 608-266-2112
Fax: 608-261-7083

Contact person: Jeff Scanlan, Bureau Director, Health Services Boards
Website: http://drl..wi.gov/

Wyoming State Board of Nursing
1810 Pioneer Avenue
Cheyenne, WY 82001

Phone: 307-777-7601
Fax: 307-777-3519

Contact person: Mary Kay Goetter, Executive Officer
Website: http://nursing.state.wy.us/

Index

A

B

How can we make this index more useful? Email us at indexes@quepublishing.com

F

G

H

J

jaundice, 319
jaw-thrust maneuver, 367
Jehovah's Witnesses, 397
Judaism, 397

K

Kasai procedure, 338
kava-kava, 39
KD (Kawasaki's disease), 353-354
Kehr's sign, 372
kernicterus, 318
ketonuria, 220
keywords, 10
kidneys
    buffer system, 91
    stones, 66-67
knee replacements, 198-199

L

L/S (lecithin/sphingomyelin) ratios, 302
lab values, therapeutic drug levels, 589-590
labor (pregnancy)
    pharmacological management, 316-317
    phases of, 312
    stages of, 311
language assessment, 387
Laparoscopic Nissen Fundoplication (LNF), 167
laryngotracheobronchitis (LTB), 347
larynx cancer, 141
laser in-situ keratomileusis (LASIK), 127
LASIK (laser in-situ keratomileusis), 127
late decelerations (fetal monitoring), 315
Latinos, cultural influences, 388-390

laws. *See* legal issues
laxatives, 19
lead poisoning, 358
lecithin/sphingomyelin (L/S) ratios, 302
left occiput anterior (LOA), 312
legal issues, 406
    case study, 414-416
    civil laws, 407
    client care management, 411-414
    common laws, 407-408
    criminal laws, 407
    legal theories, 410-411
    practice exam questions, 417-420
    resources, 420, 604
    statutory laws, 407
    terminology, 405
legal theories, 410-411
Legg-Calve-Perthes Disease, 355
Legionnaire's disease, 54-55
leukemia, 141
    pediatric care, 356
    risk factors, 141
life support guidelines (AHA), 592
lithium, 285, 589
liver cancer, 141
liver-associated diseases, 167
    cirrhosis, 172-174
    hepatitis, 167
        Hepatitis A, 168
        Hepatitis B, 169-170
        Hepatitis C, 170-171
        Hepatitis D, 171
        Hepatitis E, 171
        Hepatitis G, 171
        stages, 171-172
    pancreatitis, 174-175
LNF (Laparoscopic Nissen Fundoplication), 167
LOA (left occiput anterior), 312

M

O

How can we make this index more useful? Email us at indexes@quepublishing.com

T

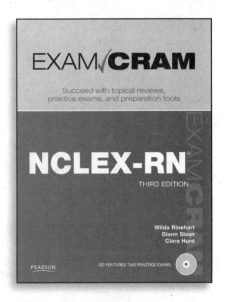

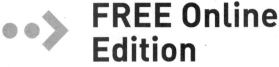

FREE Online Edition

Your purchase of **NCLEX-RN Exam Cram** includes access to a free online edition for 45 days through the Safari Books Online subscription service. Nearly every Exam Cram book is available online through Safari Books Online, along with more than 5,000 other technical books and videos from publishers such as Addison-Wesley Professional, Cisco Press, IBM Press, O'Reilly, Prentice Hall, Que, and Sams.

SAFARI BOOKS ONLINE allows you to search for a specific answer, cut and paste code, download chapters, and stay current with emerging technologies.

Activate your FREE Online Edition at www.informit.com/safarifree

> **STEP 1:** Enter the coupon code: LPGFGDB.

> **STEP 2:** New Safari users, complete the brief registration form.
> Safari subscribers, just log in.

If you have difficulty registering on Safari or accessing the online edition, please e-mail customer-service@safaribooksonline.com

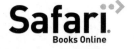

      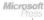